# ROLE OF BIOMARKERS IN MEDICINE

Edited by **Mu Wang** and **Frank A. Witzmann**

**Role of Biomarkers in Medicine**
http://dx.doi.org/10.5772/61449
Edited by Mu Wang and Frank A. Witzmann

**Contributors**

Ghulam Mohammad, Stefan Mircea Iencean, Andrei Stefan Iencean, Afaf El-Ansary, Suk Yu Yau, Ang Li, Xin Sun, Christine J Fontaine, Brian R Christie, Kwok-Fai So, Daniel Petrovic, Ines Cilenšek, Sara Mankoč Ramuš, Mojca Globočnik Petrovič, Hala Fawzy Mohamed Kamel, Hiba Al-Amodi, Kazumasa Matsumoto, Morihiro Nishi, Hideyasu Tsumura, Ken-Ichi Tabata, Tetsuo Fujita, Masatsugu Iwamura, Alessandra Ferlini, Chiara Scotton, Ruben Rene Gonzalez-Perez, Danielle Daley-Brown, Gabriela Oprea-Ilies, Alexander Quarshie, Sanjay K Banerjee, Ramu Adela, Monica Navarro-Meza, Jesús Manuel Alcalá-Bejarano Carrillo

**Published by InTech**

Janeza Trdine 9, 51000 Rijeka, Croatia



**Notice**

Statements and opinions expressed in the chapters are these of the individual contributors and not necessarily those of the editors or publisher. No responsibility is accepted for the accuracy of information contained in the published chapters. The publisher assumes no responsibility for any damage or injury to persons or property arising out of the use of any materials, instructions, methods or ideas contained in the book.

**Publishing Process Manager** Romina Rovan

**Technical Editor** SPi Global

**Cover** InTech Design team

First published August, 2016

Printed in Croatia

Additional hard copies can be obtained from orders@intechopen.com

Role of Biomarkers in Medicine, Edited by Mu Wang and Frank A. Witzmann

p. cm.

Print ISBN 978-953-51-2505-1
Online ISBN 978-953-51-2506-8

For EU product safety concerns:
IN TECH d.o.o., Prolaz Marije Krucifikse Kozulić 3, 51000 Rijeka, Croatia,
info@intechopen.com or visit our website at intechopen.com.

# Meet the editors

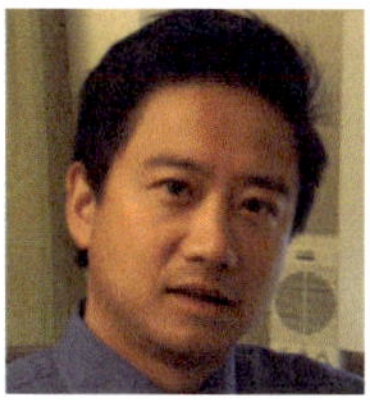

Dr. Wang is the Director of Proteomics and a tenured Associate Professor of Biochemistry and Molecular Biology at the Indiana University School of Medicine. His research centers around biomarkers and drug target discovery and deciphering the protein interaction networks in complex human diseases with use of high-throughput proteomics technologies. He has been actively collaborating with many investigators both across the United States and internationally to advance knowledge related to human health. He received numerous awards including an International Human Proteome Organization (HUPO) Young Investigator's Award in 2004. He has published more than 80 peer-reviewed articles and book chapters and served as a reviewer for many funding agencies such as the NIH and the US Department of Defense.

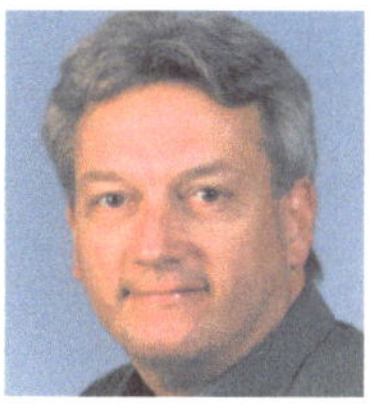

Dr. Witzmann is the Scientific Director of Proteomics and Professor of Physiology at the Indiana University School of Medicine. He has been involved in proteomics for nearly 30 years (before the term was coined), applying global protein expression analyses in various research paradigms. He currently directs the use of mass spectrometry–based proteomic approaches in a broad range of collaborative projects where both narrowly focused and comprehensive protein expression profiling and post-translational modification characterization are used to investigate the mechanistic molecular underpinnings of renal pathologies, cardiovascular disease, and biomarker discovery in various conditions. He has published more than 170 peer-reviewed articles and book chapters and served as a reviewer for many funding agencies.

# Contents

# Preface

The term "biomarkers" in medicine is defined as objective indications of medical state obtained from a patient, which can be measured accurately and reproducibly. While new technologies have accelerated the identification of disease-specific biomarkers, careful assessment of the validity of many biomarkers in risk assessment, diagnosis, prognosis, and therapeutic target identification is required with respect to the stage of disease, specificity, precision, and cost.

Biomarkers appear in various forms, including proteins, peptides, microRNAs, antibodies, cell types, metabolites, lipids, hormones, enzymes, physiological states such as blood pressure and body temperature, and imaging data. Ultimately, biomarkers are meant to be used to detect a change or changes in the physiological state of a patient that correlates well with the disease progression, with the susceptibility of a disease to a given treatment, or with the predictive treatment outcomes. In particular, biomarkers hold great promise in personalized medicine as information gained from biomarkers can be used to tailor specific treatment to the individual for highly efficient intervention in the disease process.

This book includes chapters in biomarkers of cancer, inflammation, oxidative stress, traumatic injury, autism, neurodegenerative diseases, diabetes, cardiovascular diseases, rare genetic diseases, and physical exercise–induced brain health. Although the basic principles of biomarker application are similar, the focus of each chapter rests on the practical aspects of each disease type as well as each molecular type (i.e., genes, proteins, and metabolites), enabling readers to easily acquire an understanding of useful biomarkers or potential biomarker candidates that are still under development.

Finally, we would like to thank all the contributors for their dedicated work, their time spent on their chapters, and their patience and endurance that undoubtedly is necessary for this to happen. We hope that this book will bring new insights to our readers' knowledge base and that it becomes a resource for basic science investigators and clinicians to enable appropriate application and use of biomarkers in their everyday practice.

**Mu Wang and Frank A. Witzmann**

Indiana University School of Medicine,

USA

Chapter 1

# Cancer Biomarkers

Hala Fawzy Mohamed Kamel, and
Hiba Saeed Bagader Al-Amodi

Additional information is available at the end of the chapter

http://dx.doi.org/10.5772/62421

**Abstract**

Cancer biomarkers (CB) are biomolecules produced either by the tumor cells or by other cells of the body in response to the tumor. Every cell type has its unique molecular signature and identifiable characteristics such as levels or activities of myriad of genes, proteins, or other molecular features; therefore, biomarkers can facilitate the molecular definition of cancer. Our aim was providing updated knowledge and performing detailed review about CB regarding their molecular and biochemical characterization and their clinical utility in screening, diagnosis, follow-up, or therapeutic stratification for cancer patients. Focusing on conventional, the FDA approved as well as promising future biomarkers in most common cancers. In addition, emphasizing on their prospective role may be of great value in improving the management of cancer patients. The challenge and future prospective of biomarkers, by facilitating the combination of therapeutics with diagnostics, promise to play an important role in the development of personalized medicine.

**Keywords:** cancer, biomarkers, molecular markers, prognosis, diagnosis, proteomics

## 1. Introduction

Increasing cancer burden is a major health problem; GLOBOCAN estimated nearly 8.2 million deaths and 14.1 million new cancer cases all over the world in 2012 [1] and it is expected to be 16 million new cases every year by 2020 [2]. Widespread application of existing cancer control knowledge, early detection, appropriate therapy with proper follow-up, and prediction measures through cancer biomarkers could definitely be very effective tools for the amelioration of cancer burden. Biomarkers are "Any measurable diagnostic indicator that is used to assess the risk or presence of disease" as defined by the US Food and Drugs Administration (FDA), or they would be comprehensively defined as—"A characteristic that is objectively measured and evaluated as an indicator of normal biological processes, pathogenic processes, or pharmacological responses to therapeutic intervention" [3]. Cancer biomarkers (CB) are biomolecules produced either by the tumor cells or by other cells of the body in response to the tumor, and CB could be used as screening/early detection tool of cancer, diagnostic, prognostic, or predictor for the overall outcome of a patient. Moreover, cancer biomarkers may identify subpopulations of patients who are most likely to respond to a given therapy [4]. Biomarkers can be genes, gene products, specific cells, molecules, enzymes, or hormones which can be detected in blood, urine, tissues, or other body fluid [5].

### 1.1 Historical background of cancer biomarkers

Two thousand years ago, Ancient Egyptians were the first known who try to find markers for malignancy as described in an Egyptian papyrus, they had their first attempt in distinguishing breast cancer from mastitis [6]. Use of CB in medicine then started around 170 years ago, when Sir Bence Jones described a protein in urine of multiple myeloma patients that could be identified by its special heat coagulation properties. In 1847, Bence-Jones protein was the first cancer biomarker that was discovered as a tumor-produced light chain antibody of immunoglobulin G (IgG) in multiple myeloma patients, it was excreted in urine in excess and could be identified by heat denaturation [7]. Later, in 1986, Bence-Jones protein was reported to be present also in the serum of myeloma patients [8]. Two years later, in 1988, an immunodiagnostic test was approved by the FDA for the detection of Bence-Jones protein which may aid in the diagnosis of multiple myeloma, Waldenstrom's macroglobulinemia, leukemia, and lymphoma. In 1867, amylase was introduced by Sir Michael Foster who reported the increase levels of serum amylase in patients with cancer pancreas. He suggested urinary amylase as a biomarker for cancer pancreas. Then, after years of studying pathology and physiology of pancreas, it was realized that cancer pancreas originate from ductal cells not acinar cell; the source of amylase enzyme. Therefore, elevation of amylase enzyme may occur in large tumors impinging on acinar cells [9]. During the next 100 years, numerous studies involved other CB including hormones as chorionic gonadotropin (hCG) in choriocarcinoma and catecholamines in pheochromocytoma and neuroblastoma, and enzymes as acid phosphatase in prostate cancer, and alkaline phosphatase in bone tumors [10]. Definitely, the development of the immunoassay concept in the 1950s by Yalow and Berson has very important impact on the field of CB testing using polyclonal antibodies. Later in 1970s, CEA immunoassay was commercially available. The field of cancer biomarkers showed uprising in 1975 with the development of monoclonal antibodies and in 1982 with the development of the immunemetric (sandwich) immunoassay. This leaded to feasible expansion in the introduction of several immunoassays and new tumor antigens to be used as available tests in routine clinical practice. Recombinant antibody techniques also provided better understanding of the hypothesized structure and functions of CB. Recent molecular biology techniques were the key for discovering and realizing the putative functions of CB as tumor suppresser genes, oncogenes, nuclear proteins, and telomerase [11, 12]. Unfortunately, along all these years since the discovery Bence-Jones protein, only very few CB have been approved by the FDA as diagnostic or prognostic cancer markers in spite of being extensively studied. However, emerging

http://dx.doi.org/10.5772/62421

technology of omics, such as genomics and proteomics, may indeed encourage the generation and Validation of CB [10].

### 1.2 Cancer development and mechanisms for the production of cancer biomarkers

Cancer is a multifactorial cluster of diseases reflecting fundamental abnormality involving uncontrolled cell growth and proliferation alternating the normal cell behavior. Molecular mechanisms exhibit alterations in the expression of multiple genes mostly includes: (proto) oncogenes, tumor suppressor genes, and DNA repair genes that contribute to the development of cancer genotype and phenotype with a state of dysregulation of cell proliferation events. Cancer hallmarks hypothesis has been postulated in 2000 by Hanahan and Weinberg. They initially categorized biological mechanisms for the cancer development into six processes: proliferative signaling, avoiding growth suppression, cell death resistance (immortalization), enabling of replicative immortality, induction of angiogenesis, and finally activation of invasion and metastasis [13]. Increasing evidence suggest that cancer may be triggered also by epigenetic changes as histone modification and DNA alteration of methylation causing alterations in the condensation state of chromatin [14]. Genetic alterations of cancer cells, as point mutation, gene rearrangement or amplifications, and subsequent disturbances of cell division and proliferation will be manifested by release of biomarkers of such changes in majority of patients with a specific type of cancer. Therefore, they can be used as biomarkers for the cancer detection or predicting responses to various treatments [15–17]. Comprehensive understanding of the altered molecular mechanisms and cellular processes underlying carcinogenesis or hallmarks of cancer may link cancer biomarkers and their clinical utility in

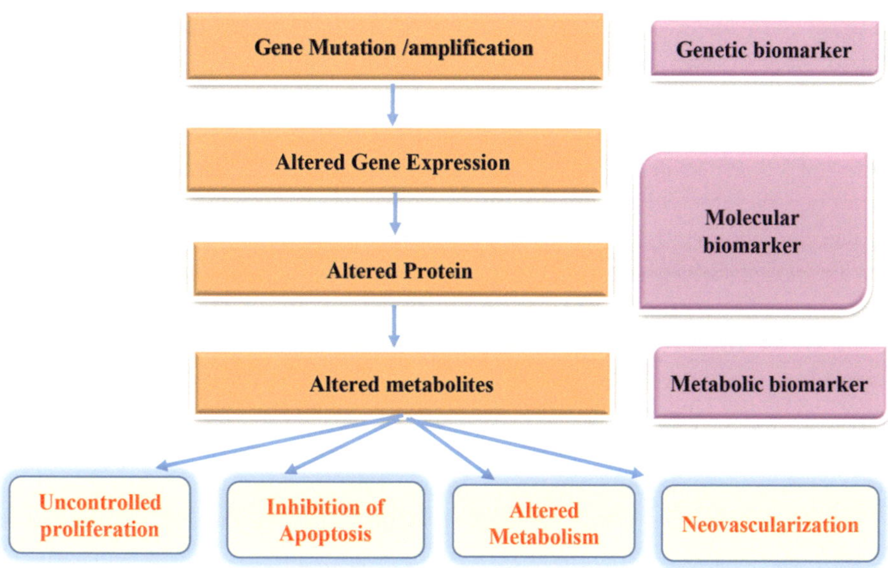


**Figure 1.** Identification of biomarkers in the process of carcinogenesis modified from Bhatt et al. [18].

cancer patient. Genetic, molecular, and metabolic biomarker may be identified through applying the sequential of events occurring in cancer cells from gene mutation following its effects on cellular proliferation and metabolism [18], as illustrated in **Figure 1**. One of the major challenges for oncology research is to establish the definite relationship between cancer biomarkers and cancer pathology, as well as, to detect cancer in early stage beside the development of targeted therapies targeting the exact altered gene or cellular process [16].

### 1.3 Serum, biological fluid, and tissue Cancer Biomarkers

Understanding mechanisms of carcinogenesis could explain the production and release of CB in cancerous cells, blood or various body fluid and hence release of those molecules and elevation during cancer initiation, development, and progression or metastasizing. Mechanisms for elevation of CB levels in any of the biological fluid could be explained by three mechanisms. The first mechanism is overexpression or amplification of gene product, or enhancement of epigenetic changes (affect gene expression) as DNA methylation with release of such CB as protein human epididymal secretory protein 4 (HE4) in ovarian cancer. HE4 is overexpressed in ovarian carcinoma and could be also detected in serum [19–21]. However, clinical evaluation of HE4 revealed that it is also overexpressed in endometrial, breast, and bronchial adenocarcinoma [22]. The second mechanism of elevation could be typically applied on serum biomarkers, which is the secretion of cellular proteins or shedding of membrane proteins. An example of such serum biomarker is alpha-fetoprotein (AFP); an oncofetal protein with altered single peptide that is elevated in circulation in patient with hepatocellular carcinoma [23] and HER2-neu, a cell membrane surface-bound tyrosine kinase, released and elevated in the serum of breast cancer patients after being cleaved by proteolysis. HER2-neu is also approved by the FDA for monitoring of metastatic cases of breast cancer [24]. The third mechanism is cell invasion and angiogenesis as occur with prostate-specific antigen (PSA). It is expressed normally by prostatic epithelium but elevation of PSA levels occurs due to distorted basement membrane of prostatic cell and lymph angiogenesis [25]. The clinical application of CB, especially circulating protein targets in cancer management, is emerging into a new era especially with the availability of promising sensitive techniques that implement the discovery of "omics" cancer biomarkers in body fluids that may represent a novel, highly sensitive diagnostic tools for the early detection of cancer. Of even much importance are hidden cancers that are not easily accessible, for example, nasopharyngeal, ovarian, and pancreatic cancers. However, there is mandatory need for validation of such biomarkers [26]. CB could be detected in cancerous cells or tissue of origin in solid tumors, bone marrow, and lymph node or as circulating cells. CB could be detected in biological body fluid such as serum, ascetic fluid, pleural fluid, or urine representing noninvasive specimens or samples. CSF fluid is a suitable candidate for brain and CNS cancer. Meanwhile, urine is one of the promising frontier for the detection of bladder cancer or for of patients' surveillance [27]. In addition, it was postulated that prostate cancer antigen 3 (PCA3) is another promising new molecular marker for diagnosis and follow-up of cancer prostate [28]. Stool for colorectal cancer, nipple aspirate fluid, ductal lavage, and cyst fluid for breast cancer are other examples for biological fluid sources for discovery or clinical application tool for CB [29].

http://dx.doi.org/10.5772/62421

## 2. Clinical applications and performance indications of Cancer Biomarkers

More than 25 years ago, the clinical usefulness of CB was limited to be an effective tool for patient's prognosis, surveillance, and therapy monitoring. Definition of tumor markers that have been adopted by the fifth International Conference on Human Tumor Markers held in Stockholm, Sweden, in 1988 stated that *"Biochemical tumor markers are substances developed in tumor cells and secreted into body fluids in which they can be quantitated by non-invasive analyses. Because of a correlation between marker concentration and active tumor mass, tumor markers are useful in the management of cancer patients. Markers, which are available for most cancer cases, are additional, valuable tools in patient prognosis, surveillance, and therapy monitoring, whereas they are presently not applicable for screening. Sero-diagnostic measurements of markers should emphasize relative trends instead of absolute values and cut-off levels."* However, CB have been reported to be used also for screening of general population or risk groups, for differential diagnosis, and for clinical staging or stratification of cancer patients. Additionally, CB are used to estimate tumor burden and to substitute for a clinical endpoint and/or to measure clinical benefit, harm or lack of benefit, or harm [4, 18, 30]. Among commonly utilized biomarkers in clinical practice are PSA, AFP, CA125, and CEA. PSA is one of the serum biomarker currently used consistently in primary care to assess the risk of underlying prostate cancer. Cancer antigen 125 (CA-125) can be a biomarker of ovarian cancer risk or an indicator of malignancy, but it has low sensitivity and specificity. CEA is another biomarker that is elevated in patients with colorectal, breast, lung, or pancreatic cancer [31]. A major challenge is to develop promising CB for the stratification of cancer patients not only to predict outcome or response for therapy, providing customized treatment, but also for personalized therapeutic strategies of cancer patients. Among promising biomarkers in that field is survivin and HER2-neu [32, 33].

### 2.1. Sensitivity and specificity for evaluation of accuracy of CB

As being released from tumor cells, or body cells in response to the tumor, CB can be detected in any of the body fluids, secretions, or tumor tissue and cells. CB can be detected in serum, plasma, or whole blood, also in whole excretions as urine, sputum, or CSF. Therefore, CB could be assessed in noninvasive and in serial manner. Evaluation of cancer biomarker in tissue or cells requires tissue biopsy or more invasive technique than serum biomarkers. CB can be detected in tissues by special techniques but in an invasive manner than serum or urine biomarkers. Genetic biomarkers could be detected in DNA derived from tumor tissue, whole blood, or buccal mucosa cells [34]. Evaluation of diagnostic value of any test or marker is usually performed with referral to the terms of sensitivity and specificity of that marker. Specificity means that ability of the marker to detect non-diseased subjects whereas sensitivity refers to the ability of that test to identify diseased subjects (patients) [35]. At definitive cutoff value, a test or biomarker may be found above that value (positive), but actually not all positives are diseased subjects. Therefore, sensitivity is calculated, as the ratio of the all positives who are found by that test, above the cutoff value to the total number of abnormals known to have the disease (true positive); simply sensitivity is the true positive rate (TPR).

Similarly, by applying the same cutoff value for the same test, some people with normal results below cutoff value are actually normal (true negative) but not all of them are not having the disease (false negative). Therefore, the true negative rate or specificity could be calculated as the ratio of the all negatives who found by the test below cutoff value to the total number of normals known not to have the disease (true negative) [36]. Therefore, a CB with 100% specificity could be used to correctly identifies all non-cancerous subjects, CB with 70% specificity could identify only 70% of the non-cancerous as being negative (true negatives), and however, 30% of non-cancerous are falsely identified positive (false positives) [37]. Supposing sensitivity of a CB is 100%, this means that it could identify all cancer patients and if another CB supposed to be with 90% sensitivity, it could detects 90% of patients with cancer (true positives) but fail to detect it only in 10% of cancer patients (false negatives). Consequently, sensitivity and specificity could be computed across all possible cutoff or threshold values and both are inversely related to each other [38].

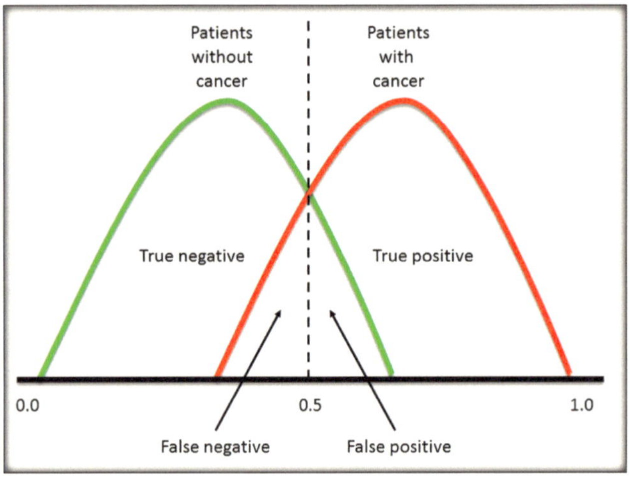


**Figure 2.** Cancer biomarker range of results among cancer and non-cancerous patients.

## 2.2. Receiver operating characteristics (ROC) curve analysis

Comparative analysis of different sensitivities and specificities at different thresholds would be very effective to judge the accuracy of diagnostic test. ROC curve was introduced by the British during World War II in order to identify accurate radar detectors and was used later in performance evaluation of radiological tests [39]. ROC curve is simply defined as performance indicator of a test or biomarker by plotting its sensitivity along the y axis and its 1-specificity or FPR (false positive rate) along the x axis to assess the diagnostic ability of such biomarker and in discrimination of the diseased from the healthy subjects [40]. ROC curves have been extensively used for evaluation of the accuracy of diagnostic tests with meaningful interpretations. Several indices could be derived from it such as the area under the curve (AUC) that determines the average of the sensitivity values for all possible specificity values and includes whole area underneath the entire ROC curve [36]. AUC could have a range between one and zero because values of the x and y axes probably having values ranging from zero to one as well. The closer the value of AUC to one the better is the clinical performance of that test [40]. Comparing AUC areas of different tests can be used to compare their diagnostic performance as AUC is a measure of their overall performance. The test with bigger AUC value is of better overall performance. On comparison of two tests and if both AUC areas are equal, this indicates same diagnostic performance of both tests, but non-necessarily mean identical ROC curves [41]. **Figure 2** represents the CB levels among cancer and non-cancer cases, while **Figure 3** illustrates ROC curve and area under the curve.

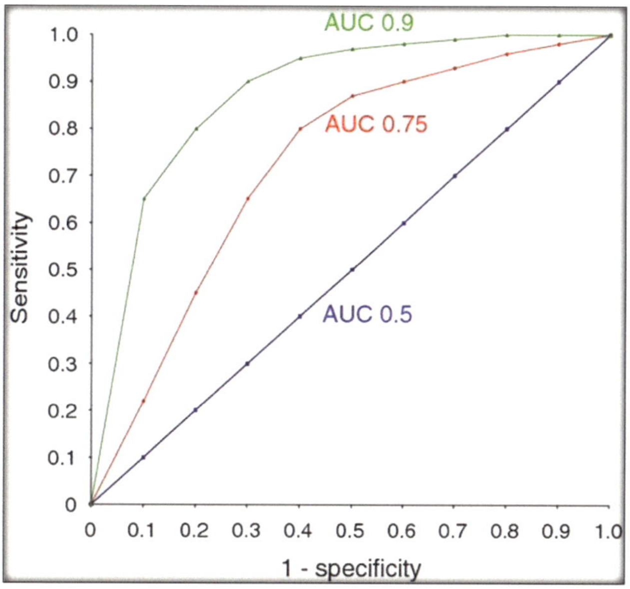


**Figure 3.** ROC curve analysis and comparison of area under the curve.

### 2.3. Ideal biomarker

Measurement of sensitivity and specificity of a biomarker at a range of cutoff values could be of an important impact for evaluation of CB as we may chose a definitive cutoff value that achieves the highest sensitivity and specificity. Increment of cutoff point will definitely lead to increase of specificity of the test or false negative patients but on the other hand, this will decrease number of false positives; this indicate a highly specific but low sensitive biomarker. Similarly, if the cutoff point is low that indicates a highly sensitive but low-specific biomarker, as there are fewer false negatives but more false positive subjects. Indeed, pairs of sensitivities and specificities may describe accuracy of the biomarker and its ability to discriminate between healthy (normal) and diseased. We can identify the threshold limit or cutoff value to a diagnostic sensitivity of 100% or less but considering the corresponding specificity for that threshold. The decision threshold must be chosen to be used in patient care, but not for assessment of accuracy. Indeed assessment for performance at definitive point may be misleading or this may results in bias for comparison between tests [42]. Ideal biomarker must be strictly able to differentiate between cancerous from benign cases, aggressive tumors from insignificant one; it should be of high specificity and sensitivity. Furthermore, it should be a noninvasive and inexpensive [30, 43]. The characteristic features of an ideal biomarker are variable and relay to some extent on the application and classification of CB. Mostly, CB have to fulfill the following general properties to be considered ideal. Obviously, no biomarker could meet these requirements all together, but these criteria should be highly considered for selection of diagnostic biomarker [44]:

- ***High clinical sensitivity:*** produced by all patients with that specific cancer (100% TPR).
- ***High clinical specificity:*** low false negative rate (100%True negative).
- ***Organ or tissue specific.***
- ***Proportional to tumor burden or volume:*** quantitatively proportionate to tumor volume or disease progression.
- ***Short half-life***: reflecting quickly any early changes in tumor burden for proper monitoring of therapy.
- ***Present (if any) at low levels in the serum of healthy individuals and those with benign disease.***
- ***Sharply discriminating metastasis.***
- ***Exist in quantitative, standardized, reproducible, and validated assay.***
- ***Inexpensive or low coasting method.***
- ***Obtained in a noninvasive manner:*** detected in serum, body fluids, or in easily accessible tissue.

## 3. Uses, clinical utility, and limitations of CB

Conventionally used tumor markers or CB may be either proteins or glycoproteins, being probably not involved in carcinogenesis or development of cancer process, rather are likely to be by-products of malignant transformation. Low molecular weight, small molecules or nucleic acids markers (as gene mutations or polymorphisms and quantitative gene expression analysis, peptides, proteins, lipids metabolites, and other small molecules are promising and recently being evaluated as potential clinically useful tumor markers, the patterns of gene expression and genetic alterations and defects may be the framework of the molecular classification of CB [11]. There are several classification s for CB depending on different aspects related to their chemical nature, proposed mechanisms for their release and applications. Six years ago, a unique classification proposed by Mishra and Verma [45] with an emphasis on clinical utility of CB. They classified CB into prediction biomarkers as DNA biomolecules,

http://dx.doi.org/10.5772/62421

detection biomarkers as RNA molecules, diagnostic biomarkers as protein biomarkers, and prognosis biomarkers as glyco-biomarkers. Clinical applications and uses of CB, as simply illustrated in **Figure 4** are screening and early detection, diagnostic confirmation, prognosis and prediction of therapeutic response, and monitoring disease and recurrence [46]. Another use of CB includes cancer susceptibility and risk assessment markers which include the identification of individuals who are at a high risk of developing cancer or candidates for screening programs and early preventive studies [47]. Risk or susceptibility assessment markers include markers of inflammation, oxidative stress and single-nucleotide polymorphisms (SNPs), and mutations in certain genes [48, 49]. **Table 1** illustrates most of traditional, the FDA approved, and clinically relevant CB with their uses in various cancer types.

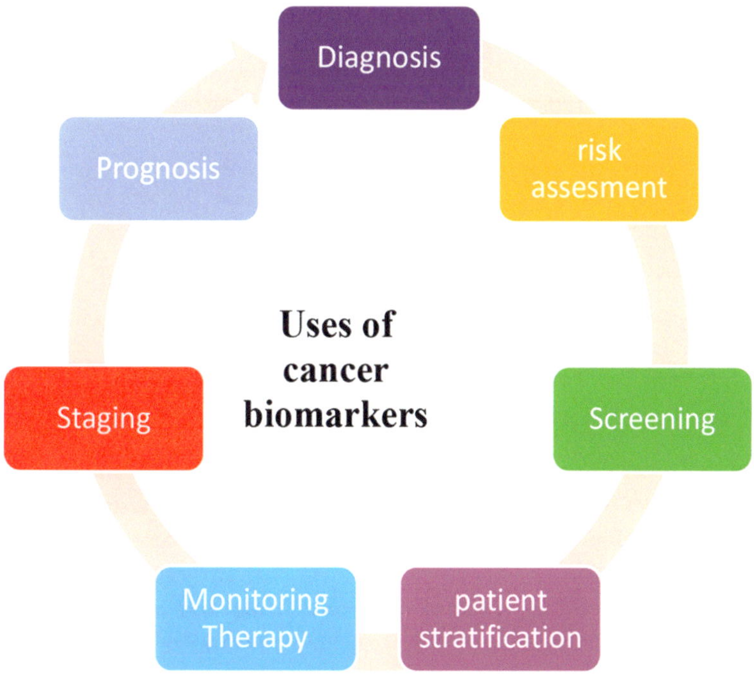


**Figure 4.** Clinical utility and uses of cancer biomarkers.

### 3.1. Screening/early detection

In 2008, Wald defined screening as "the systematic application of a test to identify subjects at sufficient risk of a specific disorder to benefit from further investigation or direct preventive action, among persons who have not sought medical attention on account of symptoms of that disorder" [50]. Earlier efficient treatment must lead to better outcome compared with the treatment available at later cancer stages or symptomatic patients. Screening aim was to detect disease when subjects are asymptomatic which differ from diagnosis of symptomatic patients. Objectives of screening and early detection of cancer were to detect cancer at curable and better

| Cancer biomarker | Organ specificity/cancer type | Application/uses | References |
|---|---|---|---|
| Prostate-specific antigen (PSA) | Prostate/BPH | Screening, diagnosis and monitoring | [86, 133] |
| Carbohydrate antigen 125 (CA125) | Ovarian | Diagnosis, prognosis, detecting recurrence and monitoring therapy | [134] |
| Carcinoembryonic antigen (CEA) | Colorectal/hepatic | Monitoring therapy | [135–137] |
| | | Prognosis | |
| | | Detecting recurrence | |
| | | Screening for hepatic metastases | |
| Carbohydrate antigen 15.3 (CA 15-3) | Breast | Monitoring therapy | [69, 138] |
| Estrogen, progesterone receptors (ER and PgR) | Breast | Stratification/select patients for endocrine therapy | [139–141] |
| HER2 | Breast | Monitoring trastuzumab therapy | [18, 32, 33, 142] |
| Carbohydrate antigen 27.29 (CA27.29) | Breast | Monitoring | [84] |
| Human chorionic gonadotropin-β (HCG-β) | Testicular | Diagnosis | [143] |
| | | Staging | |
| | | Detecting recurrence | |
| | | Monitoring therapy | |
| Alfa-fetoprotein | Hepatocellular carcinoma | Diagnosis | [144–146] |
| | | Detecting recurrence | |
| | | Monitoring therapy | |
| Calcitonin | Medullary carcinoma of thyroid | Diagnosis and monitoring therapy | [147, 148] |
| Thyroglobulin | Thyroid | Monitoring | [149] |
| CA 19-9 | Pancreatic | Monitoring therapy | [76] |
| Nuclear matrix protein 22 (NMP-22) | Bladder | Screening, monitoring and prognosis | [150] |
| Prostate cancer antigen 3 (PCA3) | Prostate | Prognostic | [151] |

**Table 1.** Current cancer biomarkers and uses in clinical practice.

outcome state and even before appearance of symptoms. Reports calculated a drop in the 5 years survival rate from being about 90%, in early localized breast cancer, to reach about 60% in local metastasizing and only 30% to distant metastasizing cases of breast cancer [51]. Therefore, screening CB should be able to detect cancer in an early stage or asymptomatic stage and consequently will result in increase of survival rate and decrease complications or morbidities. Screening test must be highly specific to minimize false positives as less as possible. High specificity is mandatory for screening biomarker because even a small false-positive rate could result in large number of unnecessary other invasive diagnostic procedures that may be unneeded with the associated psychological burden and excess costs. Ideal screening programs have to be noninvasive and inexpensive and definitely lead to obvious reduction in morbidity and mortality and increase in survival rate. Usually, screening programs are directed for highly prevalent cancers and further treatment and follow-up are mandatory [34]. Other limiting factors for screening biomarker are the low diagnostic sensitivity and specificity of most of the currently used biomarkers to serve as screening markers and being elevated later in the course of cancer. However, few biomarkers have been used as screening biomarkers as AFP in screening for hepatocellular cancer in high-risk subjects, PSA in screening for prostate cancer, CA125 in screening for ovarian cancer, and fecal occult blood testing (FOBT) in screening for colorectal cancers (CRC) and vanillymandelic acid (VMA) in screening for neuroblastoma in newborns [52]. PSA was cleared by the FDA as a screening biomarker for prostate cancer; however, false positive elevation of PSA levels can be found in individuals with benign or inflammatory conditions as benign prostatic hyperplasia and prostatitis [53]. Contribution of PSA screening in decreasing mortality is still being a matter of contraverse [54, 55].

### 3.2. Diagnosis/differential diagnosis

A diagnostic biomarker would be applied only for symptomatic patients in contrast to screening biomarker that would be applicable only for symptomatic individuals. Interestingly, the characteristics of an ideal diagnostic biomarker are similar to the characteristics for screening. Notably, most of well-established biomarkers for screening could be used as diagnostic markers and PSA is well-recognized example. PSA, in combination with a digital rectal examination (DRE), is the most commonly used diagnostic tool for prostate cancer [56]. Regarding encountered limitations for diagnostic biomarkers, current available cancer biomarkers are still having low diagnostic sensitivity and specificity; however, diagnostic biomarkers must be of high sensitivity in order to be a good diagnostic biomarker [57]. For example, Bence-Jones protein in urine remains one of the strongest, well-established diagnostic indicators of multiple myeloma [29]. Nevertheless, some CB have proved to be useful in confirming diagnosis, often in conjunction with a panel of other markers especially to identify primary tumor in metastatic cases with unknown primary and/or other clinical, imaging tools [58]. Use of panel of CB in order to increase sensitivity and specificity of CB in diagnosis has been used to confirm diagnosis of certain cancers. In 2005, Mor et al. [59] reported that a panel, consisting of 4 biomarkers: leptin, osteopontin, prolactin, and insulin-like growth factor 2, collectively had a sensitivity of 95% and a specificity of 95% for the detection of ovarian cancer. In another report, addition of two biomarkers to the previously studied panel included macrophage inhibitory factor and CA125, sensitivity was 95% and a specificity increase to 99.4% for the detection of ovarian cancer. Other attempts to improve diagnostic sensitivity and specificity included combination of CA125 with ultrasonography for diagnosis of ovarian cancer [60].

### 3.3. Prognosis/prediction

Prognosis is the probability of cure or likely outcome of any patient. A prognostic marker is a disease or patient characteristic feature at the time of diagnosis independent upon therapy; hence, prognostic marker will provide information about the natural history of the disease or the likely outcome. Meanwhile, a predictive biomarker predicts the response to different therapeutic modalities; hence, predictive biomarker is the basic concept for personalized medicine [57]. Magnitude of elevation or levels of CB usually reflects tumor burden, or mass hence higher elevation of CB level mostly reflects bad prognosis and vice versa. By reflecting the tumor burden, CB can be used in staging system for cancer or the tumor–node–metastasis (TNM) classification. For example, in testicular germ cell tumors, very high levels of a CB such as AFP, LDH, and HCG-$\beta$ may indicate an aggressive cancer with poor prognosis and outcome so such biomarkers may be used for staging in TNMS system in place with a site-specific prognostic factor (S is for site-specific prognostic factors) [61]. LDH alone has been used for staging of lymphoma as well [62]. However, the accuracy of the marker in determining tumor stage is poor. Estrogen receptor (ER) is one of the widely used prognostic and predictive tissue biomarker; as a predictive tissue biomarker, ER is used for selecting the patients likely to respond to hormonal therapy. Therefore, patients with ER positive tumors will mostly respond to selective ER modulators or aromatase inhibitors independent upon stage of breast cancer weather early or advanced [63]. ER is considered a prognostic marker as well, once ER is negative, that indicate a poor prognosis and when positive a good prognosis is likely the outcome for such patients. In spite of most of CB have some prognostic values which their specific therapeutic impact cannot be applied because of their poor predication accuracy [64]. In the same context, high serum levels of HER2 in serum of breast cancer patients correlate with poor prognosis in such patients [24]. Targeted therapy for HER-2 positive breast cancer patients, trastuzumab (Herceptin), is a recombinant monoclonal antibody against HER-2. Herceptin has been used in women with metastatic breast cancer that overexpressed HER2 and reported to increases the clinical benefit of first-line chemotherapy in those patients [65]. KRAS is a predictive biomarker for colorectal cancer, because patients with somatic mutations in KRAS have poor response to anti-epidermal growth factor receptor (EGFR)-targeting therapies [66].

### 3.4. Therapeutic monitoring/follow-up/evidence of metastasis or recurrence

Therapeutic monitoring may constitute the most common applications of CB markers in clinical practice [67]. Clinically useful biomarkers usually fluctuate in accordance with tumor behavior, size, or burden changes that are best elicited by increase in levels of CB with progressive disease, decrease with remission, and do not change significantly with stable disease. Kinetics of CB are more important than single measurement or elevated values [68]. Recurrence of cancer may be detected biochemically via rise in CB levels even before appearance of any clinical or radiological evidence of cancer recurrence. Continues follow-up for cancer patients during and after therapy can mirror their condition if the levels of CB were not elevated or remain at basal level, indicating successful therapy or remission. On the other hand, rising of CB level above the basal level indicates recurrence of the disease. CB can be a warning sign of recurrence earlier by 3–12 months before any other diagnostic methods. Many CB could be used for monitoring therapy or detection of recurrence or metastasis, for example, CEA in colorectal cancers, cancer antigen 125 (CA 125) in ovarian cancers, or PSA in prostatic cancer [69]. Some patients who encountered resistance to therapeutic modalities will experience increasing levels of CB, and in that case, reconsideration of alternative therapy is mandatory. Monitoring CB, as screening and diagnostic biomarker needs to be both diagnostically sensitive and specific to ensure proper assessment of effective therapy and continuation of such beneficial therapies and early discontinuation/replacement of ineffective therapy or resistant cancer to those therapies. A representing example of monitoring CB is carbohydrate antigen 19-9 (CA19-9) which has been used in pancreatic in CRC [70]. CA19-9 has been approved by the FDA in 2002 as a monitoring marker for pancreatic cancer. However, it is not recommended as a screening biomarker [71, 72]. Monitoring biomarkers have been extensively used in clinical practice with few limitations perhaps related to detectors' biomarkers of recurrence rather than monitoring ones. Limitations of those biomarkers probably related to short lead time and poor affection to the outcome [29].

## 4. Applications of CB in most common cancers

Cancer is an enormous health problem all over the world, over years cancer was indicated as one of the leading causes of death among males and females; an estimated 8.2 million deaths among cancer patients occurred in 2012 worldwide [73]. Over 11 million patients are diagnosed with cancer every year, and 16 million new cases will be expected yearly by 2020 [2]. According to the latest report of the International Agency for Research on Cancer (IARC), the GLOBOCAN worldwide estimates of cancer incidence and mortality published on 2015 and the most common cancers' types among males were lung, prostate, colorectal, liver, and urinary bladder. Meanwhile, breast cancer, lung, liver, ovarian cancers were among the most common cancers in females worldwide [1]. For many years ago, few CB have been used as an effective tool in clinical practice, while also promising CB were extensively studied for their clinical utility. As previously discussed, traditionally used or promising CB may be used for risk assessment for cancer, screening among asymptomatic population, confirming diagnosis or differentially discriminate benign from malignant, prediction of outcome or prognosis, and monitoring of therapy or staging of cancer applications [58].

### 4.1. Breast cancer

Breast cancer is the most common malignancy among females and the first leading cause of cancer mortality worldwide; its prevalence is surprisingly increasing at a rapid rate lately [74]. Therefore, it is critical to use all available tools for early diagnosis and proper management of cases. Clinically, symptoms are mainly breast lump, nipple discharge, or skin or nipple changes. Screening guidelines by The American Cancer Society recommend that women over 40 have to perform mammography and a yearly or every other year clinical breast exam [75]. Diagnosis mainly relies on pathological examination; however, the role of CB in breast cancer is mainly helpful with prognosis, monitoring of therapy, and for follow-up. Notably, CB does not show great utility for early diagnosis [76]. Assessment of ER and progesterone receptors (PR) in tissue for newly diagnosed breast cancers has been recommended by European Society of Medical Oncology, for predicting response to hormone therapy in early and advanced breast cancer cases [63, 77, 78]. HER-2 is another prognostic marker, most useful for selecting patients with either early or metastatic breast cancer for the treatment with Trastuzumab (Herceptin) [79] or predicting resistance to tamoxifen therapy in early stage of breast cancer [63]. Determination of risk groups for the development of breast cancer, who must be included in screening program, involves the detection of genetic mutation of BRCA 1 or BRCA 2 genes, which account for up to 5% of breast cancer cases. Due to their high susceptibility to breast and ovarian cancer, it is strongly recommended that women carrying BRCA1 or BRCA2 mutations undergo routine cancer screening [80]. It was reported that low levels of urokinase plasminogen activator (uPA) and plasminogen activator inhibitor-1 (PAI-1) correlate with a reduced risk of recurrence of breast cancer and shown to be strong independent prognostic factors of newly diagnosed lymph node-negative breast cancers [81, 82]. Serum biomarkers are mainly applicable as monitoring markers during therapy or to less extent prognostic markers and usually assisted in post-operative surveillance, and CB included under that category include CA15.3, CEA, and BR 27-29 [83, 84]. They are used in conjugation with other tools of radiological and clinical assessments to monitor chemotherapy in advanced breast cancer cases. Elevation of serum levels of these markers may indicate recurrence or progression of the disease [85].

### 4.2. Prostate cancer

Prostate cancer (PCa) is one of the most common cancer in men and most common causes of male cancer-related deaths [74]. Strong evidences suggested that PSA test revolutionized the prostate cancer screening and diagnosis landscape, and the introduction of PSA as a screening test has led to a sharp increase in the incidence of prostate cancer because there has been a shift to diagnosis at earlier stages, consequently reducing mortality from prostate cancer [86]. Later, many studies demonstrated significant improvement sensitivity of PSA as a diagnostic marker using a PSA subtractions and isoforms [−2] (proPSA) and its percentage derivative % proPSA (percent value relative to PSA) as these fraction may help for the discrimination between benign and malignant prostatic tumors in patients with PSA values ranging from 4 to 10 μg/L [87, 88]. Other novel and promising biomarkers under investigation include human kallikrein type 2, prostate cancer antigen 3 (PSA 3), and prostate stem cell antigen (PSCA) [89]. PCA3 urine assay has promising role in improving the accuracy of diagnosis in prostate cancer [90]. Elevated levels of metalloproteinase 2 and 9 (MMP-2 and MMP-9) members of protease family have been associated with prostate cancer diagnosis [91]. MMPs have been studied as biomarkers of therapeutic monitoring in prostate cancer [92].

### 4.3. Ovarian cancer

Most of the patients with epithelial ovarian cancer are diagnosed late and they have clinically advanced stage III and IV on diagnosis; therefore, ovarian cancer needs a sensitive and specific diagnostic biomarkers [93]. CA 125 is one of the most widely and conventionally used CB. It is recommended as a screening biomarker for women who have positive family history or are high risk for the development of ovarian cancer, beside CA125 has been used in conjugation with vaginal ultrasound as a well-established, diagnostic biomarker [94]. CA125 is also been used as monitoring biomarker, being decreased after starting of chemotherapy or surgery, that correlates with favorable response basal level of CA125, two weeks before starting any therapeutic intervention then follow ups and continues monitoring of its level at regular intervals are highly recommended [95]. Other biomarkers were extensively studied in monitoring of ovarian cancer and in prediction of prognosis but further studies are needed for proper confirmation of their exact role. This panel includes kallikreins (5–9), osteopontin, Her-2/neu, tumor-associated inhibin, CEA, trypsin inhibitor, hCG, interleukin-6 (IL-6), prostasin, TPA, lysophosphatidic acid, plasminogen activator inhibitor-1 (PAI-1) [95–97].

### 4.4. Colorectal cancer

CRC is ranked third among all cancers all over the world. An estimated one million new cases are diagnosed and half of a million cases died each year [1]. The most common site for colorectal carcinoma is the rectum encountering 38% of all cases followed by sigmoid accounting 29% of cases [98]. Screening program for CRC should be directed to all asymptomatic individuals above 50 years as recommended [99]. National Academy of Clinical Biochemistry (NACB) recommends that all subjects 50 years or older should undergo screening for colorectal cancer. Multiple screening procedures exist [100]. Fecal occult blood test (FOBT) is the most widely used CB in stool [101]. Testing for blood in the stools involves either detecting globin fraction of blood (hemoglobin) by fecal immunochemical test or the guaiac test which measures pseudo-peroxidase activity of heme fraction of hemoglobin. CEA was characterized and introduced into clinical practice in 1965 [76]. It is widely used as universal or non-organ, non-tissue-specific tumor marker. CEA is not used in screening of CRC due to its low sensitivity and specificity, beside the low prevalence of CRC among asymptomatic population; however, it is very efficient prognostic and therapy monitoring biomarker [102]. CEA estimation is recommended at the beginning of therapy then every 1–3 months all through the therapeutic regimen, it is also the marker of choice for metastatic cases of CRC [103]. CA19-9 has been used as prognostic marker, in surveillance of CRC after surgical resection and as monitoring marker for therapeutic intervention in advanced cases [104]. Other CB under investigation are CA242 and tissue inhibitor of metalloproteinases type 1(TIMP-1) and both may complement CEA in the surveillance of patients with colorectal cancer [105].

## 5. Discovery of new biomarkers/validation/technologies (omics)

Among hundreds of thousands of cancer biomarkers have been discovered, only few of them have been approved during the past two decades by the FDA for monitoring response, surveillance, or recurrence of cancer [106]. To be a clinically applicable and reliable biomarker, it must be of value for informing clinical decision-making to improve the patient outcome [107]. Initially, CB have to distinguish between people with cancer and those without. In fact, many biomarkers do not achieve beyond this point because the investigators are either unable to develop robust, accurate assay methods, or this biomarker lacks sufficient sensitivity and/or specificity [108]. Actually, there was very low rate (0.1%) of successful clinical translation of biomarker [109]. Developing new cancer biomarkers has been formulated in stepwise manner. About 15 years ago, Hammond and Taube proposed an approach for CB development starting from discovering the marker, developing an assay method for assessment, analyzing its clinical potential preliminarily, standardization of its assay, and finally validation of such biomarker for clinical use [110]. Structured phased model for the development evaluation, and validation of biomarkers, (shown in **Table 2**) has been proposed by Pepe et al. [111] and has been adopted and modified by others [112, 113]. This model was similar to another model commonly used in drug development strategy including five phases: preclinical exploratory studies, clinical assay and validation, retrospective longitudinal repository studies, prospective screening studies, and finally cancer control studies. Novel biomarkers must bypass an analytical validation step concerned mainly with testing and assay methods of the biomarker (technical aspects). After that, the biomarker has to be analyzed for its clinical validity for discriminating between groups independently. Finally, candidate biomarker must be assessed for clinical utility for providing additional input for patient management or aid to provide additional information helping in decision-making for patients in order to improve patient outcome [114].

| Phases | Type of studies | Outcome |
|---|---|---|
| Phase I | Preclinical exploration | Promising directions are explored and potential biomarkers identified |
| Phase II | Clinical assay and validation | Determination of the potential capacity of the biomarker to established disease |
| Phase III | Retrospective longitudinal | Determine how well biomarkers detect preclinical disease through retrospectively testing |
| Phase IV | Prospective screening | Identify the characteristics of the disease detected by the biomarker and determine the false positive rate |
| Phase V | Cancer control | Quantification of the role of the biomarkers in the reduction of disease burden through Phase 5 population screening |

**Table 2.** Structured phased model for the development evaluation, and validation of biomarkers modified from Pepe et al. [111] and Paradiso et al. [113].

### 5.1. Challenges for discovery of novel biomarkers

Development of biomarkers for cancer screening, early detection, and monitoring of treatment has both biological and economic challenges. Most detection methods currently in use identify mostly late stage or fully developed cancer, not in the premalignant or early lesions, which are amenable to resection and cure. In spite of the fact that a screening test might detect cancer at the preclinical stage, at the same time, not applicable for follow-up so it could fail to detect micrometastasis, therefore limiting the benefit of early detection and treatment [115]. Another challenge is that in many organs, for example; prostate or colon, preneoplastic lesions are much more common than aggressive cancers [116]. This creates the question of whether any screening method should just focus on early lesions or whether it should also analyze the behavior of the tumor. Another challenge for the development of CB is the nature of the cancer as being a heterogeneous disease; it is composed of many biologically different phenotypes with different responses to intervention. The nature of its heterogeneity is found between cells of a single macroscopic cancer. This heterogeneity may complicate the development of biomarkers. Therefore, the development of biomarker by genomic and proteomic means might carefully address the heterogeneity issues [117]. Detailed and comprehensive knowledge of cancer at the cellular and molecular levels has grown dramatically and exponentially in the past two decades and has resulted in significant improvement in the characterization of human tumors which in turn has catalyzed a shift toward the development of targeted therapies, the basic concept for personalized medicine [118]. Therefore, it has been recently postulated that the emergence of highly powerful "omics" technologies, such as genomics, epigenomics, transcriptomics, proteomics, and metabolomics [119]. Omics technologies may be the backbone toward the discovery of novel CB and/or panels, with distinct advantages over the currently used biomarkers. Omics have increased the number of potentially investigated biomarkers as DNA, RNA, or other protein biomolecules. The former concept of single biomarker discovery was replaced recently by multi-biomarkers discovery of panel of genes or proteins whereby, rising the query of whether the heterogeneous and multifactorial cancer may have single fingerprint.

### 5.2. Genomic technologies

Genomic technologies have been used extensively for the characterization of cancers at the molecular level hence providing better comprehensive understanding of cancer and may provide scientists the basic concepts for designing drugs that could target specific molecules or the fundamental of personalized medicine [120]. Personalized medicine has been defined by The US National Cancer Institute (NCI) as *"a form of medicine that uses information about a person's genes, proteins, and environment to prevent, diagnose, and treat disease."* [50]. Genomic alterations that may be associated with cancer include gene amplification, mutation, chromosomal rearrangements, and aberrant methylation. Molecular alterations are evolved in the content or sequence of DNA, its transcriptions mRNA or microRNA, the production of proteins, or the synthesis of various metabolites. Genomic alterations can be assessed through genome sequencing technologies or microarray for gene expression [29]. Mutation screening can be assessed by sequencing technique, while assessment of DNA copy numbers could be analyzed by DNA microarrays and DNA expression profile via PCR [120]. Genomic microarrays represent a highly powerful and sensitive technique; it can predict the clinical behavior of tumors [121]. Genomics has been extensively used for biomarker discovery and identification. Human genome accounts approximately 30,000 genes, the availability of omics techniques allows researchers to move another step further, which is designing and manufacturing of a biological drug with better understanding of pharmacogenomics, thus biomarkers allow the studying of the influence of genetic variation, providing new methods for treating patients on an individual basis. The outcome of such researches is known as personalized medicine [122].

### 5.3. Epigenomics

Epigenetics refers to heritable changes in gene expression that are not attributable to alterations in the sequence of DNA. Epigenetic changes include DNA methylation, histone modifications, and non-coding RNAs. These alterations may be present ubiquitously human malignancies and may appear in early cancer development. Therefore, they provide particularly attractive markers with broad applications in diagnostics [123]. Methylated DNA (meDNA) is a various stable carrier of epigenetic information that is directly occurred in tumor formation and progression. In fact, the inherent stability of DNA is one of the major advantages of detecting methylation. Genes that are often methylated in tumors are termed tumor biomarkers because their methylation can be used to detect the disease. Utilization of meDNA markers is superior comparing to other types of tumor biomarkers for numerous reasons including: The analysis of DNA methylation can be achieved with a wide range of methods using different types of biological material such as tissue, plasma, serum, sputum, and urine, among others [124]. Methodology of DNA methylation measurement has progressed gradually through the years. Assessment techniques for epigenetic changes may include: The bisulphate conversion of DNA followed by PCR amplification allows gene-specific methylation analysis (methylation-specific PCR, i.e., MSP), which is based on using primers and probes specific to the corresponding methylated DNA sequence [125]. This technology makes the detection of hundreds of thousands of DNA methylation signals a reality. These signals can be digitized into a long string of ones and zeros, creating a digital phenotype that reflects genetic activity in a particular cell or tissue, that is, whether it is functioning normally or whether it is abnormal. Around 200 such biomarkers have been discovered through a large-scale genome-wide screening effort of all major human tumors for DNA methylation biomarkers in bio-specimen; tissue and serum [126].

### 5.4. Proteomics

Proteomics-based strategy diseases identification is considered as one of the dynamic and innovative tools that could confirm, complement, or quite often supply more elaborate information beyond that obtained by other high-throughput approaches such as genomic, transcriptomics, and epigenomics. Despite genomic expression profiling is a highly reliable method for cancer classification and prognostication [127, 128]. The function of such genes and the data interpretation in the context of functional networks require their translation into active proteins and their analysis through the power of proteomics. Moreover, although studies focusing on detecting the differential expression of mRNA have been extremely informative, they do not necessarily correlate with the functional protein concentrations. Therefore, post genomic “proteomic” projects correlating protein expression profiles to cancer are essential for a complementary and comprehensive representation of cancer biology. Moreover, targeting-specific protein pathways involved in tumorigenesis present a realistic aim in cancer treatment, as proteins exert their effects through specific pathways rather than functioning individually [120]. Macromolecules, in general, and proteins, in particular, are highly dynamic molecules. Mechanistically, proteins can be subjected to extensive functional regulation by various processes such as proteolytic degradation, posttranslational modification, involvement in complex structures, and compartmentalization. Proteomics is concerned with studying the whole protein repertoire of a defined entity in a biological fluid, an organelle, a cell, a tissue, an organ, a system, or the whole organism. Therefore, in-depth studying of proteomics profiles of various bio-specimens obtained from cancer patients is expected to increase our understanding of tumor pathogenesis, monitoring, and the identification of novel targets for cancer therapy. In a simple way, proteins may be actively secreted or released by the tumor cells as a result of necrosis or apoptosis and released into the circulation [76]. This changes the protein profile. The difference in signal intensities may be detected by comparison with sera from normal individuals. Secretomics, a subfield of proteomics that studies secreted proteins and secretion pathways using proteomic approaches, has recently emerged as an important tool for the discovery of biomarkers. In what is now commonly referred to as proteogenomics, and proteomic technologies are further used for improving gene annotations. Parallel analysis of the genome and the proteome facilitates discovery of post-translational modifications and proteolytic events (comparative proteogenomics).

### 5.5. Metabolomics

A cancer biomarker can be a metabolite, secreted by tumor, metabolic pathway or process, and may be employed to diagnose cancer and predict patient response towards therapies and monitor recurrence. Though proteins are the key tumor markers that can be as diverse as molecular, biochemical, physiological, or anatomical [129]. Markers can be utilized for diagnosis (to identify early stage), prognosis (assess the lethality), and prediction (of patient's response to treatment) of cancer. The markers can be detected in body fluids (blood, urine, serum, stool, saliva), or tissues (tissue samples or biopsies of the cancer). Moreover, it has been shown recently that cancer volatile organic compounds (VOC) markers can be detected in breath [130]. However, detecting the markers is a sophisticated process and metabolomics is one of the omic technologies. Among genome, transcriptome, proteome, and metabolome, the latter is the powerful representative of the phenotype [131]. Exploring the cancer metabolome seems to be an effective way to study the phenotypic changes associated with tumor. Screening biomarkers by recruiting an array of analytical techniques has been emphasized [132]. Rather than a single metabolite, a pattern is believed to be more indicative of cancer status. Metabolomic approach makes it feasible to detect an array of metabolites in a single assay. The principal analytical tools employed for metabolome analysis are mass spectrometry (MS) and nuclear magnetic resonance spectroscopy (NMR).

## 6. Conclusion and prospective

Cancer biomarkers play an important role in the field of oncology and in clinical practice for risk assessment, screening, diagnosis integrated with other diagnostic tools and mostly for the determination of prognosis and response to treatment and/or relapse. Cancer biomarkers can also facilitate the molecular definition of cancer. It is necessary for clinicians and researchers to have a comprehensive understanding of molecular aspects, clinical utility, and reliability of biomarkers in order to determine whether and in what setting a biomarker is clinically useful for the patient care, or additional evaluation is required before integration into routine medical practice. The challenge and future prospective of biomarkers, by facilitating the combination of therapeutics with diagnostics, promise to play an important role in the development of personalized medicine.

## Author details

Hala Fawzy Mohamed Kamel,[1,2*] and Hiba Saeed Bagader Al-Amodi[1]

*Address all correspondence to: kamelhala@msn.com; dr.halakamel@gmail.com

1 Biochemistry Department, Faculty of Medicine Umm AL Qura University, Makkah, KSA

2 Medical Biochemistry Department, Faculty of Medicine, Ain Shams University, Cairo, Egypt

## References

[1] Ferlay J, Soerjomataram I, Dikshit R, Eser S, Mathers C, Rebelo M, et al. Cancer incidence and mortality worldwide: sources, methods and major patterns in GLOBOCAN 2012. International Journal of Cancer Journal International du Cancer 2015;136:E359–86.

[2] Cho WC. Contribution of oncoproteomics to cancer biomarker discovery. Molecular Cancer 2007;6:25.

[3] Ilyin SE , Belkowski SM, Plata-Salaman CR. Biomarker discovery and validation: technologies and integrative approaches. Trends in Biotechnology 2004;22:411–6.

[4] Goossens N , Nakagawa S, Sun X, Hoshida Y. Cancer biomarker discovery and validation. Translational Cancer Research 2015;4:256–69.

[5] Rhea JM , Molinaro RJ. Cancer biomarkers: surviving the journey from bench to bedside. MLO: Medical Laboratory Observer 2011;43:10–2, 6, 8; quiz 20, 2.

[6] Pandha HS , Waxman J. Tumour markers. QJM: Monthly Journal of the Association of Physicians 1995;88:233–41.

[7] Kyle RA. Multiple myeloma: how did it begin? Mayo Clinic Proceedings 1994;69:680–3.

[8] Sinclair D , Dagg JH, Smith JG, Stott DI. The incidence and possible relevance of Bence-Jones protein in the sera of patients with multiple myeloma. British Journal of Haematology 1986;62:689–94.

[9] Schwartz MK. Enzymes in cancer. Clinical Chemistry 1973;19:10–22.

[10] Pritzker KP. Cancer biomarkers: easier said than done. Clinical Chemistry 2002;48:1147–50.

[11] Johnson PJ. A framework for the molecular classification of circulating tumor markers. Annals of the New York Academy of Sciences 2001;945:8–21.

[12] Suresh MR. Classification of tumor markers. Anticancer Research 1996;16:2273–7.

[13] Hanahan D , Weinberg RA. The hallmarks of cancer. Cell 2000;100:57–70.

[14] Baylin SB , Ohm JE. Epigenetic gene silencing in cancer—a mechanism for early oncogenic pathway addiction? Nature Reviews Cancer 2006;6:107–16.

[15] Weissleder R , Ntziachristos V. Shedding light onto live molecular targets. Nature Medicine 2003;9:123–8.

[16] Sidransky D. Emerging molecular markers of cancer. Nature Reviews Cancer 2002;2:210–9.

[17] Vogelstein B , Kinzler KW. Cancer genes and the pathways they control. Nature Medicine 2004;10:789–99.

[18] Bhatt AN , Mathur R, Farooque A, Verma A, Dwarakanath BS. Cancer biomarkers—current perspectives. The Indian Journal of Medical Research 2010;132:129–49.

[19] Welsh JB , Zarrinkar PP, Sapinoso LM, Kern SG, Behling CA, Monk BJ,. Analysis of gene expression profiles in normal and neoplastic ovarian tissue samples identifies candidate molecular markers of epithelial ovarian cancer. Proceedings of the National Academy of Sciences of the United States of America 2001;98:1176–81.

[20] Hellstrom I , Raycraft J, Hayden-Ledbetter M, Ledbetter JA, Schummer M, McIntosh M,. The HE4 (WFDC2) protein is a biomarker for ovarian carcinoma. Cancer Research 2003;63:3695–700.

[21] Chang X , Ye X, Dong L, Cheng H, Cheng Y, Zhu L,. Human epididymis protein 4 (HE4) as a serum tumor biomarker in patients with ovarian carcinoma. International Journal of Gynecological Cancer: Official Journal of the International Gynecological Cancer Society 2011;21:852–8.

[22] Galgano MT , Hampton GM, Frierson HF Jr. Comprehensive analysis of HE4 expression in normal and malignant human tissues. Modern Pathology: An Official Journal of the United States and Canadian Academy of Pathology, Inc 2006;19:847–53.

[23] Abelev GI , Eraiser TL. Cellular aspects of alpha-fetoprotein reexpression in tumors. Seminars in Cancer Biology 1999;9:95–107.

[24] Molina R , Jo J, Filella X, Zanon G, Pahisa J, Munoz M,. C-erbB-2 oncoprotein in the sera and tissue of patients with breast cancer. Utility in Prognosis. Anticancer Research 1996;16:2295–300.

[25] Stacker SA , Achen MG, Jussila L, Baldwin ME, Alitalo K. Lymphangiogenesis and cancer metastasis. Nature Reviews Cancer 2002;2:573–83.

[26] Wulfkuhle JD , Liotta LA, Petricoin EF. Proteomic applications for the early detection of cancer. Nature Reviews Cancer 2003;3:267–75.

[27] Xylinas E , Kluth LA, Rieken M, Karakiewicz PI, Lotan Y, Shariat SF. Urine markers for detection and surveillance of bladder cancer. Urologic Oncology 2014;32:222–9.

[28] Locke JA , Black PC. Next generation biomarkers in prostate cancer. Frontiers in Bioscience 2016;21:328–42.

[29] Kulasingam V , Diamandis EP. Strategies for discovering novel cancer biomarkers through utilization of emerging technologies. Nature Clinical Practice Oncology 2008;5:588–99.

[30] Levenson VV. Biomarkers: diagnostic highlights and surrogate end points. Cambridge Healthtech Institute's biomarker series: biomarker validation: bringing discovery to the clinic & cancer biomarkers: from discovery to clinical practice. May 3–5, 2004, Philadelphia, Pennsylvania, USA. Pharmacogenomics 2004;5:459–61.

[31] Nolen B. The expansion and advancement of cancer biomarkers. Cancer Biomarkers: Section A of Disease Markers 2011;10:61–2.

[32] Ross JS , Slodkowska EA, Symmans WF, Pusztai L, Ravdin PM, Hortobagyi GN. The HER-2 receptor and breast cancer: ten years of targeted anti-HER-2 therapy and personalized medicine. The Oncologist 2009;14:320–68.

[33] Span PN , Sweep FC, Wiegerinck ET, Tjan-Heijnen VC, Manders P, Beex LV,. Survivin is an independent prognostic marker for risk stratification of breast cancer patients. Clinical Chemistry 2004;50:1986–93.

[34] Duffy MJ. Clinical uses of tumor markers: a critical review. Critical Reviews in Clinical Laboratory Sciences 2001;38:225–62.

[35] Swets JA. Measuring the accuracy of diagnostic systems. Science 1988;240:1285–93.

[36] Zweig MH , Campbell G. Receiver-operating characteristic (ROC) plots: a fundamental evaluation tool in clinical medicine. Clinical Chemistry 1993;39:561–77.

[37] Begg CB. Advances in statistical methodology for diagnostic medicine in the 1980s. Statistics in Medicine 1991;10:1887–95.

[38] Camp BW. What the clinician really needs to know: questioning the clinical usefulness of sensitivity and specificity in studies of screening tests. Journal of Developmental and Behavioral Pediatrics: JDBP 2006;27:226–30.

[39] Obuchowski NA. Receiver operating characteristic curves and their use in radiology. Radiology 2003;229:3–8.

[40] Kumar R , Indrayan A. Receiver operating characteristic (ROC) curve for medical researchers. Indian Pediatrics 2011;48:277–87.

[41] DeLong ER , DeLong DM, Clarke-Pearson DL. Comparing the areas under two or more correlated receiver operating characteristic curves: a nonparametric approach. Biometrics 1988;44:837–45.

[42] Robertson EA , Zweig MH, Van Steirteghem AC. Evaluating the clinical efficacy of laboratory tests. American Journal of Clinical Pathology 1983;79:78–86.

[43] Biomarkers Definitions Working G. Biomarkers and surrogate endpoints: preferred definitions and conceptual framework. Clinical Pharmacology and Therapeutics 2001;69:89–95.

[44] Cooner WH. Definition of the ideal tumor marker. The Urologic Clinics of North America 1993;20:575–9.

[45] Mishra A , Verma M. Cancer biomarkers: are we ready for the prime time? Cancers 2010;2:190–208.

[46] Schrohl AS , Holten-Andersen M, Sweep F, Schmitt M, Harbeck N, Foekens J,. Tumor markers: from laboratory to clinical utility. Molecular & Cellular Proteomics: MCP 2003;2:378–87.

[47] Greenwald P. Cancer risk factors for selecting cohorts for large-scale chemoprevention trials. Journal of Cellular Biochemistry Supplement 1996;25:29–36.

[48] Fagan P , Moolchan ET, Pokhrel P, Herzog T, Cassel KD, Pagano I,. Biomarkers of tobacco smoke exposure in racial/ethnic groups at high risk for lung cancer. American Journal of Public Health 2015;105:1237–45.

[49] Goodman M , Bostick RM, Kucuk O, Jones DP. Clinical trials of antioxidants as cancer prevention agents: past, present, and future. Free Radical Biology & Medicine 2011;51:1068–84.

[50] Wald NJ. Guidance on terminology. Journal of Medical Screening 2008;15:50.

[51] Weigelt B , Peterse JL, van't Veer LJ. Breast cancer metastasis: markers and models. Nature Reviews Cancer 2005;5:591–602.

[52] Duffy MJ. Use of biomarkers in screening for cancer. Advances in Experimental Medicine and Biology 2015;867:27–39.

[53] Catalona WJ , Smith DS, Ratliff TL, Dodds KM, Coplen DE, Yuan JJ,. Measurement of prostate-specific antigen in serum as a screening test for prostate cancer. The New England Journal of Medicine 1991;324:1156–61.

[54] Andriole GL , Crawford ED, Grubb RL 3rd, Buys SS, Chia D, Church TR,. Mortality results from a randomized prostate-cancer screening trial. The New England Journal of Medicine 2009;360:1310–9.

[55] Schroder FH , Hugosson J, Roobol MJ, Tammela TL, Ciatto S, Nelen V,. Screening and prostate-cancer mortality in a randomized European study. The New England Journal of Medicine 2009;360:1320–8.

[56] Heidenreich A , Bellmunt J, Bolla M, Joniau S, Mason M, Matveev V,. EAU guidelines on prostate cancer. Part I: screening, diagnosis, and treatment of clinically localised disease. Actas urologicas espanolas 2011;35:501–14.

[57] Pavlou MP , Diamandis EP, Blasutig IM. The long journey of cancer biomarkers from the bench to the clinic. Clinical Chemistry 2013;59:147–57.

[58] Henry NL , Hayes DF. Cancer biomarkers. Molecular Oncology 2012;6:140–6.

[59] Mor G , Visintin I, Lai Y, Zhao H, Schwartz P, Rutherford T,. Serum protein markers for early detection of ovarian cancer. Proceedings of the National Academy of Sciences of the United States of America 2005;102:7677–82.

[60] Visintin I , Feng Z, Longton G, Ward DC, Alvero AB, Lai Y,. Diagnostic markers for early detection of ovarian cancer. Clinical Cancer Research: An Official Journal of the American Association for Cancer Research 2008;14:1065–72.

[61] Szymendera JJ , Zborzil J, Sikorowa L, Kaminska JA, Gadek A. Value of five tumor markers (AFP, CEA, hCG, hPL and SP1) in diagnosis and staging of testicular germ cell tumors. Oncology 1981;38:222–9.

[62] Swan F Jr. , Velasquez WS, Tucker S, Redman JR, Rodriguez MA, McLaughlin P,. A new serologic staging system for large-cell lymphomas based on initial beta 2-microglobulin and lactate dehydrogenase levels. Journal of Clinical Oncology: Official Journal of the American Society of Clinical Oncology 1989;7:1518–27.

[63] Duffy MJ. Predictive markers in breast and other cancers: a review. Clinical Chemistry 2005;51:494–503.

[64] Hanstein B , Djahansouzi S, Dall P, Beckmann MW, Bender HG. Insights into the molecular biology of the estrogen receptor define novel therapeutic targets for breast cancer. European Journal of Endocrinology/European Federation of Endocrine Societies 2004;150:243–55.

[65] Burstein HJ , Kuter I, Campos SM, Gelman RS, Tribou L, Parker LM,. Clinical activity of trastuzumab and vinorelbine in women with HER2-overexpressing metastatic breast cancer. Journal of Clinical Oncology: Official Journal of the American Society of Clinical Oncology 2001;19:2722–30.

[66] Allegra CJ , Jessup JM, Somerfield MR, Hamilton SR, Hammond EH, Hayes DF,. American Society of Clinical Oncology provisional clinical opinion: testing for KRAS gene mutations in patients with metastatic colorectal carcinoma to predict response to anti-epidermal growth factor receptor monoclonal antibody therapy. Journal of Clinical Oncology: Official Journal of the American Society of Clinical Oncology 2009;27:2091–6.

[67] Sharma S. Tumor markers in clinical practice: general principles and guidelines. Indian Journal of Medical and Paediatric Oncology: Official Journal of Indian Society of Medical & Paediatric Oncology 2009;30:1–8.

[68] Basuyau JP , Leroy M, Brunelle P. Determination of tumor markers in serum. Pitfalls and good practice. Clinical Chemistry and Laboratory Medicine 2001;39:1227–33.

[69] Bast RC Jr. , Ravdin P, Hayes DF, Bates S, Fritsche H Jr., Jessup JM,. 2000 update of recommendations for the use of tumor markers in breast and colorectal cancer: clinical practice guidelines of the American Society of Clinical Oncology. Journal of Clinical Oncology: Official Journal of the American Society of Clinical Oncology 2001;19:1865–78.

[70] Koprowski H , Steplewski Z, Mitchell K, Herlyn M, Herlyn D, Fuhrer P. Colorectal carcinoma antigens detected by hybridoma antibodies. Somatic Cell Genetics 1979;5:957–71.

[71] Rosty C , Goggins M. Early detection of pancreatic carcinoma. Hematology/Oncology Clinics of North America 2002;16:37–52.

[72] Locker GY , Hamilton S, Harris J, Jessup JM, Kemeny N, Macdonald JS,. ASCO 2006 update of recommendations for the use of tumor markers in gastrointestinal cancer. Journal of Clinical Oncology: Official Journal of the American Society of Clinical Oncology 2006;24:5313–27.

[73] Bray F , Jemal A, Grey N, Ferlay J, Forman D. Global cancer transitions according to the Human Development Index (2008–2030): a population-based study. The Lancet Oncology 2012;13:790–801.

[74] Pisani P , Bray F, Parkin DM. Estimates of the world-wide prevalence of cancer for 25 sites in the adult population. International Journal of Cancer Journal International du Cancer 2002;97:72–81.

[75] Sabatino SA , White MC, Thompson TD, Klabunde CN, Centers for Disease C, Prevention. Cancer screening test use—United States, 2013. MMWR Morbidity and Mortality Weekly Report 2015;64:464–8.

[76] Ludwig JA , Weinstein JN. Biomarkers in cancer staging, prognosis and treatment selection. Nature Reviews Cancer 2005;5:845–56.

[77] Mirza AN , Mirza NQ, Vlastos G, Singletary SE. Prognostic factors in node-negative breast cancer: a review of studies with sample size more than 200 and follow-up more than 5 years. Annals of Surgery 2002;235:10–26.

[78] Duffy MJ. Estrogen receptors: role in breast cancer. Critical Reviews in Clinical Laboratory Sciences 2006;43:325–47.

[79] Ross JS , Fletcher JA, Linette GP, Stec J, Clark E, Ayers M,. The Her-2/neu gene and protein in breast cancer 2003: biomarker and target of therapy. The Oncologist 2003;8:307–25.

[80] Vietri MT , Molinari AM, Laura De Paola M, Cantile F, Fasano M, Cioffi M. Identification of a novel in-frame deletion in BRCA2 and analysis of variants of BRCA1/2 in

Italian patients affected with hereditary breast and ovarian cancer. Clinical Chemistry and Laboratory Medicine 2012;50:2171–80.

[81] Harbeck N , Kruger A, Sinz S, Kates RE, Thomssen C, Schmitt M,. Clinical relevance of the plasminogen activator inhibitor type 1—a multifaceted proteolytic factor. Onkologie 2001;24:238–44.

[82] Andres SA , Edwards AB, Wittliff JL. Expression of urokinase-type plasminogen activator (uPA), its receptor (uPAR), and inhibitor (PAI-1) in human breast carcinomas and their clinical relevance. Journal of Clinical Laboratory Analysis 2012;26:93–103.

[83] Molina R , Jo J, Filella X, Zanon G, Pahisa J, Mu noz M, et al. c-erbB-2 oncoprotein, CEA, and CA 15.3 in patients with breast cancer: prognostic value. Breast Cancer Research and Treatment 1998;51:109–19.

[84] Jensen JL , Maclean GD, Suresh MR, Almeida A, Jette D, Lloyd S,. Possible utility of serum determinations of CA 125 and CA 27.29 in breast cancer management. The International Journal of Biological Markers 1991;6:1–6.

[85] Sparano JA. TAILORx: trial assigning individualized options for treatment (Rx). Clinical Breast Cancer 2006;7:347–50.

[86] Bjartell AS. Next-generation prostate-specific antigen test: ready to use? European Urology 2013;64:700–2.

[87] Gao CL , Rawal SK, Sun L, Ali A, Connelly RR, Banez LL,. Diagnostic potential of prostate-specific antigen expressing epithelial cells in blood of prostate cancer patients. Clinical Cancer Research: An Official Journal of the American Association for Cancer Research 2003;9:2545–50.

[88] Steuber T , Niemela P, Haese A, Pettersson K, Erbersdobler A, Felix Chun KH,. Association of free-prostate specific antigen subfractions and human glandular kallikrein 2 with volume of benign and malignant prostatic tissue. The Prostate 2005;63:13–8.

[89] Haese A , Vaisanen V, Lilja H, Kattan MW, Rittenhouse HG, Pettersson K,. Comparison of predictive accuracy for pathologically organ confined clinical stage T1c prostate cancer using human glandular kallikrein 2 and prostate specific antigen combined with clinical stage and Gleason grade. The Journal of Urology 2005;173:752–6.

[90] Marks LS , Fradet Y, Deras IL, Blase A, Mathis J, Aubin SM,. PCA3 molecular urine assay for prostate cancer in men undergoing repeat biopsy. Urology 2007;69:532–5.

[91] Moses MA , Wiederschain D, Loughlin KR, Zurakowski D, Lamb CC, Freeman MR. Increased incidence of matrix metalloproteinases in urine of cancer patients. Cancer Research 1998;58:1395–9.

[92] Morgia G , Falsaperla M, Malaponte G, Madonia M, Indelicato M, Travali S,. Matrix metalloproteinases as diagnostic (MMP-13) and prognostic (MMP-2, MMP-9) markers of prostate cancer. Urological Research 2005;33:44–50.

[93] Coticchia CM , Yang J, Moses MA. Ovarian cancer biomarkers: current options and future promise. Journal of the National Comprehensive Cancer Network: JNCCN 2008;6:795–802.

[94] Duffy MJ , Bonfrer JM, Kulpa J, Rustin GJ, Soletormos G, Torre GC,. CA125 in ovarian cancer: European Group on Tumor Markers guidelines for clinical use. International Journal of Gynecological Cancer: Official Journal of the International Gynecological Cancer Society 2005;15:679–91.

[95] Morgan RJ Jr., Alvarez RD, Armstrong DK, Boston B, Chen LM, Copeland L, . Ovarian cancer. Clinical Practice Guidelines in Oncology. Journal of the National Comprehensive Cancer Network: JNCCN 2008;6:766–94.

[96] Chambers SK , Gertz RE Jr., Ivins CM, Kacinski BM. The significance of urokinase-type plasminogen activator, its inhibitors, and its receptor in ascites of patients with epithelial ovarian cancer. Cancer 1995;75:1627–33.

[97] Coppola D , Szabo M, Boulware D, Muraca P, Alsarraj M, Chambers AF,. Correlation of osteopontin protein expression and pathological stage across a wide variety of tumor histologies. Clinical Cancer Research: An Official Journal of the American Association for Cancer Research 2004;10:184–90.

[98] Davies RJ , Miller R, Coleman N. Colorectal cancer screening: prospects for molecular stool analysis. Nature Reviews Cancer 2005;5:199–209.

[99] Smith RA , von Eschenbach AC, Wender R, Levin B, Byers T, Rothenberger D,. American Cancer Society guidelines for the early detection of cancer: update of early detection guidelines for prostate, colorectal, and endometrial cancers. Also: update 2001–testing for early lung cancer detection. CA: A Cancer Journal for Clinicians 2001;51:38–75; quiz 7–80.

[100] Allison JE. Colon Cancer Screening Guidelines 2005: the fecal occult blood test option has become a better FIT. Gastroenterology 2005;129:745–8.

[101] Allison JE , Sakoda LC, Levin TR, Tucker JP, Tekawa IS, Cuff T,. Screening for colorectal neoplasms with new fecal occult blood tests: update on performance characteristics. Journal of the National Cancer Institute 2007;99:1462–70.

[102] Duffy MJ. Carcinoembryonic antigen as a marker for colorectal cancer: is it clinically useful? Clinical Chemistry 2001;47:624–30.

[103] Benson AB 3rd , Schrag D, Somerfield MR, Cohen AM, Figueredo AT, Flynn PJ, . American Society of Clinical Oncology recommendations on adjuvant chemotherapy for stage II colon cancer. Journal of Clinical Oncology: Official Journal of the American Society of Clinical Oncology 2004;22:3408–19.

[104] Reiter W , Stieber P, Reuter C, Nagel D, Lau-Werner U, Lamerz R. Multivariate analysis of the prognostic value of CEA and CA 19-9 serum levels in colorectal cancer. Anticancer Research 2000;20:5195–8.

[105] Holten-Andersen MN , Christensen IJ, Nielsen HJ, Stephens RW, Jensen V, Nielsen OH,. Total levels of tissue inhibitor of metalloproteinases 1 in plasma yield high diagnostic sensitivity and specificity in patients with colon cancer. Clinical Cancer Research: An Official Journal of the American Association for Cancer Research 2002;8:156–64.

[106] Anderson NL , Anderson NG. The human plasma proteome: history, character, and diagnostic prospects. Molecular & Cellular Proteomics: MCP 2002;1:845–67.

[107] Sawyers CL , van't Veer LJ. Reliable and effective diagnostics are keys to accelerating personalized cancer medicine and transforming cancer care: a policy statement from the American association for cancer research. Clinical Cancer Research: An Official Journal of the American Association for Cancer Research 2014;20:4978–81.

[108] Srivastava S , Verma M, Henson DE. Biomarkers for early detection of colon cancer. Clinical Cancer Research: An Official Journal of the American Association for Cancer Research 2001;7:1118–26.

[109] Poste G. Bring on the biomarkers. Nature 2011;469:156–7.

[110] Hammond ME , Taube SE. Issues and barriers to development of clinically useful tumor markers: a development pathway proposal. Seminars in Oncology 2002;29:213–21.

[111] Pepe MS , Etzioni R, Feng Z, Potter JD, Thompson ML, Thornquist M,. Phases of biomarker development for early detection of cancer. Journal of the National Cancer Institute 2001;93:1054–61.

[112] Bensalah K , Montorsi F, Shariat SF. Challenges of cancer biomarker profiling. European Urology 2007;52:1601–9.

[113] Paradiso A , Mangia A, Orlando C, Verderio P, Belfiglio M, Marchetti A,. The Integrated Oncology Program of the Italian Ministry of Health. Analytical and clinical validation of new biomarkers for early diagnosis: network, resources, methodology, quality control, and data analysis. The International Journal of Biological Markers 2009;24:119–29.

[114] Teutsch SM , Bradley LA, Palomaki GE, Haddow JE, Piper M, Calonge N,. The Evaluation of Genomic Applications in Practice and Prevention (EGAPP) Initiative: methods of the EGAPP Working Group. Genetics in Medicine: Official Journal of the American College of Medical Genetics 2009;11:3–14.

[115] Pollak MN , Foulkes WD. Challenges to cancer control by screening. Nature Reviews Cancer 2003;3:297–303.

[116] Neugut AI , Jacobson JS, Rella VA. Prevalence and incidence of colorectal adenomas and cancer in asymptomatic persons. Gastrointestinal Endoscopy Clinics of North America 1997;7:387–99.

[117] Wagner PD , Verma M, Srivastava S. Challenges for biomarkers in cancer detection. Annals of the New York Academy of Sciences 2004;1022:9–16.

[118] Diamandis EP. Towards identification of true cancer biomarkers. BMC Medicine 2014;12:156.

[119] Kulasingam V , Pavlou MP, Diamandis EP. Integrating high-throughput technologies in the quest for effective biomarkers for ovarian cancer. Nature Reviews Cancer 2010;10:371–8.

[120] Sawyers CL. The cancer biomarker problem. Nature 2008;452:548–52.

[121] Tran B , Dancey JE, Kamel-Reid S, McPherson JD, Bedard PL, Brown AM,. Cancer genomics: technology, discovery, and translation. Journal of Clinical Oncology: Official Journal of the American Society of Clinical Oncology 2012;30:647–60.

[122] Arteaga CL , Baselga J. Impact of genomics on personalized cancer medicine. Clinical Cancer Research: An Official Journal of the American Association for Cancer Research 2012;18:612–8.

[123] Gibney ER , Nolan CM. Epigenetics and gene expression. Heredity 2010;105:4–13.

[124] Nogueira da Costa A , Herceg Z. Detection of cancer-specific epigenomic changes in biofluids: powerful tools in biomarker discovery and application. Molecular Oncology 2012;6:704–15.

[125] Herman JG , Graff JR, Myohanen S, Nelkin BD, Baylin SB. Methylation-specific PCR: a novel PCR assay for methylation status of CpG islands. Proceedings of the National Academy of Sciences of the United States of America 1996;93:9821–6.

[126] Booth MJ , Branco MR, Ficz G, Oxley D, Krueger F, Reik W,. Quantitative sequencing of 5-methylcytosine and 5-hydroxymethylcytosine at single-base resolution. Science 2012;336:934–7.

[127] Zeidan BA , Townsend PA. SELDI-TOF proteomic profiling of breast carcinomas identifies clinicopathologically relevant groups of patients similar to previously defined clusters from cDNA expression. Breast Cancer Research: BCR 2008;10:107.

[128] Curtis C , Shah SP, Chin SF, Turashvili G, Rueda OM, Dunning MJ,. The genomic and transcriptomic architecture of 2,000 breast tumours reveals novel subgroups. Nature 2012;486:346–52.

[129] Winter PM , Caruthers SD, Kassner A, Harris TD, Chinen LK, Allen JS,. Molecular imaging of angiogenesis in nascent Vx-2 rabbit tumors using a novel alpha(nu)beta3-targeted nanoparticle and 1.5 tesla magnetic resonance imaging. Cancer Research 2003;63:5838–43.

[130] Westhoff M , Litterst P, Freitag L, Urfer W, Bader S, Baumbach JI. Ion mobility spectrometry for the detection of volatile organic compounds in exhaled breath of patients with lung cancer: results of a pilot study. Thorax 2009;64:744–8.

[131] Holmes E , Wilson ID, Nicholson JK. Metabolic phenotyping in health and disease. Cell 2008;134:714–7.

[132] Spratlin JL , Serkova NJ, Eckhardt SG. Clinical applications of metabolomics in oncology: a review. Clinical Cancer Research An Official Journal of the American Association for Cancer Research 2009;15:431–40.

[133] Vickers AJ , Brewster SF. PSA Velocity and Doubling Time in Diagnosis and Prognosis of Prostate Cancer. British Journal of Medical & Surgical Urology 2012;5:162–8.

[134] van Nagell JR , Jr., DePriest PD, Reedy MB, Gallion HH, Ueland FR, Pavlik EJ, et al. The efficacy of transvaginal sonographic screening in asymptomatic women at risk for ovarian cancer. Gynecologic Oncology 2000;77:350–6.

[135] Koizumi F , Odagiri H, Fujimoto H, Kawamura T, Ishimori A. Clinical evaluation of four tumor markers (CEA, TPA, CA50 and CA72-4) in colorectal cancer. Rinsho Byori: The Japanese Journal of Clinical Pathology 1992;40:523–8.

[136] Matsuoka Y. Basic and clinical aspects of tumor markers–with special reference to CEA. Rinsho Byori: The Japanese Journal of Clinical Pathology 1990;38:31–4.

[137] von Kleist S. The clinical value of the tumor markers CA 19/9 and carcinoembryonic antigen (CEA) in colorectal carcinomas: a critical comparison. The International Journal of Biological Markers 1986;1:3–8.

[138] Molina R , Barak V, van Dalen A, Duffy MJ, Einarsson R, Gion M,. Tumor markers in breast cancer-European Group on Tumor Markers recommendations. Tumour Biology: The Journal of the International Society for Oncodevelopmental Biology and Medicine 2005;26:281–93.

[139] McGuire WL , Horwitz KB, Pearson OH, Segaloff A. Current status of estrogen and progesterone receptors in breast cancer. Cancer 1977;39:2934–47.

[140] Colleoni M , Viale G, Zahrieh D, Pruneri G, Gentilini O, Veronesi P,. Chemotherapy is more effective in patients with breast cancer not expressing steroid hormone receptors: a study of preoperative treatment. Clinical Cancer Research: An Official Journal of the American Association for Cancer Research 2004;10:6622–8.

[141] Paik S , Tang G, Shak S, Kim C, Baker J, Kim W,. Gene expression and benefit of chemotherapy in women with node-negative, estrogen receptor-positive breast cancer. Journal of Clinical Oncology: Official Journal of the American Society of Clinical Oncology 2006;24:3726–34.

[142] Varadan V , Kamalakaran S, Gilmore H, Banerjee N, Janevski A, Miskimen KL,. Brief-exposure to preoperative bevacizumab reveals a TGF-beta signature predictive of

response in HER2-negative breast cancers. International Journal of Cancer Journal International du Cancer 2016;138:747–57.

[143] Kurtzman JT , Wilson H, Rao CV. A proposed role for hCG in clinical obstetrics. Seminars in Reproductive Medicine 2001;19:63–8.

[144] Chen L , Ho DW, Lee NP, Sun S, Lam B, Wong KF,. Enhanced detection of early hepatocellular carcinoma by serum SELDI-TOF proteomic signature combined with alpha-fetoprotein marker. Annals of Surgical Oncology 2010;17:2518–25.

[145] Johnson PJ , Williams R. Serum alpha-fetoprotein estimations and doubling time in hepatocellular carcinoma: influence of therapy and possible value in early detection. Journal of the National Cancer Institute 1980;64:1329–32.

[146] Minami T , Tateishi R, Kondo M, Nakagomi R, Fujiwara N, Sato M,. Serum alpha-fetoprotein has high specificity for the early detection of hepatocellular carcinoma after hepatitis C virus eradication in patients. Medicine 2015;94:e901.

[147] Bae YJ , Schaab M, Kratzsch J. Calcitonin as biomarker for the medullary thyroid carcinoma. Recent results in cancer research Fortschritte der Krebsforschung Progres dans les recherches sur le cancer 2015;204:117–37.

[148] van Veelen W , de Groot JW, Acton DS, Hofstra RM, Hoppener JW, Links TP,. Medullary thyroid carcinoma and biomarkers: past, present and future. Journal of Internal Medicine 2009;266:126–40.

[149] Mazzaferri EL , Robbins RJ, Spencer CA, Braverman LE, Pacini F, Wartofsky L,. A consensus report of the role of serum thyroglobulin as a monitoring method for low-risk patients with papillary thyroid carcinoma. The Journal of Clinical Endocrinology and Metabolism 2003;88:1433–41.

[150] Kibar Y , Goktas S, Kilic S, Yaman H, Onguru O, Peker AF. Prognostic value of cytology, nuclear matrix protein 22 (NMP22) test, and urinary bladder cancer II (UBC II) test in early recurrent transitional cell carcinoma of the bladder. Annals of Clinical and Laboratory Science 2006;36:31–8.

[151] van Gils MP, Cornel EB, Hessels D, Peelen WP, Witjes JA, Mulders PF, et al. Molecular PCA3 diagnostics on prostatic fluid. The Prostate 2007;67:881–7.

Chapter 2

# Dynamics of Cancer-Related Proteins in Patients with Bladder Cancer

Kazumasa Matsumoto, Morihiro Nishi,
Hideyasu Tsumura, Ken-ichi Tabata,
Tetsuo Fujita and Masatsugu Iwamura

Additional information is available at the end of the chapter

http://dx.doi.org/10.5772/62525

**Abstract**

Bladder cancer (BC) is the second most common malignancy in the urologic field. Preoperative predictive biomarkers of cancer progression and prognosis are imperative for optimizing appropriate treatment for patients with BC. The prediction of patient outcomes before initial treatment would enable physicians to choose better modalities and avoid unnecessary aggressive treatments. In addition, preoperative molecular markers are expected to be a minimally invasive tool for predicting precise prognosis and progression in patients with BC. The proteins secreted from the tumor cells reflect various states of tumors in real time and at given conditions, and those expression patterns are different from normal cell components. Approximately 20–25% of cellular proteins are in extracellular spaces, and these proteins have important roles in invasion, angiogenesis, regulation of cell-to-cell interactions, and metastasis. It has been suggested that tumor-secreting proteins are a promising source for tumor diagnostic biomarkers. Proteomic analysis was utilized to identify the secreted proteins in sera from patients with BC. Several biomarkers associated with BC are reviewed here.

**Keywords:** bladder cancer, urothelial carcinoma, diagnosis, protein, biomarker

## 1. Introduction

Bladder cancer (BC) is one of the most common malignancies of the urinary tract and results in significant morbidity and mortality worldwide. Approximately 75–85% of BC cases are diagnosed as nonmuscle-invasive bladder cancer (NMIBC) at the first diagnosis, and approximately 70% of cases present as pTa, 20% present as pT1, and 10% present as carcinoma in situ (CIS) lesions [1]. NMIBC has a tendency to recur (50–70%) and may progress (10–20%) to a higher grade and/or muscle-invasive BC (MIBC) in time, which can lead to high cancer-specific mortality [2].

Histological tumor grade is one of the clinical factors associated with outcomes of patients with NMIBC. High-grade NMIBC generally exhibits more aggressive behavior than low-grade NMIBC, and it increases the risk of a poorer prognosis [3, 4]. Due to the unfavorable prognosis of high-grade NMIBC, a differential diagnosis between high-grade and low-grade NMIBC might be crucial for more appropriate follow-up and aggressive treatment. Cystoscopy and urine cytology are commonly used techniques for the diagnosis and surveillance of BC. Cystoscopy can identify the most papillary and solid lesions, but this is highly invasive for the patients; however, urine cytology is limited by examiner experience and low sensitivity. For these reasons, some tumor markers have been investigated (e.g., BTAstat, NMP22), but their sensitivity and specificity are limited [5] and they are unable to predict the clinical outcome of BC patients.

Preoperative predictive biomarkers for cancer progression and prognosis are imperative for optimizing appropriate treatment for patients with BC. The prediction of patient outcomes before initial treatment would enable physicians to choose better modalities and avoid unnecessary aggressive treatments [6, 7]. Various predictive models have been widely investigated to reduce BC-related deaths. One of the challenges is precisely predicting the pathological stage, which is a reliable and established factor connected to disease prognosis [8, 9]. Although preoperative computed tomography and magnetic resonance imaging for BC staging are undergoing development, their accuracy for predicting pathological stage varies between 40% and 90% [10, 11]. To overcome these limitations, preoperative molecular markers are expected to be a minimally invasive tool for predicting precise prognosis and progression in patients with BC.

Numerous efforts have been made to identify tumor markers. In recent years, a vast array of tumor antigens and their products have been identified. Hegele et al. investigated the serum levels of carcinoembryonic antigen (CEA) and carbohydrate-antigen 19-9 (CA19-9) in patients with BC [12]. They concluded that the serum levels of CEA and CA19-9 are associated with tumor invasiveness and pathologic grade. Another study of the serum level of CEA, CA19-9, and soluble cytokeratin 19 fragment (CYFRA21-1) in BC patients indicated that CYFRA21-1 is relatively useful for monitoring BC and predicting its prognosis [13]. These serum materials might be useful for monitoring and staging BC. However, a serum marker that can serve as a reliable detection marker for BC has yet to be identified.

The proteins secreted from the tumor cells reflect various states of the tumor in real time and at given conditions, and those expression patterns are different from normal cell components. Thus, the proteins secreted into body fluids, such as serum, urine, cerebrospinal fluid, tears, and saliva, from tumor cells and conditioned media of cultured tumor cells have been investigated. Approximately 20–25% of cellular proteins are in extracellular spaces, and these proteins have important roles in differentiation, invasion, metastasis, angiogenesis, and regulation of cell-to-cell and cell-to-extracellular matrix interactions [3, 14, 15]. It has been suggested that tumor-secreting proteins are a promising source for tumor diagnostic biomarkers. Proteomic analysis was utilized to identify the secreted proteins in sera from patients with BC. Several biomarkers and their association with BC are reviewed here [4, 5, 16, 17].

## 2. Candidates for a serum biomarker in patients with bladder cancer

### 2.1. Uroplakin III

Uroplakin plays a key role in urothelial functions, including participation in the permeability barrier, adjustment of urothelial surface area, stabilization of the urothelial surface, and development of the urinary tract [18]. Because of their specific expression in the urothelium, uroplakin has been investigated as a potential immunohistochemical marker for primary lesions and for identification of the primary cancer in patients with metastases of unknown origin [19]. The uroplakin family comprises a group of four transmembrane proteins, including Ia (27 kDa), Ib (28 kDa), II (15 kDa), and III (47 kDa) [20]. Uroplakin III is the largest protein in the uroplakin family and has been exclusively investigated by immunohistochemical staining. In a previous study, the loss of uroplakin III expression in pathological specimens is associated with biologically aggressive BC and poor prognosis for patients who underwent radical cystectomy [3]. However, the utility of serum uroplakin III (e.g., predictive models of disease outcome) in patients with BC is unknown.

Serum uroplakin III levels were investigated in patients with BC and healthy controls utilizing dot blot analysis to demonstrate the role of preoperative serum uroplakin III levels as a potential biomarker for BC (**Table 1**) [17]. The uroplakin III levels in serum in patients with NMIBC, in those with MIBC, and in healthy controls were 1.3, 2.8, and 0.7, respectively. The serum uroplakin III levels in patients with NMIBC and MIBC were significantly higher than those in healthy controls ($P = 0.04$ and $P < 0.001$, respectively). Comparison of BC groups with the control group yielded the area under the curve-receiver operating characteristics (AUC-ROC) levels for NMIBC and MIBC of 0.62 and 0.88, respectively. The sensitivity and specificity for NMIBC, using a cut-point of 2.1, were 29% and 96%, respectively. The sensitivity and specificity for MIBC, using a cut-point of 2.0, were 67% and 96%, respectively. There was a significantly greater increase in serum uroplakin III levels in patients with MIBC than in those with NMIBC ($P = 0.003$). Preoperative serum uroplakin III levels were significantly higher in patients with positive lymphovascular invasion and pathological grade 3 disease than in those with negative lymphovascular invasion and grade 1 or grade 2 disease. There were no significant differences in other factors, including gender, age, and lymph node status. Survival analysis showed that patients with high serum uroplakin III had a significantly increased probability of cancer-specific death ($P = 0.04$). However, there was no factor associated with an increased risk for cancer-specific death in multivariate Cox proportional hazards regression analysis. These findings suggest that serum uroplakin III is one of the candidates for a predictive biomarker for prognosis of patients with BC.

| | N of patients (%) | Serum uroplakin III level | | P* |
|---|---|---|---|---|
| | | Median | Range | |
| Sex | | | | 0.41 |
| Male | 44 (85) | 1.8 | 0.0–6.9 | |
| Female | 8 (15) | 1.7 | 0.02–3.2 | |
| Age (years) | | | | 0.72 |
| <65 | 18 (35) | 1.6 | 0.0–6.9 | |
| ≥65 | 34 (65) | 1.8 | 0.0–6.0 | |
| Pathological stage | | | | 0.003 |
| <pT2 | 28 (54) | 1.3 | 0.66–6.0 | |
| ≥pT2 | 24 (46) | 2.8 | 0.0–6.9 | |
| Pathological grade | | | | 0.005 |
| Grade 1 or 2 | 27 (52) | 1.3 | 0.0–5.4 | |
| Grade 3 | 25 (48) | 2.5 | 0.25–6.9 | |
| Lymphovascular invasion | | | | 0.02 |
| Negative | 35 (67) | 1.3 | 0.0–6.9 | |
| Positive | 17 (33) | 2.5 | 0.66–6.0 | |
| Lymph node metastases | | | | 0.4 |
| Negative | 46 (88) | 1.7 | 0.0–6.9 | |
| Positive | 6 (12) | 2.6 | 0.74–5.4 | |

*Mann-Whitney *U* test.

**Table 1.** Serum uroplakin III levels in patients with bladder cancer.

Other investigators have evaluated the role of the uroplakin family in blood samples from patients with BC [21, 22]. Circulating uroplakin II mRNA-positive cells in blood samples were detected using a nested reverse-transcription polymerase chain reaction assay, as reported by Lu et al. [22]. The detection rate was associated with pathological stage, and positive rates of uroplakin II mRNA were increased with disease extension. Li et al. [21] investigated expression levels of uroplakin II–positive cells in sequential blood samples from patients with metastatic BC. After chemotherapeutic treatment, patients responded well to chemotherapy and uroplakin II–positive cells disappeared. These previous studies showed that uroplakin II in peripheral blood might be used as a biomarker for cancer stage and treatment response.

http://dx.doi.org/10.5772/62525

Although none of the biomarkers detected prognosis for patients with BC, reliable biomarkers will lead to avoidance of unnecessary chemotherapy and radiation and will help physicians choose intensive treatment for the appropriate patients. Expression levels of serum uroplakin III could be used as a predictive biomarker for patients who are at increased risk for worse prognosis. This would help physicians make decisions regarding individual treatment.

## 2.2. Periplakins

The plakin family mediates tissue filaments that represent the cell cytoskeleton in cell-to-cell junctions mediated by cadherin, and it is able to withstand mechanical stimulation and provide integrity of tissues [23, 24]. Dysfunctional plakin proteins show diverse diseases, and autoantibodies (AAb) and mutations perturb their activities with profound consequences. Seven plakin proteins are currently reported. For example, envoplakin, desmoplakin, and periplakin are related to desmosomes in various tissues. A proteomics technique like two-dimensional gel electrophoresis (2-DE) plus immunoblot analysis has been demonstrated to identify tumor-associated proteins for BC [4]. The 195-kDa membrane-associated protein periplakin is involved in cellular movement and attachment [25]. Loss of periplakin expression determined using immunohistochemical staining was associated with biological aggressiveness of BC [26]. In addition, the majority of BC cases showed loss or decreased expression patterns compared with normal or benign lesions on pathological slides. Another study determined whether the dynamics of serum periplakin would detect BC and predict the prognosis of patients with BC (**Table 2**) [16].

| | N of patients (%) | Serum periplakin levels | | P* |
|---|---|---|---|---|
| | | Median | Range | |
| Sex | | | | 1 |
| Male | 43 (86) | 0.23 | 0.0–4.4 | |
| Female | 7 (14) | 0.32 | 0.0–20.5 | |
| Age (years) | | | | 0.4 |
| <65 | 16 (32) | 0 | 0.0–7.0 | |
| ≥65 | 34 (68) | 0.51 | 0.0–20.5 | |
| Pathological stage | | | | 0.03 |
| <pT2 | 27 (54) | 0 | 0.0–4.1 | |
| ≥pT2 | 23 (46) | 1.5 | 0.0–20.5 | |
| Pathological grade | | | | 0.4 |
| Grade 1 or 2 | 26 (52) | 0 | 0 0–7.9 | |
| Grade 3 | 24 (48) | 0.98 | 0.0–20.5 | |
| Lymphovascular invasion | | | | 0.4 |
| Negative | 33 (67) | 0.043 | 0.0–7.0 | |

| | N of patients (%) | Serum periplakin levels | | P* |
|---|---|---|---|---|
| | | Median | Range | |
| Positive | 17 (33) | 0.74 | 0.0–20.5 | |
| Lymph node metastases | | | | 0.4 |
| Negative | 44 (88) | 0.50 | 0.0–3.8 | |
| Positive | 6 (12) | 0.16 | 0.0–20.5 | |

*Mann-Whitney *U* test.

**Table 2.** Serum periplakin levels in patients with bladder cancer.

The median levels of serum periplakin in patients with BC were significantly less than those of healthy controls (0.3 and 5.7, respectively; $P < 0.0001$). The AUC-ROC level for the comparison between the BC group and the control group was 0.85. The sensitivity and specificity for BC, using a cut-off point of 4.0, were 84% and 73%, respectively. The levels of serum periplakin were higher in patients with MIBC than in those with NMIBC (0 and 1.5, respectively; $P = 0.03$). However, serum periplakin levels were not associated with other factors, including gender, age, pathological grade, lymphovascular invasion, and lymph node status. Survival analyses using the log-rank test showed no significant differences in terms of progression and cancer-specific survival. Using multivariate Cox proportional hazards regression analysis, it was determined that none of the factors was associated with an increased risk for progression or cancer-specific survival.

Recent studies described the biological role of periplakin in cancer. Decreased expression of periplakin was associated with the progression of esophageal squamous cell carcinoma [27, 28]. Cyclin A2–induced upregulation of periplakin was associated with poor prognosis as well as cisplatin resistance in endometrial cancer cells [29]. Periplakin silencing reduced migration and attachment of pharyngeal squamous cancer cells [30]. Periplakin silencing in triple-negative breast cancer cells increased cell growth and reduced cell motility [31]. The loss of periplakin expression determined using immunohistochemical staining was associated with pathological stage and cancer-specific survival in patients with BC [26]. Periplakin is imperative for maintaining epithelial cell barriers, cellular movement, and attachment in normal physiology [23–25].

Patients with BC showed significantly decreased expression of serum periplakin protein compared with normal controls. It may be suitable as an adjunct to urine cytology and cystoscopy as a noninvasive diagnostic modality.

### 2.3. S100A6

The S100 protein family contains more than 20 low-molecular-weight $Ca^{2+}$-binding proteins [32]. Most of the genes encoding S100 proteins are located as a cluster on chromosome 1 in the human genome [32, 33]. These proteins are localized in the cytoplasm and nucleus of a wide range of cells and help regulate many cellular processes, such as cell-cycle progression and differentiation [33]. Therefore, the S100 protein family is emerging as a potentially important group of markers in multiple types of tumors. One of these proteins, S100A6, was reported to regulate the actin cytoskeleton function, ubiquitin ligase action, cell proliferation, and apoptosis [32]. S100A6 overexpression has been frequently reported under stress conditions [34] and in various types of cancers, including melanoma, colon, pancreatic, gastric cancer, and BC [5].

The levels of S100A6 expression in sera of healthy controls and BC patients were investigated [5]. There was a significant difference between BC patients and healthy controls (P = 0.001; **Figure 1**). Serum S100A6 expression in NMIC patients was significantly higher than that of healthy controls (P = 0.04). Serum S100A6 in patients with MIBC was significantly higher than that in NMIBC patients (P = 0.004). Serum S100A6 in BC patients was associated with pathological grade (P = 0.001). However, there was no association between lymph node status and serum S100A6. At a cut-off point of 0.5, the sensitivity and specificity of S100A6 expression as a marker for BC were 48% and 93%, respectively. As a detection marker for MIBC, at a cut-off point of 0.4, the sensitivity and specificity were 80% and 63%, respectively. The AUC-ROC levels were 0.73 and 0.73, respectively.

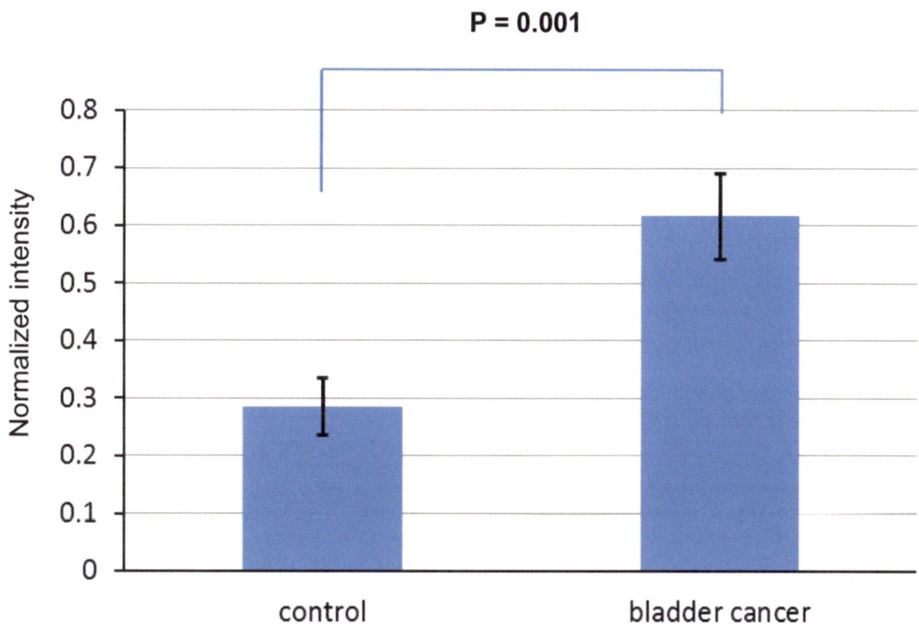


**Figure 1.** Levels of serum S100A6 in healthy controls and bladder cancer patients. There was statistical significance between groups.

S100A6, a member of the S100 family of calcium-binding proteins, is expressed in BC tissue [35], and immunohistochemical staining of S100A6 showed localization mainly in the cytoplasm of tumor cells [36]. The expression patterns of S100A2 and S100A4, also members of the S100 family, correlated well with pathological stage and prognosis [14]. This finding demonstrated that only one clinical aspect represented postoperative outcomes. It is difficult to determine which S100 protein is better for BC in terms of biological markers; however, serum markers are potentially useful in clinical practice both preoperatively and postoperatively. Cai et al. reported an association between increased serum S100A6 levels and acute coronary syndrome [37]. S100A6 levels were significantly increased and correlated with tumor necrosis factor (TNF)-$\alpha$ levels in patients with coronary events. They concluded that a close relationship exists between S100A6 and TNF-$\alpha$-mediated inflammation. Another study reported the expressions of TNF-$\alpha$ and pigment epithelium-derived factor (PEDF), which are highly selective in inhibiting remodeling vessels by inducing apoptosis of endothelial cells in healthy urothelium and in patients with urothelial carcinoma. Decreased PEDF expression and increased TNF-$\alpha$ expression were identified in tumorous tissue compared with healthy urothelium, and the authors concluded that decreased PEDF or increased TNF-$\alpha$ expression is related to differentiation, invasiveness, and angiogenesis of BC [38]. In a study using immunohistochemical staining of 83 patients who underwent radical cystectomy, univariate and multivariate analyses showed that overall survival was significantly greater among patients with lower S100A6 expression [36]. Although the precise mechanism underlying the correlation of S100A6 expression with pathological stage remains to be clarified, serum S100A6 may reveal its role in the biological aggressiveness of BC.

Serum levels of S100A6 in BC patients were significantly higher than in healthy controls. In addition, serum level of S100A6 was associated with pathological stage. By applying this serum marker in clinical practice, patients would benefit from experiencing less invasive examinations and it would allow detection of life-threatening cancer earlier than current modalities.

## 3. Future Potential

BC ranks as one of the most prevalent newly diagnosed cancers. High-risk NMIBC revealed high rates (up to 90%) of recurrence [39]. It is important to diagnose BC accurately and quickly with the help of a simple and cost-effective method. Although histological examination remains the gold standard, urine cytology is helpful as a noninvasive method of early diagnosis of BC [40]. With the currently available modalities, there is no reliable biochemical or molecular examination that can be used as a universal screening tool for BC.

Tumor-associated antigens released into the bloodstream could induce a humoral immune response and generate AAb. The immune response to such antigens generates remarkable biological amplification, although tumor-associated antigens are undetectable in sera during the early stage of tumorigenesis [41]. Therefore, hundreds of tumor-associated antibodies have been identified as potential AAb biomarkers that could be useful for cancer diagnosis [42]. In addition, recent studies based on AAb profiling of cancer patients have suggested diagnostic and prognostic biomarker potential of AAb [43].

Immunoblot analysis combined with 2-DE can identify tumor-associated secreted antigenic proteins that elicit a humoral response in sera of BC patients. By comparing immunoreactive patterns from sera of patients with high-grade and low-grade BC, tumor markers associated with histological grade were obtained. The proteins extracted from culture supernatants of BC cell lines were separated by 2-DE and transferred onto the polyvinylidene difluoride membranes, and they reacted with mixed sera of patients with high-grade BC or low-grade BC. Results indicated that serum IgG levels of anti-calreticulin (CALR) and matrix metalloproteinase (MMP)-2 AAb were significantly higher in BC patients than in normal controls ($P < 0.01$) [4]. In the ROC analysis for anti-CALR AAb, the diagnostic sensitivity and specificity for BC patients were 64% and 60%, respectively. In terms of anti-MMP AAb, sensitivity and specificity for BC patients were 60% and 62%, respectively. The AUC-ROC levels were 0.65 and 0.59, respectively. AAb against tumor-associated antigens have been identified in sera from patients with various cancers, including BC [4]. The application of the humoral immune response for the detection of cancer biomarkers has great potential [42, 43]. Furthermore, the immune system is especially well adapted for early detection of cancer because AAb can be detected before the appearance of other biomarkers or phenotypic alternations at an early stage of tumorigenesis [41].

Although the prostate-specific antigen test is utilized for the detection of prostate cancer, a diagnosis of BC still relies on imaging modality and cystoscopy because effective and simple screening biomarkers are lacking. Further research is warranted to clarify the availability and limits of the aforementioned serum markers in patients with BC.

## Acknowledgements

This study was supported in part by a Grant-in-Aid for Scientific Research C (15K10607) from The Japan Society for Promotion of Science (to K. Matsumoto).

## Author details

Kazumasa Matsumoto*, Morihiro Nishi, Hideyasu Tsumura, Ken-ichi Tabata, Tetsuo Fujita and Masatsugu Iwamura

*Address all correspondence to: kazumasa@cd5.so-net.ne.jp

Department of Urology, Kitasato University School of Medicine, Minami-ku, Sagamihara, Kanagawa, Japan

## References

[1] Kirkali Z, Chan T, Manoharan M, Algaba F, Busch C, et al. Bladder cancer: epidemiology, staging and grading, and diagnosis. Urology. 2005; 66: 4–34. DOI: 10.1016/j.urology.2005.07.062

[2] Witjes JA, Hendricksen K. Intravesical pharmacotherapy for non-muscle-invasive bladder cancer: a critical analysis of currently available drugs, treatment schedules, and long-term results. Eur Urol. 2008; 53: 45–52. DOI: 10.1016/j.eururo.2007.08.015

[3] Matsumoto K, Satoh T, Irie A, Ishii J, Kuwao S, et al. Loss expression of uroplakin III is associated with clinicopathologic features of aggressive bladder cancer. Urology. 2008; 72: 444–449. DOI: 10.1016/j.urology.2007.11.128

[4] Minami S, Nagashio R, Ueda J, Matsumoto K, Goshima N, et al. Detection of tumor-associated antigens in culture supernatants using autoantibodies in sera from patients with bladder cancer. Biomed Res. 2014; 35: 25–35.

[5] Nishi M, Matsumoto K, Kobayashi M, Yanagita K, Matsumoto T, et al. Serum expression of S100A6 is a potential detection marker in patients with urothelial carcinoma in the urinary bladder. Biomed Res. 2014; 35: 351–356. DOI: 10.2220/biomedres.35.351

[6] Otunctemur A, Koklu I, Ozbek E, Dursun M, Sahin S, et al. Are bladder neoplasms more aggressive in patients with a smoking-related second malignancy? Asian Pac J Cancer Prev. 2014; 15: 4025–4028.

[7] Ikeda M, Matsumoto K, Nishi M, Tabata K, Fujita T, et al. Comparison of radical cystectomy and chemoradiotherapy in patients with locally advanced bladder cancer. Asian Pac J Cancer Prev. 2014; 15: 6519–6524.

[8] Ghafouri-Fard S, Nekoohesh L, Motevaseli E. Bladder cancer biomarkers: review and update. Asian Pac J Cancer Prev. 2014; 15: 2395–2403.

[9] Wang HF, Wang JS. Research progress in potential urinary markers for the early detection, diagnosis and follow-up of human bladder cancer. Asian Pac J Cancer Prev. 2012; 13: 1723–1726.

[10] El-Assmy A, Abou-El-Ghar ME, Mosbah A, El-Nahas AR, Refaie HF, et al. Bladder tumour staging: comparison of diffusion- and T2-weighted MR imaging. Eur Radiol. 2009; 19: 1575–1581. DOI: 10.1007/s00330-009-1340-7

[11] Takeuchi M, Sasaki S, Ito M, Okada S, Takahashi S, et al. Urinary bladder cancer: diffusion-weighted MR imaging—accuracy for diagnosing T stage and estimating histologic grade. Radiology. 2009; 251: 112–121. DOI: 10.1148/radiol.2511080873

[12] Hegele A, Mecklenburg V, Varga Z, Olbert P, Hofmann R, Barth P. CA19.9 and CEA in transitional cell carcinoma of the bladder: serological and immunohistochemical findings. Anticancer Res. 2010; 30: 5195–5200.

[13] Washino S, Hirai M, Matsuzaki A, Kobayashi Y. Clinical usefulness of CEA, CA19-9, and CYFRA 21-1 as tumor markers for urothelial bladder carcinoma. Urol Int. 2011; 87: 420–428. DOI: 10.1159/000327517

[14] Matsumoto K, Irie A, Satoh T, Ishii J, Iwabuchi K, et al. Expression of S100A2 and S100A4 predicts for disease progression and patient survival in bladder cancer. Urology. 2007; 70: 602–607. DOI: 10.1016/j.urology.2007.04.007

[15] Matsumoto K, Shariat SF, Casella R, Wheeler TM, Slawin KM, Lerner SP. Preoperative plasma soluble E-cadherin predicts metastases to lymph nodes and prognosis in patients undergoing radical cystectomy. J Urol. 2003; 170: 2248–2252. DOI: 10.1097/01.ju.0000094189.93805.17

[16] Matsumoto K, Ikeda M, Matsumoto T, Nagashio R, Nishimori T, et al. Serum periplakin as a potential biomarker for urothelial carcinoma of the urinary bladder. Asian Pac J Cancer Prev. 2014; 15: 9927–9931.

[17] Tsumura H, Matsumoto K, Matsumoto T, Ikeda M, Satoh T, et al. Increased expression of serum uroplakin III is associated with the detection and pathological features of aggressive bladder cancer. Eur Urol Suppl. 2014; 13: e48.

[18] Huang HY, Shariat SF, Sun TT, Lepor H, Shapiro E, et al. Persistent uroplakin expression in advanced urothelial carcinomas: implications in urothelial tumor progression and clinical outcome. Hum Pathol. 2007; 38: 1703–1713. DOI: 10.1016/j.humpath.2007.04.003

[19] Xu X, Sun TT, Gupta PK, Zhang P, Nasuti JF. Uroplakin as a marker for typing metastatic transitional cell carcinoma on fine-needle aspiration specimens. Cancer. 2001; 93: 216–221.

[20] Wu XR, Lin JH, Walz T, Haner M, Yu J, et al. Mammalian uroplakins. A group of highly conserved urothelial differentiation-related membrane proteins. J Biol Chem. 1994; 269: 13716–13724.

[21] Li SM, Zhang ZT, Chan S, McLenan O, Dixon C, et al. Detection of circulating uroplakin-positive cells in patients with transitional cell carcinoma of the bladder. J Urol. 1999; 162: 931–935.

[22] Lu JJ, Kakehi Y, Takahashi T, Wu XX, Yuasa T, et al. Detection of circulating cancer cells by reverse transcription-polymerase chain reaction for uroplakin II in peripheral blood of patients with urothelial cancer. Clin Cancer Res. 2000; 6: 3166–3171.

[23] Jefferson JJ, Leung CL, Liem RK. Plakins: goliaths that link cell junctions and the cytoskeleton. Nat Rev Mol Cell Biol. 2004; 5: 542–553. DOI: 10.1038/nrm1425

[24] Sonnenberg A, Liem RK. Plakins in development and disease. Exp Cell Res. 2007; 313: 2189–2203. DOI: 10.1016/j.yexcr.2007.03.039

[25] Nagata Y, Karashima T, Watt FM, Salmhofer W, Kanzaki T, Hashimoto T. Paraneoplastic pemphigus sera react strongly with multiple epitopes on the various regions of envoplakin and periplakin, except for the c-terminal homologous domain of periplakin. J Invest Dermatol. 2001; 116: 556–563. DOI: 10.1046/j.1523-1747.2001.01263.x

[26] Matsumoto K, Ikeda M, Sato Y, Kuruma H, Kamata Y, et al. Loss of periplakin expression is associated with pathological stage and cancer-specific survival in patients with urothelial carcinoma of the urinary bladder. Biomed Res. 2014; 35: 201–206.

[27] Hatakeyama H, Kondo T, Fujii K, Nakanishi Y, Kato H, et al. Protein clusters associated with carcinogenesis, histological differentiation and nodal metastasis in esophageal cancer. Proteomics. 2006; 6: 6300–6316. DOI: 10.1002/pmic.200600488

[28] Nishimori T, Tomonaga T, Matsushita K, Oh-Ishi M, Kodera Y, et al. Proteomic analysis of primary esophageal squamous cell carcinoma reveals downregulation of a cell adhesion protein, periplakin. Proteomics. 2006; 6: 1011–1018. DOI: 10.1002/pmic.200500262

[29] Suzuki A, Horiuchi A, Ashida T, Miyamoto T, Kashima H, et al. Cyclin A2 confers cisplatin resistance to endometrial carcinoma cells via up-regulation of an Akt-binding protein, periplakin. J Cell Mol Med. 2010; 14: 2305–2317. DOI: 10.1111/j.1582-4934.2009.00839.x

[30] Tonoike Y, Matsushita K, Tomonaga T, Katada K, Tanaka N, et al. Adhesion molecule periplakin is involved in cellular movement and attachment in pharyngeal squamous cancer cells. BMC Cell Biol. 2011; 12: 41. DOI: 10.1186/1471-2121-12-41

[31] Choi YK, Woo SM, Cho SG, Moon HE, Yun YJ, et al. Brain-metastatic triple-negative breast cancer cells regain growth ability by altering gene expression patterns. Cancer Genomics Proteomics. 2013; 10: 265–275.

[32] Lesniak W, Slomnicki LP, Filipek A. S100A6 - new facts and features. Biochem Biophys Res Commun. 2009; 390: 1087–1092. DOI: 10.1016/j.bbrc.2009.10.150

[33] Shiota M, Tsunoda T, Song Y, Yokomizo A, Tada Y, et al. Enhanced S100 calcium-binding protein P expression sensitizes human bladder cancer cells to cisplatin. BJU Int. 2011; 107: 1148–1153. DOI: 10.1111/j.1464-410X.2010.09535.x

[34] Lesniak W, Szczepanska A, Kuznicki J. Calcyclin (S100A6) expression is stimulated by agents evoking oxidative stress via the antioxidant response element. Biochim Biophys Acta. 2005; 1744: 29–37. DOI: 10.1016/j.bbamcr.2004.11.003

[35] Cross SS, Hamdy FC, Deloulme JC, Rehman I. Expression of S100 proteins in normal human tissues and common cancers using tissue microarrays: S100A6, S100A8, S100A9 and S100A11 are all overexpressed in common cancers. Histopathology. 2005; 46: 256–269. DOI: 10.1111/j.1365-2559.2005.02097.x

[36] Shah CH, Viktorsson K, Kanter L, Sherif A, Asmundsson J, et al. Vascular endothelial growth factor receptor 2, but not S100A4 or S100A6, correlates with prolonged survival in advanced urothelial carcinoma. Urol Oncol. 2014; 32: 1215–1224. DOI: 10.1016/j.urolonc.2014.04.015

[37] Cai XY, Lu L, Wang YN, Jin C, Zhang RY, et al. Association of increased S100B, S100A6 and S100P in serum levels with acute coronary syndrome and also with the severity of

myocardial infarction in cardiac tissue of rat models with ischemia-reperfusion injury. Atherosclerosis. 2011; 217: 536–542. DOI: 10.1016/j.atherosclerosis.2011.05.023

[38] Feng CC, Wang PH, Ding Q, Guan M, Zhang YF, et al. Expression of pigment epithelium-derived factor and tumor necrosis factor-alpha is correlated in bladder tumor and is related to tumor angiogenesis. Urol Oncol. 2013; 31: 241–246. DOI: 10.1016/j.urolonc.2010.12.001

[39] Shelley MD, Mason MD, Kynaston H. Intravesical therapy for superficial bladder cancer: a systematic review of randomised trials and meta-analyses. Cancer Treat Rev. 2010; 36: 195–205. DOI: 10.1016/j.ctrv.2009.12.005

[40] Matsumoto K, Ikeda M, Hirayama T, Nishi M, Fujita T, et al. Clinical value of dividing false positive urine cytology findings into three categories: atypical, indeterminate, and suspicious of malignancy. Asian Pac J Cancer Prev. 2014; 15: 2251–2255.

[41] Heo CK, Bahk YY, Cho EW. Tumor-associated autoantibodies as diagnostic and prognostic biomarkers. BMB Rep. 2012; 45: 677–685.

[42] Hanash S. Harnessing immunity for cancer marker discovery. Nat Biotechnol. 2003; 21: 37–38. DOI: 10.1038/nbt0103-37

[43] Kobold S, Luetkens T, Cao Y, Bokemeyer C, Atanackovic D. Prognostic and diagnostic value of spontaneous tumor-related antibodies. Clin Dev Immunol. 2010; 2010: 721531. DOI: 10.1155/2010/721531

Chapter 3

# Emerging Biomarkers and Clinical Implications in Endometrial Carcinoma

Danielle Daley-Brown, Gabriela Oprea-Ilies,
Alexander Quarshie and
Ruben Rene Gonzalez-Perez

Additional information is available at the end of the chapter

http://dx.doi.org/10.5772/62772

## Abstract

Endometrial cancer (EmCa) is the most common type of gynecological cancer. EmCa is the fourth most common cancer in the United States, which has been linked to increased incidence of obesity. EmCa can be classified into two main types: Type I and Type II, which include the major histological subtypes. Type I EmCa is hormonally driven, less aggressive, and has a more favorable prognosis. In contrast, Type II EmCa grows independently of hormonal signals, is more aggressive, and generally has an unfavorable prognosis. Various tumor biomarkers [*i.e.*, tumor suppressor p53, hypoxia-inducible factor 1-alpha (HIF1-$\alpha$), human epidermal growth factor receptor 2 (HER2/neu), and vascular endothelial growth factor (VEGF)] have been identified in EmCa. Biomarkers of treatment effectiveness involve immunosuppressive factors targeted by microRNA (miRNA)-based therapy. However, there are no reliable biomarker tests for early detection of EmCa and treatment effectiveness. A potential new biomarker is Notch, Interleukin-1, leptin crosstalk outcome (NILCO) that could affect the progression of Type II EmCa. NILCO expression in EmCa might be dependent on patient's obesity status. This chapter presents updated information on these, and other potential emerging biomarkers for EmCa, and discusses current challenges and clinical implications on this area of research.

**Keywords:** Endometrial cancer, Biomarkers, NILCO, Leptin, Obesity

# 1. Introduction

## 1.1. Endometrium

The uterus is a pear-shaped hollow organ, with a virtual cavity, composed of the cervix and corpus (body of uterus). The corpus has three tissue layers: the endometrium, myometrium, and the perimetrium. The endometrium is the innermost layer, is comprised of endometrial glands, stroma, and blood vessel, and is the most active layer in responding to cyclic hormonal cues. The endometrium is essential for reproductive function (**Figure 1**) [1]. The myometrium or the muscle layer comprises interwoven spirals of smooth muscle fibers more compactly arranged adjacent to mucosa as visualized by magnetic resonance imaging (MRI) studies [2]. It

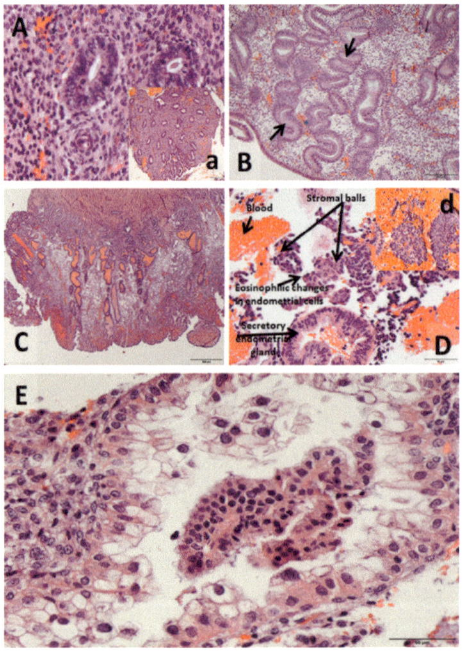


**Figure 1. Representative pictures from hematoxylin and eosin staining of endometrial tissue from different menstrual phases and pregnancy.** (**A**) Proliferative-phase endometrium shows round to oval endometrial glands lined by columnar cells with basally located nuclei. Multiple mitoses are present during the proliferative phase (40×). (**a**) The thumb image is a lower magnification of proliferative-phase endometrium revealing the evenly spaced round-to-oval glands within the endometrial stroma (10×). (**B**) Early secretory endometrium that shows the saw-tooth appearance of endometrial glands during secretory phase; some of the subnuclear secretions of the early phase are marked with short arrows (10×). (**C**) Secretory-phase endometrium that shows the basalis and functional layers. Upper arrows: basalis. Lower arrow: functionalis, composed of compact layer, situated ad-luminal, formed by the necks of endometrial glands and spongy layer underlies the compact layer, and is formed by the tortuous endometrial glands (10×). (**D**) Menstrual endometrium. The functionalis layer sheds during menstruation. The endometrial glands shed and may show eosinophilic change. The stromal cells condensate and form "stromal balls" a characteristic finding in shedding endometrium. A residual secretory gland is also visible. The background is blood (10×). (**d**) Stromal balls are depicted in the thumb image. (**E**) Pregnancy endometrium: Arias-Stella reaction showing enlarged endometrial glands with abundant clear or eosinophilic cytoplasm and marked nuclear changes. The nuclei are large, hyperchromatic, pleomorphic, and smudged). Rare mitotic figures may be found. The stroma is decidualized (40×).

is responsible for uterine contractions that occur during the entire menstrual cycle, varying in frequency and intensity during the follicular and luteal phase and at the time of menstruation and delivery [2, 3]. The outer most layer, the perimetrium, oftentimes referred to as the (tunica) serosa lines the entire uterus and consists of a thin layer or epithelial cells [1]. The uterus functions in receiving the embryo, housing the fetus throughout pregnancy and labor and delivery of the infant [3]. Implantation occurs in the endometrium layer and its function, and morphology is dependent on the release of sexual hormones. The morphology of the endometrium in the absence of hormonal influence (*i.e.*, pre-pubescent females and postmenopausal women) is constant and maintains a certain thickness. After the onset of menarche, the uterus prepares to receive a fertilized oocyte during the menstrual cycle. If implantation fails to occur, the functional layer of the endometrium sheds which leads to menstruation [4].

### 1.2. Menstrual cycle

At puberty, females undergo monthly cyclic changes controlled by the hypothalamus. The hypothalamus produces and releases gonadotropin-releasing hormone (GnRH), which acts on the anterior pituitary gland to stimulate the release of follicle stimulating hormone (FSH) and luteinizing hormone (LH) to initiate and control these cyclic changes [4]. Throughout the menstrual cycle, estrogen and progesterone are responsible for the morphological and biological changes that occur in the endometrium, cervix, and vagina. Additionally, estrogen and progesterone are responsible for the feedback of FSH and LH secretion [5].

The phases of the menstrual cycle are as follows: menstrual phase, proliferative or follicular phase, ovulation, and luteal or secretory phase [4]. The first day of the menstrual cycle begins with menstrual bleeding due to the regression and shedding of the outer layer of the endometrium, which is the functional layer. The menstrual period or menses typically lasts 3–4 days. The proliferative phase or follicular phase lasts on average 8–10 days. During the follicular phase, ovarian follicles begin to develop and secrete 17β-estradiol. In addition, FSH and LH receptors are upregulated in ovarian theca and granulosa cells. FSH stimulates rapid growth of ovarian follicles. An increase in 17β-estradiol induces cell proliferation of the endometrium and reconstructing the outer layer lost during menstruation [6]. Ovulation occurs on day 14 and is followed by an increase in estradiol secretion at the end of the proliferative phase. A surge in FSH and LH causes ovulation of the ovum. Estradiol levels decrease shortly after ovulation and increase during the luteal phase. The luteal phase or secretory phase begins after ovulation where the formation of the corpus luteum is evident [6]. The corpus luteum synthesizes and secretes estradiol and progesterone. Progesterone increases the vascularity of the endometrium and prepares the endometrium to receive the fertilized ovum with the endometrium reaching its maximum thickness. If fertilization does not occur, the corpus luteum regresses, thus decreasing the levels of estradiol and progesterone in circulation [5]. Menses follows for the beginning of the next menstrual cycle (see **Figure 1**).

### 1.3. Menopause

The menstrual cycle occurs in women of reproductive age and continues until the onset of menopause. Menopause usually occurs between the ages of 45–55, but can begin as early as

40. The age of onset could be determined by various factors such as genetics, diet, hysterectomy, or damage to ovary due to the chemotherapy or radiation. Common symptoms associated with menopause include as follows: irregular vaginal bleeding, hot flashes, changes in mood, and urinary and vaginal symptoms [7, 8].

Menopause is defined as the permanent cessation of menstruation, which results from the loss of ovarian function [7]. In other words, the ovaries become less sensitive to gonadotropin stimulation, which is associated with follicular attrition. Throughout a woman's life, oocytes undergo atresia, which results in the decline of the quality and quantity of ovarian follicles. Normally, follicles mature and release their ova for the purpose of ovulation and secretion hormones; and the failure to ovulate alters the menstrual pattern immensely. During menopause, estrogen levels decline dramatically, leading to a decrease in the number and size of ovarian follicles. As a consequence of declining estrogen levels, FSH and LH levels are elevated during menopause due to the follicular changes in sensitivity to gonadotropins and negative endocrine feedback [5]. Then, menopause is characterized by the loss of progesterone synthesis, and the increase in body weight and androgen levels [9].

The surge of androgens augments aromatization and production of estrogen by adipose tissue that further increases EmCa risk. In addition, estrogen can be produced by the aromatization of androgens in the ovarian stroma as well as in other tissues and organs such as bone, muscle, bone marrow, liver, fibroblasts, and hair roots [10]. Consequently, estrogen production that is accompanied by sharp decrease of progesterone leads to an unopposed estrogen status. This can result in endometrial hyperplasia that could possibly develop into EmCa [10, 11]. Also, postmenopausal women having increased levels of estrone are also under EmCa risk. Furthermore, there is evidence that chronic hyperinsulinemia is an EmCa risk factor [9]. The unopposed estrogen hypothesis proposes that EmCa is a result of the mitogenic effects of unbalanced estrogens. Then, situations showing chronic anovulation and progesterone deficiency lead to hyperandrogenism, which together with nutritional lifestyle factors increase EmCa risk. Indeed, pre- and postmenopausal women having elevated plasma androstenedione and testosterone also have increased EmCa risk. Approximately 75% of women with EmCa are postmenopausal; the most common symptom is postmenopausal bleeding [9].

## 2. Endometrial cancer

EmCa is a malignancy of the endometrial glands of the uterus and is the most frequent malignancy of the female pelvic reproductive tract [12]. EmCa comprises a series of malignant diseases of the endometrium with diverse phenotypes. Although it is not categorical, EmCa can be subdivided into two main different types based on the histologic examination: endometrioid and non-endometrioid with their variants [12]. EmCa may also be classified based on epidemiological, histologic, and behavioral information into two types: Type I EmCa and Type II EmCa (**Figure 2**) [12]. Type I EmCa comprising the endometrioid carcinomas is the most common type of adenocarcinoma. Then, Type I accounts for 85% of all EmCa cases and is more common than Type II EmCa (non-endometrioid carcinoma) [12]. Type I EmCa is dependent on estrogen hormonal stimulation, less aggressive, and shows a favorable prog-

http://dx.doi.org/10.5772/62772

nosis [12, 13]. Endometrioid carcinoma is well differentiated, closely resembles the endometrial glands and can be developed from atypical hyperplasia [14]. A common variant of Type I EmCa displays squamous cells adjacent to glandular elements, representing a tumor with squamous differentiation. Rare variants of endometrioid carcinomas are ciliated carcinoma, secretory carcinoma, and villoglandular adenocarcinoma [13]. Type II EmCas are the non-endometrioid type. Type II EmCa includes serous adenocarcinoma, clear cell carcinoma, uterine carcinosarcoma, mucinous adenocarcinoma, squamous cell carcinoma, mixed type of carcinoma, and undifferentiated carcinoma [14]. Type II EmCa is high grade and stage, independent of estrogen stimulation, poorly differentiated, and more aggressive with a poor prognosis. Most Type II EmCas have metastasized outside the uterus at the time of diagnosis [13, 14].

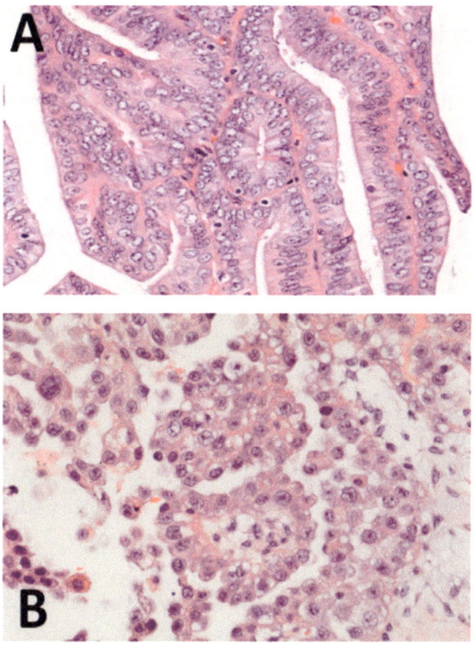


**Figure 2. Histopathological features of endometrial cancer**. (**A**) Type I (endometrioid) endometrial carcinoma: This is a 40× magnification of an H&E stain revealing columnar cells with basally located nuclei. This tumor shows slender villous architecture (better seen at the right of the picture) as well as glandular architecture (central). (**B**) Type II (serous) endometrial carcinoma. This 40× magnification of an H&E stain shows a high-grade tumor with micropapillary architecture. The nuclei are enlarged with irregular nuclear membrane, often protruding, giving a "hob nail" appearance. They show hyperchromasia or most often nuclear clearing with prominent, sometimes multiple nucleoli.

According to the system of the International Federation of Gynecology and Obstetrics (FIGO), grading of EmCa is determined by how closely similar the cancer forming glands appear when compared to benign endometrium [13]. Low-grade tumors form more glands and are well differentiated whereas high-grade tumors do not form glands, and are poorly differentiated [13]. Grade 1 tumors have well-formed glands with roughly 95% of the cancer forming glands and no more than 5% of solid non-squamous areas [13]. Grade 2 tumors have 50–94% of cancerous forming glands, while Grade 3 tumors have less than 50% of cancerous forming glands. Grade 3 tumors are considered high-grade and are more aggressive than lower-grade tumors [14]. Similarly, the FIGO system is also used for staging [15]. According to the National Cancer Institute (NCI), Stage I cancer is limited to the uterus; Stage II extends into the cervix; Stage III cancer has spread outside of the uterus, but is limited to the pelvic region; Stage IV cancer invades the bladder, bowel, and distant locations [16]. Staging is further stratified (*i.e.*, IA, IIB, IIIC) based on myometrial invasiveness [17].

In the United States, EmCa is the fourth most common cancer among women after breast, lung and bronchus, and colorectal cancer. In 2015, there were approximately 54,870 new EmCa cases diagnosed in the United States with roughly 10,170 estimated deaths. The overall 5-year survival rate is 96% when diagnosed at the local site, and 67% when diagnosed at the regional area [18]. The survival rate drastically decreases to 16% when diagnosed at a distant site.

The incidence of EmCa has been steady since 2004 for most ethnic groups, but is increasing by 1.9% in African-American women. The incidence rates in Caucasian women are the highest when compared to all ethnic groups. In Caucasian women, the incidence rate is 24.8/100,000 when compared to African-American women at 21.8/100,000 [19]. Even though the incidence of EmCa is higher in Caucasian women, the mortality rates are more than two times higher in African-American women (3.9/100,000 and 7.3/100,000, respectively). When comparing the survival rates between both ethnic groups, Caucasian women exceed that for African-American women roughly by 7% at each stage of diagnosis. Possible multifactorial reasons for EmCa health disparities usually include socioeconomic status, limited access to healthcare, comorbidities, etc., but the exact causes for this disparity are unknown [20].

### 2.1. Risks factors

A major role in endometrial carcinogenesis is represented by estrogen actions, both endogenous and exogenous. Increased exposure to estrogen augments the risk of EmCa. Postmenopausal women on estrogen replacement therapy have an increased risk of developing EmCa, and the risk further increases with the duration of replacement therapy use [21]. It has been reported that the relative risk of developing EmCa rises to 9.5:1 when the use of exogenous unopposed estrogen last for 10 years or longer [21]. Moreover, EmCa risk in these women persists for several years after estrogen discontinuation [22].

Tamoxifen is widely used as an adjuvant therapy in patients with estrogen receptor positive breast cancer. However, tamoxifen use also increases EmCa risk due to its agonistic effects on the endometrium [23]. However, the majority of tamoxifen-related carcinomas present mainly at early stages and show low grade [23, 24].

Ovarian tumors and conditions, such as granulosa cell tumor, thecoma, polycystic ovary disease, and hyperthecosis, causing prolonged unopposed estrogen production may lead to endometrial hyperplasia, and usually low-grade endometrioid carcinoma. Granulosa cell tumor is a relatively uncommon sex cord–stromal tumor, which affects mainly perimenopausal women. These tumors are associated with increased estrogen production. EmCa occur in 9–13% of women with granulosa cell tumors [25]. Thecomas are benign ovarian neoplasms developed by ovarian theca cells, which affect women of any age, but predominantly in women older than 40 years of age. EmCa have been reported in up to 21% of women with thecomas [26]. Polycystic ovarian disease (PCOD) occurs in young, usually infertile women with menstrual irregularities. Multiple cysts, stromal hyperplasia, and hyperthecosis enlarge the ovaries. These conditions show elevated estrogen and androgen serum levels. However, endometrioid carcinoma may occur in less than 5% of these women [27]. Hyperthecosis may occur independently for PCOD and may be associated with increased androgen production and virilization, or it may produce estrogen. Data from a small series of patients showed that a third of them have developed EmCa [28].

Major endogenous risk factors associated with EmCa are as follows: age, obesity, hypertension, and reproductive characteristics (late menopause, low parity and infertility). These conditions are associated with increased levels of estrogen.

Most women diagnosed with EmCa are postmenopausal or 50 years and older [20]. Approximately 15% of women diagnosed with EmCa are younger than 50 years of age, while 5% are diagnosed before the age of 40 [29]. Metabolic syndrome including obesity, hypertension, insulin resistance, diabetes, and dyslipidemia increase the risk of developing multiple malignancies, particularly EmCa [30]. Younger women diagnosed with EmCa are usually obese, and their carcinomas show a well-differentiated histology [20]. Obesity is a major risk factor for EmCa [12]. EmCa incidence is higher in well-developed countries where obesity is on the rise [18]. Hypertension has been linked to an increase in the incidence of EmCa, but it is unclear whether it is an independent risk factor or could be related to comorbidities of conditions and diseases (*i.e.,* obesity and diabetes) [31].

Lastly, as it was mentioned, infertility, late age onset of menopause, early age of menarche, and nulliparity increase EmCa risk. However, smoking decreases the risk of developing EmCa as well as oral contraceptive use lowers the risk [20, 32]. In regards to smoking, the anti-EmCa effect is probably related to its actions on estrogen metabolism. This anti-EmCa effect is primarily found in postmenopausal women, with current smokers showing the greatest risk reduction, in contrast to former smokers [32]. The greatest extent of risk reduction for EmCa is reported in postmenopausal, multiparous, obese, women who had no exogenous hormones [33]. Additionally, about 50% of women that used combined oral contraceptives (COCs, which is related to use of progestins and estrogens) show decrease EmCa risk. In most of these studies, this protective effect persisted for more than 15–20 years after cessation of the COC [34]. The adverse effects of oral contraceptive have been investigated extensively, whereas their non-contraceptive benefits have been underestimated. COC therapy could also reduce the risk of developing EmCa after menopause [35].

## 3. Endometrial cancer biomarkers

A biomarker is a characteristic or substance that can be quantified or measured objectively, and predicts the incidence and outcome of disease or normal biological function/process [36]. Cancer and non-malignant cells produce tumor markers. Biomarkers are molecules produced by cancer or non-cancer cells in response to malignant or benign conditions. Tumor markers are expressed higher under cancerous conditions. They can be present in urine, tumor tissue, blood, and bodily fluids. Most biomarkers are of protein origin (*i.e.*, growth and angiogenic factors, oncogenes, tumor suppressor, cytokines, and serum proteins, etc.). Recent studies have shown that alterations in DNA and gene expression can also be used as tumor markers (*i.e.*, mRNA, miRNA) (**Figure 3**) [12, 36].

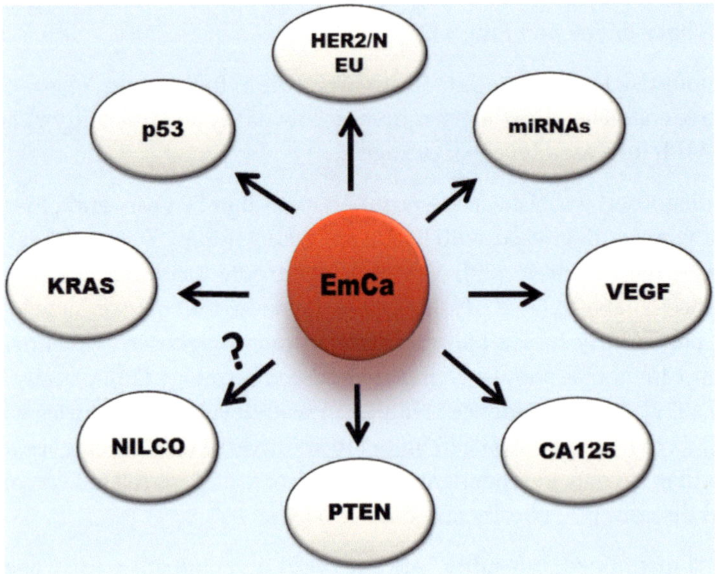


**Figure 3.** Main biomarkers of endometrial cancer (EmCa).

Tumor biomarkers have been instrumental in designing treatments of certain types of cancer. Tumor markers can be used for early detection, screening, diagnosis and prognosis, recurrence of cancer, and response to therapy. Studies on serum and plasma biomarkers are emerging and promising areas of research for early screening, treatment effectiveness, and recurrence in EmCa. Although these molecules have potential for the early detection of this disease, the impact of risk factors on EmCa and biomarkers is an area of promising research.

### 3.1. Tumor suppressors

Normally, tumor suppressor genes act to inhibit or arrest cell proliferation and tumor development [37]. However; when mutated, tumor suppressors become inactive, thus permitting tumor growth. For example, mutations in p53 have been determined in various cancers such as breast, colon, lung, endometrium, leukemias, and carcinomas of many tissues. These p53 mutations are found in approximately 50% of all cancers [38]. Roughly 10–20% of endometrial carcinomas exhibit p53 mutations [37]. Additionally, overexpression of mutated tumor suppressor p53 has been associated with Type II EmCa (poor histologic grade, non-endometrioid histology, advanced stage, and poor survival). African-American women present with stage I EmCa are three times more likely to have overexpression of mutant p53 and also have higher recurrence with poor survival rates when compared to Caucasian women [20]. Similarly, the tumor suppressor phosphatase and tensin homolog (PTEN) is the natural inhibitor of PI3K/AKT, which is involved in the progression of many cancers. PTEN can affect the regulation of cell cycle; enabling apoptosis and inhibiting the AKT survival pathway. Therefore, mutated PTEN causes an increase in cell proliferation, survival, and angiogenesis of cancer cells. PTEN mutations occur in 83% of all EmCa and are typically associated with Type I EmCa, which shows a more favorable prognosis and less aggressiveness [12]. Caucasian women have higher PTEN mutations, which may be related to a better overall survival rate when compared to African-American women [20].

### 3.2. Oncogenes

Oncogenes have the capacity to accelerate cell-cycle progression and induce the expression of several factors that induce tumor growth. These proteins are highly mutated and are overexpressed in many cancers. Oncogenes come from proto-oncogenes, which are involved in cell growth and differentiation [39]. For example, the overexpression of the oncogene HER2/neu (human epidermal growth factor receptor 2) has been associated with poor prognosis and resistance to treatment in breast, ovary, and EmCa [20]. Indeed, HER2/neu is involved in 20% of endometrioid (Type I EmCa) and serous carcinomas (Type II EmCa) [12]. In a study, African-American women with uterine papillary serous carcinoma showed three times higher HER2/neu overexpression when compared to Caucasian women showing this disease [20].

RAS (Rat Sarcoma Viral Oncogene Homolog) gene encodes GTPases involved in signal transduction [40]. Mutations in Kirsten mutated RAS (KRAS) have been associated with the progression of many malignancies [12]. An estimated 10–30% of EmCa cases exhibit RAS mutations that are predominantly observed in Type I EmCa, and also in non-malignant conditions such as endometrial hyperplasia. [40].

### 3.3. Vascular endothelial growth factor

Angiogenesis is important for tumor growth and the development of metastases [41]. Angiogenesis is controlled by pro-angiogenic and anti-angiogenic factors. An important angiogenic factor is vascular endothelial growth factor (VEGF), which was firstly identified by Senger et al. [42]. The overexpression of VEGF by cancer cells enhances tumor growth and metastasis of colorectal, head and neck, ovarian, and EmCa [41]. Elevated levels of VEGF and other angiogenic markers are associated with poor survival rates in EmCa [43]. Therapeutic targets for VEGF such as bevacizumab (anti-VEGF antibody) could be promising in inhibiting tumor growth in EmCa [44].

### 3.4. Hypoxia-inducible factor-$1\alpha$

Hypoxia-inducible factor 1 (HIF-$1\alpha$) is a major regulator of cellular processes that constitutes a biological response to hypoxic conditions. During hypoxia, HIF-$1\alpha$ is produced and accumulated within cells. HIF-$1\alpha$ is translocated to the nucleus, where it binds to hypoxia response elements (HREs), in the promoter region of several genes (*i.e.*, VEGF), thus activating angiogenesis and other processes that facilitate adaptation and survival of cells and the whole organism from normoxia. To date, there are more than one hundred HIF-1$\alpha$ downstream genes identified with varying functions, including erythropoiesis/iron metabolism, angiogenesis, vascular tone, matrix and glucose metabolism, cell proliferation/survival, and apoptosis [45]. In a study, HIF-1$\alpha$ expression was detected in approximately 49% of EmCa. Additionally, a strong correlation between HIF-1$\alpha$ and well-differentiated EmCa was found.

Since hypoxia enhances tumor progression and is a major obstacle for chemotherapy and radiation, HIF1-$\alpha$ could be used as a useful tool to predict patient outcome after surgery and radiation [46].

### 3.5. Serum markers

Several serum tumor markers have been identified as potential useful tools for detecting early relapse and monitoring response to therapy. Increased levels of Cancer Antigen 125 (CA 125) have been detected in many malignancies and are associated with endometrial proliferation and EmCa [47]. Approximately 11–33.9% of EmCa patients have increased CA 125 levels (>35 U/ml) [47]. Moreover, CA 125 is positively correlated with tumor size and stage in EmCa and is significantly associated with poorer survival rates in EmCa patients [48].

Other tumor-associated serum markers for EmCa include CA 15.3 and CA 19.9 that are detected in 24–32.1 and 22.3% of EmCa cases, respectively [48]. Surprisingly, 47% of patients with occult stage III EmCa exhibit elevated levels of CA 15.3 levels (>30 U/ml) when compared to stage I–II in which 18% of this tumor marker was observed [5]. CA 125 levels in combination with CA 19.9 levels could be used as a predictor of recurrence [49].

### 3.6. Epigenetic markers

The epigenetic change associated with gene regulation is an emerging area of research. MiRNAs or microRNAs regulates gene expression by binding to target mRNAs, resulting in the degradation of RNA or the repression of mRNA expression. MiRNAs can influence signaling pathways by functioning as a promoter or repressor in tumor cells and are involved in cell proliferation, migration, apoptosis, and differentiation. Targeting altered expression patterns of microRNAs could prove valuable in correcting abnormal signaling pathways observed in EmCa [50]. There are several miRNAs that might be used as biomarkers of EmCa: miR-99a, miR-199b, miR-205, miR-125b, miR-194, and miR-181b [51].

Some miRNAs have been found differentially expressed in the less aggressive endometrioid EmCa (Type I) versus the more aggressive serous papillary EmCa (Type II). MiR-99a and miR-199b expression levels were upregulated in Type I EmCa, and the combination of these two miRNAs with miR-100 could be used as diagnostic factors in the less aggressive Type I EmCa [51]. Interestingly, miR-205 levels are also increased in Type I EmCa. MiRNA-205 is a target for PTEN and is associated with poor survival [52]. In addition, miR-129-2 is involved in DNA methylation of the mismatch repair gene: human mutL homolog 1 (hMLH1) that is observed in the progression of Type I EmCa [51]. Moreover, methylated hMLH1 occurs frequently in EmCa and could induce mutations in certain cancer associated genes, which includes type II transforming growth factor-beta (TGF-βII), PTEN, Bcl2-associated X protein (BAX) and mutS homolog 6 (hMSH6) [51, 53].

In contrast, several miRNAs positively or negatively correlate with the progression of Type II EmCa. For example, miR-125b is significantly upregulated in Type II EmCa and targets Tumor protein p53 inducible nuclear protein1 (TP53INP1) gene and V-erb-b2 erythroblast leukemia viral oncogene homolog 2 (ERBB2) gene-inducing cancer cell proliferation and invasion [54, 55]. Conversely, decreased expression levels of miR-194 were correlated with advanced stage and poor survival in Type II EmCa [51]. Studies have demonstrated the administration of miR-194 in EmCa cells targets the B cell-specific Moloney murine leukemia virus integration site 1 (BMI1) gene, which is a cell-cycle regulator, and subsequently results in the inhibition of EMT phenotype and cell invasion in EmCa [56]. Similarly, miR-181b is downregulated in cancers with RAS mutations; hence, miR-181b could be a potential prognostic marker for Type II EmCa [57].

The use of miRNAs seems to be promising as biomarkers of EmCa. However, miRNA has limitations for cancer treatment, mainly due to the lack of effective transport of miRNAs in to cells [51].

Therefore, there is an unmet need to find novel biomarkers for EmCa diagnosis, prognosis, and treatment outcome. For example, NILCO (Notch, Interleukin-1, leptin crosstalk outcome; refer to Obesity and Cancer Section, page 21) may be used as a potential biomarker. NILCO has been associated with cell proliferation, metastasis, invasion, and overall decreased survival in breast cancer patients [58, 59]. Also, NILCO overexpression has been detected in the more aggressive Type II EmCa. Thus, it may be used a biomarker of EmCa aggressive phenotype.

## 4. Obesity and cancer

Obesity is a global epidemic and a major risk factor for several cancers, including EmCa [60, 61]. Obesity is defined as a condition of abnormal or excessive accumulation of fat in adipose tissue and a body mass index (BMI) of 30 kg/m$^2$ or higher [60]. Remarkably, several studies have shown that EmCa has the strongest correlation with obesity when comparing to diverse obesity-related cancers in women [62, 63]. Roughly, half of the EmCa cases are linked to obesity. Obese women are four times more likely to develop EmCa when compared to normal weight women [61]. Noticeably, it is known that African-American women have the higher incidence of obesity in the United States. Albeit EmCa rates are slightly higher among Caucasian than African-American women, they are less likely to die from EmCa compared to African-American women. The causes of this health disparity have not yet been determined, but the gap of the mortality rates between the two ethnic groups seems to be increasing [64].

Additionally, other populations also show strong correlations between obesity and EmCa. A case–control study performed in Europe that included 305 EmCa patients and 574 matched controls showed a significant increase in the risk of EmCa in patients with elevated levels of CRP, IL-6, and IL-1Ra. However, after adjustment for BMI, the estimates were strongly reduced and became non-significant. Nevertheless, the study provided epidemiological evidence that chronic inflammation might mediate the association between obesity and EmCa and that endometrial carcinogenesis could be promoted by an inflammatory milieu [65].

Obesity is characterized by high serum leptin levels in circulation [66]. Leptin is a 16 KD hormone (main adipokine) secreted by adipose tissue. Leptin regulates food intake, reproduction, body weight, inflammatory response, hematopoiesis, angiogenesis, bone formation, and wound healing [66]. Although leptin is mainly from adipose tissue origin, the stomach, mammary epithelium, placenta and heart, and several cancer cell types also produce this hormone. Leptin crosses the blood brain barrier and cerebrospinal fluid to bind receptors in the hypothalamus to carry out its energy-balance regulatory functions [67].

Obese individuals oftentimes exhibit resistance to leptin and show high levels of the adipokine in blood, which is known as leptin resistance [66]. The precise mechanisms involved in leptin resistance are ambiguous. One possible cause could be due to over-eating, which causes higher leptin levels in circulation. The prolonged exposure of leptin damages the hypothalamus causing it to become insensitive to the effects of leptin [68, 69]. Additionally, leptin resistance could be due to a defect in the transport system of leptin across the blood brain barrier [66].

Leptin receptor obese receptor (OB-R) has several molecular isoforms due to the posttranscriptional splicing. The long OB-R isoform (OB-RL or OB-Rb) has full signaling capabilities and is expressed in the hypothalamus and peripheral tissues [67]. The short isoform of the receptor (OB-Rb) has limited signaling capabilities and is more abundant in EmCa tissues. Evidence shows that leptin is an important pro-inflammatory, pro-angiogenic, and mitogenic factor for cancer. Leptin produced by cancer cells acts in an autocrine and paracrine manner to promote tumor cell proliferation, migration and invasion, pro-inflammation, and angiogenesis [58, 70]. High levels of leptin and OB-R are associated with metastasis and decreased survival rates in breast cancer patients [58].

Obesity is a known risk factor for several cancers, including EmCa, but there are scarce reports on the identification and detection of specific biomarkers for obesity-related EmCa. Our lab is currently investigating the relationship between an adipokine (leptin) and its crosstalk with other oncogenic factors in EmCa [12, 19].

### 4.1. Leptin signaling

Leptin binding to the extracellular region of OB-Rb activates Janus-activated kinase 2 (JAK2) proteins. JAK2 binding leads to the phosphorylation of tyrosine residues (Tyr985, Tyr1077, and Tyr1138) on the intracellular side of Ob-R. Phosphorylation of Tyr1138 recruits STAT3 (signal transducers and activators of transcription proteins), forming a dimer that is translocated to the nucleus to initiate transcription of target genes [71]. Additionally, JAK2 binding to OB-R causes auto-phosphorylation of JAK2 which can lead to the phosphorylation of insulin receptor proteins, recruitment of PI3K, and MAPK to activate a cascade of signaling mechanisms of downstream targets [72].

On the other hand, leptin-binding OB-R and the recruitment of JAK2 allow for the activation of tyrosine residue Tyr 985 on OB-R [71]. Src homology 2 (SH2) proteins are recruited and activated that allows the binding of growth factor receptor-bound protein 2 (Grb-2). Grb-2 is involved in the activation of ERK in the MAPK signaling [72]. Overexpression or mutations in these signaling mechanisms can lead to malignancies [71]. Obesity and leptin significantly alter the profiles of numerous proteins linked to cellular processes in cancerous tissues such as Notch and Interleukin-1 (IL-1) [71, 77].

### 4.2. Notch signaling

Notch signaling is an embryonic signaling pathway also involved in various cellular processes in adult cells, some of which include: proliferation, apoptosis, cell survival, epithelial–mesenchymal transition (EMT), differentiation, and angiogenesis [74, 75]. Notch Signaling is initiated through receptor–ligand interaction expressed in adjacent cells. Currently, four Notch receptors have been identified in mammals (Notch 1–4) [76]. Each receptor consists of an extracellular domain, which is involved in ligand binding, and a cytoplasmic domain involved in signal transduction [74]. Five ligands for Notch have been identified: Jagged (JAG1 and JAG2) and Delta-like (DLL1, DLL3, and DLL4) [76]. Once the ligand binds to its receptor, the Notch receptor is proteolitically cleaved at the extracellular domain by an $\alpha$-secretase (ADAM10), which is subsequently followed by the cleavage of the receptor's intracellular domain by $\gamma$-secretase, resulting in the formation of the intracellular domain of Notch (NICD or Notch-IC) [71]. The cleaved NICD then translocate to the nucleus to bind CSL transcription factor (CBF or RBP-JK) and initiate transcription of target genes such as survivin and hairy/enhancer-of-split related with YRPW motif 2 (Hey2), among others [74]. Aberrant activation of Notch signaling can lead to various pathological conditions such as cancer [74, 77]. In tumorigenesis, aberrant Notch activation can be initiated through the abnormal expression of Notch ligands, receptors, and target genes, all of which have been reported in many solid tumors, including breast, prostate, and pancreatic tumors [76]. The Notch signaling pathway exhibits oncogenic properties in some tumors and suppressive properties in others, which suggests a dual role in carcinogenesis [78]. Remarkably, we have identified leptin as an important regulator of Notch in breast cancer [58, 73, 79].

The role of Notch is poorly understood in EmCa. However, our recent research shows that leptin and Notch signaling may crosstalk in EmCa [12, 19]. Additionally, leptin upregulates IL-1 in breast and EmCa cells cultured in vitro, indicating that leptin and IL-1 could also crosstalk in these cancer types [58, 80, 81].

### 4.3. IL-1 system

The IL-1 system actively participates in inflammation. This system is composed of ligands (IL-1$\alpha$ and IL-1$\beta$), two membrane-bound receptors (IL-1RtI and IL-1RtII), and a soluble antagonist (IL-1Ra) derived from the extracellular domain of the IL-1R. IL-1$\beta$ is an inflammatory and pro-angiogenic cytokine that represents the more abundant ligand, which preferably binds IL-1RtI in normal and cancer cells [80, 81]. The IL-1 system is involved in various roles in both physiological and pathological states [80]. In cancer cells, IL-1 promotes inflammation, angiogenesis, tumor growth, and metastasis [81]. IL-1 is known to be upregulated in many tumor types. Indeed, the presence of IL-1 in some human cancers is associated with aggressive tumor biology [80]. IL-1 has been shown to upregulate leptin levels in some cancer cells. Overexpression of IL-1 is seen in breast cancer and linked to proliferation of breast cancer cells [83].

Interestingly, leptin was shown to upregulate the IL-1 system in endometrial cancer (EmCa) cells in a biunivocal manner [81] Additionally, it has been shown that IL-1 upregulates leptin and OB-R, and both cytokines upregulate β3-integrin in endometrial epithelial cells [84]. Moreover, an active leptin-IL-1 crosstalk seems to be involved in embryonic implantation [85]. Similarly, an active crosstalk between leptin, Notch, and IL-1 could lead to cancer progression [58, 59, 80, 81].

### 4.4. NILCO and cancer

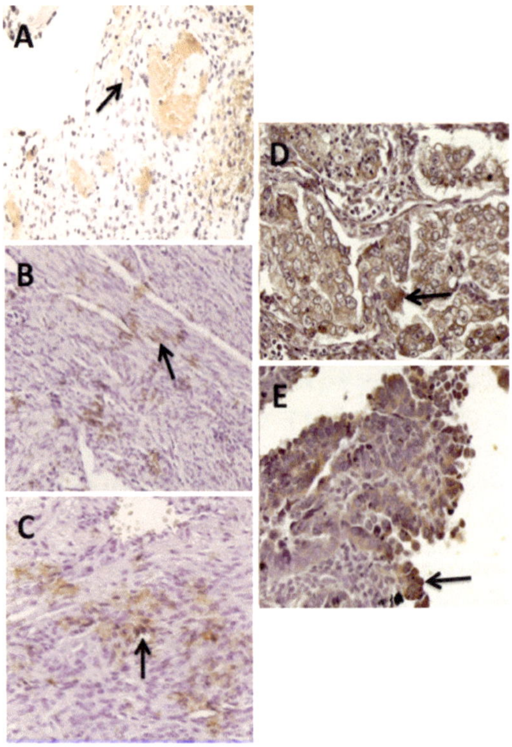


**Figure 4.** Immunohistochemistry (IHC) detection of NILCO in Type II endometrial cancer (Type II EmCa). Representative pictures for the IHC staining of: (**A**) Notch1, (**B**) Notch2, (**C**) Notch3, (**D**) Notch4, and (**E**) OB-R in Type II EmCa. Arrows indicate specific brown staining of NILCO antigens (40×).

A leptin-signaling crosstalk has been established in breast cancer among known pro-angiogenic factors, NILCO: Notch, IL-1, and leptin crosstalk outcome [58]. Signals triggered by these factors induce the expression of VEGF/VEGFR2 system, which is a main driver of tumor angiogenesis and tumor progression [58]. Notably, the overexpression of Notch, IL-1, and leptin has been associated with poor outcomes in breast cancer [59]. NILCO is involved in tumor cell proliferation and migration. Indeed, (NILCO) is correlated with decreased survival rates in breast cancer patients. Earlier studies from the Gonzalez–Perez's lab demonstrated that leptin induces Notch signaling in breast cancer [58]. Leptin was early identified as an upregulator of the IL-1 system in breast and EmCa [81, 86]. Similarly, leptin upregulates VEGF/VEGFR2 [87] and can also upregulate VEGF/VEGFR2 via IL-1 and Notch [58]. In addition, VEGF signaling could also upregulate Notch signaling in breast cancer [87]. However, these interactions have not been previously determined in EmCa.

Although obesity is a risk factor for cancer, the precise mechanisms involved in obesity-related cancer have not been explored. For the first time, our lab has shown that NILCO components are differentially expressed in EmCa, which correlated with the progression of the more aggressive Type II EmCa (**Figure 4**). NILCO components expressed in EmCa include Notch receptors (Notch1–4), ligands (DLL4 and JAG1), and targets (OB-R, IL-1RtI, Survivin, and Hey2).

Our studies have shown that in African-American (n = 20) and Chinese women (n = 75: in duplicate) suffering from EmCa, higher expression of several NILCO components was found in Type II EmCa patients compared to Type I EmCa (**Table 1**). These results suggest that the more aggressive non-hormonal responsive form of EmCa (Type II) could be more dependent on leptin signaling [12]. This would imply that Type II could be more affected by obesity than Type I EmCa.

| **African American Women** | | | | | | | |
|---|---|---|---|---|---|---|---|
| | Type I (n=12) | Type II (n=17) | | | Type I (n=12) | Type II (n=17) | |
| NILCO | | | | NILCO | | | |
| IHC | H SCORE | H SCORE | P-value | WB | Protein Expression | Protein Expression | P-value |
| Notch1 | 1.19 | 1.80 | <0.01 | Notch1 | 48 | 58 | <0.05 |
| Notch2 | 1.10 | 1.30 | =0.05 | Notch2 | 38 | 36 | >0.05 |
| Notch3 | 1.15 | 1.45 | >0.05 | Notch3 | 48 | 44 | >0.05 |
| Notch4 | 1.50 | 1.96 | <0.01 | Notch4 | 44 | 98 | <0.01 |
| JAG1 | 1.36 | 2.20 | <0.01 | JAG1 | 140 | 172 | <0.05 |
| DLL4 | 1.80 | 2.49 | <0.01 | DLL4 | 40 | 115 | <0.01 |
| Survivin | 1.20 | 1.96 | <0.01 | Survivin | 131 | 230 | <0.05 |
| OB-R | 1.60 | 1.73 | <0.01 | OB-R | 25 | 70 | <0.01 |
| IL-1R tI | 1.28 | 2.00 | <0.01 | IL-1R tI | 59 | 109 | <0.05 |
| Hey2 | 1.14 | 1.45 | <0.01 | Hey2 | 46 | 100 | >0.01 |
| Chinese Women | | | | | | | |
| | Type I (n=97) | Type II (n=23) | | NILCO qPCR | mRNA Expression | mRNA Expression | P-value |

**African American Women**

NILCO

| IHC | H SCORE | H SCORE | P-value | Notch1 | 1.00 | 1.30 | <0.01 |
|---|---|---|---|---|---|---|---|
| | | | | Notch3 | 0.45 | 0.80 | <0.05 |
| Notch1 | 1.00 | 1.78 | <0.01 | Notch4 | 0.80 | 1.40 | <0.01 |
| Notch2 | 1.00 | 1.15 | >0.05 | JAG1 | 0.05 | 0.52 | <0.01 |
| Notch3 | 1.10 | 1.20 | >0.05 | DLL4 | 1.10 | 1.50 | <0.01 |
| Notch4 | 1.10 | 1.58 | <0.05 | Survivin | 0.48 | 0.51 | <0.05 |
| JAG1 | 1.30 | 1.87 | <0.01 | OB-R | 0.45 | 0.65 | >0.05 |
| DLL4 | 1.31 | 1.80 | <0.01 | IL-1R tI | 0.82 | 1.56 | <0.01 |
| Survivin | 1.17 | 1.60 | <0.01 | Hey2 | 0.03 | 0.62 | <0.01 |
| OB-R | 1.10 | 1.50 | <0.05 | | | | |
| IL-1R tI | 1.40 | 1.73 | <0.05 | | | | |

IHC: immunohistochemistry; H SCORE[59]: semi-quantitative value calculated for each antigen and is determined by the equation HSCORE = $\sum$ pi (i + 1); WB: western blot; qPCR: Real-time polymerase chain reaction; Notch 1–4: transmembrane receptors; JAG1: Jagged 1; DLL4: Delta like-4 protein: Notch ligands; survivin: a cell survival factor and Notch target; OB-R: leptin receptor; IL-1R tI: interleukin 1 receptor type I; Hey2: hes-related family BHLH transcription factor with YRPW motif 2 and Notch target. Statistical significance set at $P < 0.05$.

**Table 1.** Expression of NILCO components in African-American and Chinese women suffering from endometrial cancer.

Our data further suggest that an active-signaling crosstalk (NILCO) triggered by obesity signals (leptin) occurs in EmCa, which might lead to the identification of novel biomarkers, particularly for Type II EmCa. NILCO investigations could lead to the identification of novel biological determinants of EmCa health disparity in African-American women [12]. However, a limitation to our preliminary data is that validation of this idea will require a larger sample size which is necessary to assess more conclusive statements.

## 5. Conclusions

Various biomarkers have been identified in EmCa; however, present targeted therapies have not been established in clinical practice. Clinical studies involving particular biomarkers such as VEGF and HER2 in EmCa resulted in minimal effects. Targeted therapies remain an obstacle due to the lack of specificity in EmCa cells. Therefore, more specific therapies are needed to target EmCa cells that overexpress tumor surface markers to avoid potential adverse effects on normal cells. The use of targeting epigenetic regulatory mechanisms involving miRNA biomarkers seems promising, but a more expansive approach is necessary to target the multiple signaling pathways involved in EmCa. Prognostic factors with a specific molecular biological signature may contribute to enhance tumor characterization in order to predict the

http://dx.doi.org/10.5772/62772

clinical behavior of such factors. Hence, the identification of novel biomarkers could prove effective in predicting disease outcome and links to risk factors (*i.e.*, obesity). One such potential new biomarker could be NILCO, particularly for Type II EmCa. Moreover, if further proven, NILCO association with obesity-related EmCa and perhaps with race may provide new molecular evidences on the impact of chronic mild inflammation (obesity) and leptin signaling on EmCa and health disparities. Additionally, targeting NILCO could be a novel and effective way to prevent and treat EmCa, especially in obese patients.

## 6. Future directions

It seems that histological classifications and discoveries of reliable EmCa markers will depend heavily on molecular study findings. Establishing NILCO's role in EmCa might allow early disease detection and provide new targets for some or all components of the crosstalk. In this respect, specific and potent leptin-signaling inhibitors (*i.e.*, leptin peptide receptor antagonists: LPrA1 and LPrA2) may be used for this purpose. LPrAs for the abrogation of leptin signaling have been successfully used in several disease scenarios [84, 88]. Additionally, inhibition of IL-1 signaling via specific antibodies or the natural inhibitor, IL-1Ra, has produced satisfactory results in situations where this cytokine plays an essential role [89]. Furthermore, several inhibitors of Notch signaling have been developed and tested (*i.e.*, DAPT and other $\gamma$-secretase inhibitors) [90]. However, with the exception of LPrAs, these compounds have off target effects that could jeopardize their clinical use. LPrAs specifically block OB-R signaling, are not toxic, and have no effect on general health status, body weight, and appetite when were tested in a large number of mice. Therefore, LPrA may prove to be effective biological to disrupt NILCO and progression of EmCa.

## Acknowledgements

This work was supported in part by the National Cancer Institute at the National Institutes of Health (NIH 1R41 CA183399-01A1, 5U54 CA118638 Pilot Project Award and UAB/UMN SPORE in Pancreatic Cancer) and the Congressionally Directed Medical Research Programs-Department of Defense (CDMRP DOD W81XWH-13-1-0382) to R.R.G.P.; and NCI S21 MD000101, 5G12 MD0076021, G12 RR026250-03, NIH RR03034 and 1C06 RR18386 to Morehouse School of Medicine, and the National Center for Advancing Translational Sciences of the NIH Award 5T32HL103104-04 (MPI) to D.D-B.

## Author details

Danielle Daley-Brown[1], Gabriela Oprea-Ilies[2], Alexander Quarshie[3] and Ruben Rene Gonzalez-Perez[1*]

*Address all correspondence to: rgonzalez@msm.edu

1 Department of Microbiology, Biochemistry and Immunology, Morehouse School of Medicine, Atlanta, GA, USA

2 Department of Pathology and Laboratory Medicine, Emory University School of Medicine, Atlanta, GA, USA

3 Department of Community Health and Preventative Medicine, Morehouse School of Medicine, Atlanta, GA, USA

## References

[1] Sadler T, Langman J. Medical Embryology. 12. 2012. Philadelphia: Wolters Kluwer Health/Lippincott Williams & Williams.

[2] Brosens J, Souza NM, Barker FG, Paraschos T, Winston RM. Endovaginal ultrasonography in the diagnosis of adenomyosis uteri: identifying the predictive characteristics. BJOG: An International Journal of Obstetrics & Gynaecology 1995;102(6):471–4.

[3] Novellas S, Chassang M, Delotte J, Toullalan O, Chevallier A, Bouaziz J, et al. MRI Characteristics of the Uterine Junctional Zone: From Normal to the Diagnosis of Adenomyosis. American Journal of Roentgenology 2011;196(5):1206–13.

[4] Maggi R, Cariboni AM, Montagnani Marelli M, Moretti RM, Andre V, Marzagalli M, et al. GnRH and GnRH receptors in the pathophysiology of the human female reproductive system. Human Reproduction Update 2015.

[5] Costanzo L. Physiology. Philadelphia: Saunders/Elsevier; 2014.

[6] Mescher A. Junqueira's Basic Histology: Text and Atlas, 12th Edition. New York: McGraw-Hill Education; 2009.

[7] Encyclopædia Britannica Online. Menopause. Encyclopaedia Britannica Online. 2-6-2016. Encyclopædia Britannica Online, Encyclopædia Britannica Inc.

[8] Burger HG, Hale GE, Robertson DM, Dennerstein L. A review of hormonal changes during the menopausal transition: focus on findings from the Melbourne Women's Midlife Health Project. Human Reproduction Update 2007;13(6):559–65.

[9] Kaaks R, Lukanova A, Kurzer MS. Obesity, endogenous hormones, and endometrial cancer risk: a synthetic review. Cancer Epidemiology Biomarkers & Prevention 2002;11(12):1531–43.

[10] Santoro N, Randolph Jr JF. Reproductive Hormones and the Menopause Transition. Obstetrics and Gynecology Clinics of North America 2011;38(3):455–66.

[11] Management of symptomatic vulvovaginal atrophy: (2013). position statement of The North American Menopause Society. Menopause 2013;., 20(9).

[12] Daley-Brown D, Oprea-Ilies G, Lee R, Pattillo R, Gonzalez R. Molecular cues on obesity signals, tumor markers and endometrial cancer. Hormone Molecular Biology and Clinical Investigation 2016;21(1):89–106.

[13] Amant Fdr, Floquet A, Friedlander M, Kristensen G, Mahner S, Nam EJ, et al. Gynecologic Cancer InterGroup (GCIG) Consensus Review for Endometrial Stromal Sarcoma. International Journal of Gynecological Cancer 2014;24(9).

[14] American Cancer Society. Endometrial Cancer Facts 2016. 2016. Atlanta, GA:American Cancer Society, Inc. 1-25-2016.

[15] Percorelli S. Revised FIGO staging for carcinoma of the vulva, cervix, and endometrium. International Journal of Gynaecology and Obstetrics 2009;105(2):103–4.

[16] National Cancer Institute. Endometrial Cancer. 2016. National Cancer Institute. 1-28-2016.

[17] Abu-Rustum NR, Zhou Q, Iasonos A, Alektiar KM, Leitao MMJ, Chi DS, et al. The Revised 2009 FIGO Staging System for endometrial cancer: Should the 1988 FIGO Stages IA and IB be altered? International Journal of Gynecological Cancer 2011;21(3).

[18] Siegel RL, Miller KD, Jemal A. Cancer statistics, 2015. CA: A Cancer Journal for Clinicians 2015;65(1):5–29.

[19] Lipsey C, Harbuzariu A, Daley-Brown D. Oncogenic role of leptin and Notch Interleukin-1 leptin crosstalk outcome (NILCO) in Cancer. World Journal of Methodology 2016.

[20] Collins Y, Holcomb K, Chapman-Davis E, Khabele D, Farley JH. Gynecologic cancer disparities: A report from the Health Disparities Taskforce of the Society of Gynecologic Oncology. Gynecologic Oncology 2014; 133(2):353–61.

[21] Grady D, Gebretsadik T, Ernster V, Petitti D. Hormone replacement therapy and endometrial cancer risk: a meta-analysis. Obstetrics and Gynecology 1995;85(2):304–13.

[22] Green P, Weiss N, McKnight B, Voigt L, Beresford S. Risk of endometrial cancer following cessation of menopausal hormone use (Washington, United States). Cancer Causes Control 1996;7(6):575–80.

[23] Jordan V, Assikis V. Endometrial carcinoma and tamoxifen: clearing up a controversy. Clinical Cancer Research 1995;1(5):467–72.

[24] Moberger B, Fornander T, Hellstrom AC. VI.3 DNA content in tamoxifen-induced endometrial carcinoma. European Journal of Cancer 34:S64.

[25] Malmstrom H, Hogberg T, Risberg Br, Simonsen E. Granulosa cell tumors of the ovary: prognostic factors and outcome. Gynecologic Oncology 1994;52(1):50–5.

[26] Bjorkholm E, Silfversward C. Theca-cell tumors: clinical features and prognosis. Acta Radilogica - Oncology 1980;19(4):241–4.

[27] Scully RE, Young RH, Clement PB. Atlas of Tumor Pathology: Tumors of the Ovary, Maldeveloped Gonads, Fallopian Tube and Broad Ligament. 3rd Series ed. Washington, D.C.: Armed Forces Institute of Pathology; 1998. p. 409–50.

[28] Sasano H, Fukunaga M, Rojas M, Silverberg SG. Hyperthecosis of the ovary: clinicopathologic study of 19 cases with immunohistochemical analysis of steroidogenic enzymes. International Journal of Gynecological Pathology 1989;8(4).

[29] Howlader N, Noone A, Krapcho M, Neyman N, Aminou R, et al. SEER Cancer Statistics Review. 2016. Bethesda, MD: National Cancer Institute. 1-29-2016.

[30] Friedenreich CM, Biel RK, Lau DCW, Csizmadi I, Courneya KS, Magliocco AM, et al. Case ▪ control study of the metabolic syndrome and metabolic risk factors for endometrial cancer. Cancer Epidemiology Biomarkers & Prevention 2011;20(11):2384–95.

[31] Soler M, Chatenoud L, Negri E, Parazzini F, Franceschi S, La Vecchia C. Hypertension and hormone-related neoplasms in women. Hypertension 1999;34(2):320–5.

[32] Austin H, Drews C, Partridge EE. A case-control study of endometrial cancer in relation to cigarette smoking, serum estrogen levels, and alcohol use. American Journal of Obstetrics & Gynecology 1993;169(5):1086–91.

[33] Brinton LA, Barrett RJ, Berman ML, Mortel R, Twiggs LB, Wilbanks GD. Cigarette smoking and the risk of endometrial cancer. American Journal of Epidemiology 1993;137(3):281–91.

[34] Mueck AO, Seeger H, Rabe T. Hormonal contraception and risk of endometrial cancer: a systematic review. Endocrine-Related Cancer 2010;17(4):R263-R271.

[35] Caserta D, Ralli E, Matteucci E, Mallozzi M, Oscarini M. Combined oral contraceptives: health benefits beyond contraception. Panminerva Med2014;56(3):233–44.

[36] Strimbu K, Tavel JA. What are biomarkers? Current Opinion in HIV and AIDS 2010;5(6).

[37] Kohler MF, Berchuck A, Davidoff AM, Humphrey PA, Dodge RK, Iglehart JD, et al. Overexpression and mutation of p53 in endometrial carcinoma. Cancer Research 1992;52(6):1622–7.

[38] Cooper G. The Cell: A Molecular Approach. Tumor Suppressor Genes. Sunderland (MA): Sinauer Associates; 2000.

[39] Moasser MM. The oncogene HER2: Its signaling and transforming functions and its role in human cancer pathogenesis. Oncogene 2007;26(45):6469–87.

[40] Ito K, Watanabe K, Nasim S, Sasano H, Sato S, Yajima A, et al. K-ras point mutations in endometrial carcinoma: effect on outcome is dependent on age of patient. Gynecologic Oncology 1996;63(2):238–46.

[41] Kamat AA, Merritt WM, Coffey D, Lin YG, Patel PR, Broaddus R, et al. Clinical and biological significance of vascular endothelial growth factor in endometrial cancer. Clinical Cancer Research 2007;13(24):7487–95.

[42] Senger DR, Water L, Brown LF, Nagy JA, Yeo KT, Yeo TK, et al. Vascular permeability factor (VPF, VEGF) in tumor biology. Cancer and Metastasis Reviews 1993;12(3):303–24.

[43] Sanseverino F, Santopietro R, Torricelli M, D'Andrilli G, Cevenini G. pRb2/p130 and VEGF expression in endometrial carcinoma in relation to angiogenesis and histopathologic tumor grade. Cancer Biology & Therapy 2006;5(1):84–8.

[44] Davies S, Dai D, Pickett G, Thiel K, Korovkina VP, Leslie KK. Effects of bevacizumab in mouse model of endometrial cancer: defining the molecular basis for resistance. Oncology Reports 2011;25(3):855–62.

[45] Ke Q, Costa M. Hypoxia-inducible factor-1 (HIF-1). Molecular Pharmacology 2006;70(5):1469–80.

[46] Espinosa I, Jose Carnicer M, Catasus L, Canet Bn, D'Angelo E, Zannoni GF, et al. Myometrial invasion and lymph node metastasis in endometrioid carcinomas: tumor-associated macrophages, microvessel density, and HIF1A have a crucial role. The American Journal of Surgical Pathology 2010;34(11).

[47] Gadducci A, Cosio S, Carpi A, Nicolini A, Genazzani AR. Serum tumor markers in the management of ovarian, endometrial and cervical cancer. Biomedicine & Pharmacotherapy 2004;58(1):24–38.

[48] Linkov F, Edwards R, Balk J, Yurkovetsky Z, Stadterman B, Lokshin A, et al. Endometrial hyperplasia, endometrial cancer and prevention: gaps in existing research of modifiable risk factors. European Journal of Cancer 44(12):1632–44.

[49] Lo SST, Cheng DKL, Ng TY, Wong LC, Ngan HYS. Prognostic significance of tumour markers in endometrial cancer. Tumor Biology 1997;18(4):241–9.

[50] Dong P, Masanori K, Hidemichi W, Satoko S, Noriaki S. Emerging therapeutic biomarkers in endometrial cancer. BioMed Research International 2013;2013.

[51] Megumi Y, Kouji B, Miho I, Haruko I, Kiyoko U, et al. MicroRNAS in endometrial cancer: recent advances and potential clinical applications. EXCLI Journal 2015;(14): 190–8.

[52] Tsukamoto O, Miura K, Mishima H, Abe S, Kaneuchi M, Higashijima A, et al. Identification of endometrioid endometrial carcinoma-associated microRNAs in tissue and plasma. Gynecologic Oncology 2014;132(3):715–21.

[53] Banno K, Kisu I, Yanokura M, Masuda K, Ueki A, Kobayashi Y, et al. Epigenetics and genetics in endometrial cancer: new carcinogenic mechanisms and relationship with clinical practice. Epigenomics 2012;4(2):147–62.

[54] Jiang F, Liu T, He Y, Yan Q, Chen X, Wang H, et al. MiR-125b promotes proliferation and migration of type II endometrial carcinoma cells through targeting TP53INP1 tumor suppressor in vitro and in vivo. BMC Cancer 2011;11(1):1–12.

[55] Chao S, Yan-ming L, Li-rong M. MicroRNA-125b downregulation mediates endometrial cancer invasion by targeting ERBB2. Medical Science Monitor 2012;18(4):149–55.

[56] Dong P, Kaneuchi M, Watari H, Hamada J, Sudo S, Ju J, et al. MicroRNA-194 inhibits epithelial to mesenchymal transition of endometrial cancer cells by targeting oncogene BMI-1. Molecular Cancer 2011;10(1):1–9.

[57] Larissa L, Elena R, Mohamed U, Kathryn W, Marta B, Kathryn G, et al. The KRAS-variant and miRNA expression in RTOG endometrial cancer clinical trials 9708 and 9905. PLoS One 2014;9(4).

[58] Shanchun G, Ruben G-P. Notch, IL-1 and Leptin Crosstalk Outcome (NILCO) is critical for leptin-induced proliferation, migration and VEGF/VEGFR-2 expression in breast cancer. PLoS One 2016;6(6).

[59] Colbert LS, Wilson K, Kim S, Liu Y, Oprea-Ilies G, Gillespie C, et al. NILCO biomarkers in breast cancer from Chinese patients. BMC Cancer 2014;14(1):1–12.

[60] Ofei F. Obesity-a preventable disease. Ghana Medical Journal 2005;39(3):98–101.

[61] Lu L, Risch H, Irwin ML, Mayne ST, Cartmel B, Schwartz P, et al. Long-term overweight and weight gain in early adulthood in association with risk of endometrial cancer. International Journal of Cancer 2011 ;129(5):1237–43.

[62] Renehan AG, Tyson M, Egger M, Heller RF, Zwahlen M. Body-mass index and incidence of cancer: a systematic review and meta-analysis of prospective observational studies. The Lancet 2008;371(9612):569–78.

[63] Calle EE, Kaaks R. Overweight, obesity and cancer: epidemiological evidence and proposed mechanisms. Nature Reviews Cancer 2004;4(8):579–91.

[64] Williamson DF, Kahn HS, Byers T. The 10-y incidence of obesity and major weight gain in black and white US women aged 30-55 y. The American Journal of Clinical Nutrition 1991;53(6):1515S–8S.

[65] Dossus L, Rinaldi S, Becker S, Lukanova A, Tjonneland A, Olsen A, et al. Obesity, inflammatory markers, and endometrial cancer risk: a prospective case–control study. Endocrine-Related Cancer 2010;17(4):1007–19.

[66] Klok MD, Jakobsdottir S, Drent ML. The role of leptin and ghrelin in the regulation of food intake and body weight in humans: a review. Obesity Reviews 2007;8(1):21–34.

[67] Gonzalez RR, Simon C, Caballero-Campo P, Norman R, Chardonnens D, Devoto L, et al. Leptin and reproduction. Human Reproduction Update 2000;6(3):290–300.

[68] Levine JA, Eberhardt NL, Jensen MD. Leptin responses to overfeeding: relationship with body fat and nonexercise activity thermogenesis. The Journal of Clinical Endocrinology & Metabolism 1999;84(8):2751–4.

[69] Kolaczynski JW, Ohannesian JP, Considine RV, Marco CC, Caro JF. Response of leptin to short-term and prolonged overfeeding in humans. The Journal of Clinical Endocrinology & Metabolism 1996;81(11):4162–5.

[70] Carino C, Olawaiye AB, Cherfils S, Serikawa T, Lynch MP, Rueda BR, et al. Leptin regulation of proangiogenic molecules in benign and cancerous endometrial cells. International Journal of Cancer 2008;123(12):2782–90.

[71] Newman G, Gonzalez-Perez RR. Leptin–cytokine crosstalk in breast cancer. Molecular and Cellular Endocrinology 2014;382(1):570–82.

[72] Yang R, Barouch LA. Leptin Signaling and obesity: cardiovascular consequences. Circulation Research 2007;101(6):545–59.

[73] Battle M, Gillespie C, Quarshie A, Lanier V, Harmon T, Wilson K, et al. Obesity induced a leptin-Notch signaling axis in breast cancer. International Journal of Cancer 2014;134(7):1605–16.

[74] Guo S, Liu M, Gonzalez-Perez RR. Role of Notch and its oncogenic signaling crosstalk in breast cancer. Biochimica et Biophysica Acta (BBA)—Reviews on Cancer 2011;1815(2):197–213.

[75] Borggrefe T, Lauth M, Zwijsen A, Huylebroeck D, Oswald F, Giaimo BD. The Notch intracellular domain integrates signals from Wnt, Hedgehog, TGF/BMP and hypoxia pathways. Biochimica et Biophysica Acta (BBA)—Molecular Cell Research 2016;1863(2):303–13.

[76] Mitsuhashi Y, Horiuchi A, Miyamoto T, Kashima H, Suzuki A, Shiozawa T. Prognostic significance of Notch signalling molecules and their involvement in the invasiveness of endometrial carcinoma cells. Histopathology 2012;60(5):826–37.

[77] Jonusiene V, Sasnauskiene A, Lachej N, Kanopiene D, Dabkeviciene D, Sasnauskiene S, et al. Down-regulated expression of Notch signaling molecules in human endometrial cancer. Medical Oncology 2013;30(1):1–7.

[78] Kitagawa M. Notch signalling in the nucleus: roles of Mastermind-like (MAML) transcriptional coactivators. Journal of Biochemistry 2015.

[79] Gillespie C, Quarshie A, Penichet M, Gonzalez-Perez R. Potential role of leptin signaling in DMBA-induced mammary tumors by non-responsive C57BL/6J mice fed a high-fat diet. Journal of Carcinogenesis & Mutagenesis 2012;3:132.

[80] Elaraj DM, Weinreich DM, Varghese S, Puhlmann M, Hewitt SM, Carroll NM, et al. The role of interleukin 1 in growth and metastasis of human cancer xenografts. Clinical Cancer Research 2006;12(4):1088–96.

[81] Gonzalez RR, Leary K, Petrozza JC, Leavis PC. Leptin regulation of the interleukin1 system in human endometrial cells. Molecular Human Reproduction 2003;9(3):151–8.

[82] Yang W, Yu XH, Wang C, He WS, Zhang SJ, Yan YG, et al. Interleukin-1 in intervertebral disk degeneration. Clinica Chimica Acta 2015;450:262–72.

[83] Singer CF, Hudelist G, Gswchwantler-Kaulich D, Fink-Retter A, Mueller R, Walter I, et al. Interleukin1 protein secretion in breast cancer is associated with poor differentiation and estrogen receptor negativity. International Journal of Gynecological Cancer 2006;16(s2):556–9.

[84] Gonzalez RR, Leavis P. Leptin upregulates beta3-integrin expression and interleukin-1 upregulates leptin and leptin receptor expression in human endometrial epithelial cell cultures. Endocrine 2001;16(1):21–8.

[85] Ramos MP, Rueda BR, Leavis PC, Gonzalez RR. Leptin serves as an upstream activator of an obligatory signaling cascade in the embryo-implantation process. Endocrinology 2005;146(2):694–701.

[86] Zhou W, Guo S, Gonzalez-Perez RR. Leptin pro-angiogenic signature in breast cancer is linked to IL-1 signalling. British Journal of Cancer 2011 Jan 4;104(1):128–37.

[87] Gonzalez-Perez RR, Xu Y, Guo S, Watters A, Zhou W, Leibovich SJ. Leptin upregulates VEGF in breast cancer via canonic and non-canonical signalling pathways and NFκB/HIF-1$\alpha$ activation. Cellular Signalling 2010;22(9):1350–62.

[88] Gonzalez RR, Cherfils S, Escobar M, Yoo JH, Carino C, Styer AK, et al. Leptin signaling promotes the growth of mammary tumors and increases the expression of vascular endothelial growth factor (VEGF) and its receptor type two (VEGF-R2). Journal of Biological Chemistry 2006;281(36):26320–8.

[89] Voronov E, Shouval DS, Krelin Y, Cagnano E, Benharroch D, Iwakura Y, et al. IL-1 is required for tumor invasiveness and angiogenesis. Proceedings of the National Academy of Sciences 2003;100(5):2645–50.

[90] Espinoza I, Miele L. Notch inhibitors for cancer treatment. Pharmacology & Therapeutics 2013;139(2):95–110.

Chapter 4

# Oxidative Stress Biomarkers for Diabetic Retinopathy and Medical Management Affecting Oxidative Stress

Ines Cilenšek, Sara Mankoč Ramuš,
Mojca Globočnik Petrovič and Daniel Petrovič

Additional information is available at the end of the chapter

http://dx.doi.org/10.5772/63353

**Abstract**

Changes in dietary habits and lifestyles associated with rapid economic growth have dramatically increased the incidence of diabetes and related vascular complications. Diabetic retinopathy (DR), a microvascular complication of diabetes, is associated with both environmental and genetic factors. Several metabolic abnormalities are implicated in its pathogenesis; however, the exact mechanism remains to be determined. Among them, oxidative stress is expected to play an important role.

Environmental, genetic, and epigenetic factors affecting the oxidative stress responsible for DR are reviewed in this paper. The knowledge about genetic biomarkers of DR is quite extensive, whereas the awareness about epigenetics and epigenetic markers is only beginning to be understood.

Modulation of epigenetic changes by pharmaceutical means may provide a potential strategy to retard the progression of DR. In addition to the intense medical management, these strategies include dietary measures (antioxidants) and the introduction of epigenetic drugs, such as inhibitors of DNA methylation and histone demethylases.

**Keywords:** oxidative stress, diabetic retinopathy, gene polymorphisms, epigenetics, medical management

## 1. Introduction

Diabetes mellitus is a group of metabolic diseases characterized by hyperglycemia resulting from defects in insulin secretion, insulin action, or both [1]. The prevalence of diabetes has reached global epidemic proportions. According to the Internal Diabetes Federal (IDF) data, there were 382 million people living with diabetes in 2013, whereas a further 316 million with impaired glucose tolerance are at high risk of the disease—an alarming number that is set to reach 471 million by 2035. Type 2 diabetes (T2DM) is the most prevalent type of diabetes. It is by far the most common form of diabetes in elderly people, but is increasingly seen in children and adolescents IDF, 2013 as well. The causes of the T2DM epidemic are embedded in a very complex group of genetic and epigenetic systems interacting within an equally complex societal framework that determines behavior and environmental influences [2]. The chronic hyperglycemia of diabetes is associated with long-term damage, dysfunction, and failure of various organs, especially the eyes, kidneys, nerves, heart, and blood vessels [1].

## 2. Pathogenesis of DR

Chronic elevation in circulating blood glucose damages blood vessels, which results in many micro- and macrovascular complications. DR is one of the major microvascular complications affecting the vision and is the leading cause of blindness in working-age adults [3]. It progresses from mild nonproliferative abnormalities, characterized by increased vascular permeability, to nonproliferative diabetic retinopathy (NPDR), characterized by vascular closure, to proliferative diabetic retinopathy (PDR), characterized by the growth of new blood vessels in the retina and the posterior surface of the vitreous [4] (**Figure 1**).

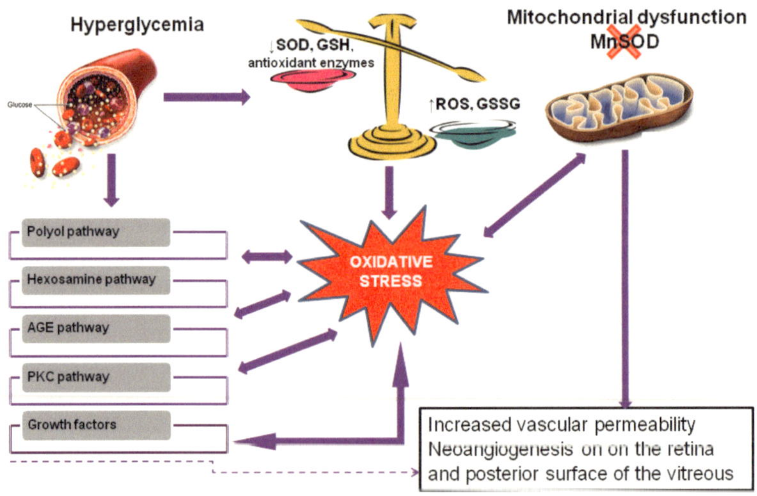


**Figure 1.** Major pathways implicated in the development of diabetic retinopathy.

It is a multifactorial condition for which the pathophysiology is incompletely understood [5]. There are many pathophysiological mechanisms through which diabetes might affect the initiation and promotion of the many underlying pathologies associated with DR [6]. The strong impact of hyperglycemia on DR incidence was confirmed by the Diabetes Control and

Complications Trial (DCCT) and the UK Prospective Diabetes Study (UKPDS) clinical trials [7,8]. Hyperglycemia activates several well-characterized biochemical pathways that play a significant role in the development of DR [9]. Major pathways implicated in the development of DR are the polyol pathway, protein kinase C (PKC) activation, accumulation of advanced glycation end products (AGEs), oxidative stress, activation of the hexosamine biosynthesis pathway, and growth factors (**Figure 1**) [3,6,9–11]. The activation of these pathways, in turn, leads to the secondary production of reactive oxygen species (ROS) and the consequent increase in oxidative stress that affects carbohydrates, lipids, proteins, and nucleic acids [9]. The oxidative stress plays a pivotal role in cellular injury from hyperglycemia.

## 3. Biomarkers

A biomarker is a measurable indicator of a specific biological state, usually one relevant to the risk, presence, severity, prognosis, or predicted therapeutic response of the disease. In medicine, biomarkers are often compounds isolated from serum, urine, or other fluids that can be used as an indicator of the presence or severity of a particular disease state. Molecular biomarkers can themselves take many forms, and as a consequence there are many strategies available for their discovery and validation. Transcriptional profiling, DNA methylation studies, and kinase sequencing have shown a strong potential for biomarker discovery in several disorders; metabolomics approaches are beginning to show promise for metabolic diseases, such as DR. Molecular biomarkers (DNA gene polymorphisms, RNA gene polymorphisms, proteins) hold special promise for a wide range of clinical and biomedical applications in several disorders, including DR [12].

## 4. Oxidative stress and its role in the development of DR

Oxidative stress may be defined as an imbalance between the level of ROS or oxygen radicals and the antioxidant defenses in a biological system [10]. The term "ROS" includes all unstable metabolites of molecular oxygen ($O_2$) that have a higher reactivity than $O_2$, such as the superoxide radical ($O_2'^{\bullet}$) and the hydroxyl radical ($HO^{\bullet}$), and nonradical molecules, such as hydrogen peroxide ($H_2O_2$) [13]. To counteract the harmful effects of ROS, the cell has developed antioxidant defense mechanisms. Antioxidants may be classified according to their structure (enzymes or small nonenzymatic protein molecules) and antioxidants according to their source (endogenous or exogenous). There are many enzymes with an antioxidant role in the organism, such as superoxide dismutase (SOD), catalase (CAT), glutathione peroxidase (GPx), glutathione S-transferases (GSTs), and the thioredoxin (Trx) system [14,15].

Increasing data indicate that oxidative stress is involved in the development of DR [16–19]. The retina has a high content of polyunsaturated fatty acids and has the highest oxygen uptake and glucose oxidation relative to any other tissue. This phenomenon renders the retina more susceptible to oxidative stress [20]. Oxidative stress-induced biochemical changes contribute to either functional or structural changes in the microvasculature in the retina [6]. Structural changes range from basement membrane thickening and microvascular cell loss to capillary closure and acellular capillary formation [6]. ROS mediate these changes by both direct and indirect mechanisms. Structural changes may both contribute to and result from functional changes, such as altered blood flow, loss of intercellular junctions, and increased vessel permeability. Thus, oxidative stress-induced structural and functional changes appear to be highly interrelated in the pathogenesis of diabetic retinopathy (DR) [6].

Since long-term exposure to oxidative stress is strongly implicated in the pathogenesis of diabetic complications, polymorphic genes of detoxifying enzymes may be involved in the development of DR.

## 5. Polymorphisms in oxidative stress genes and risk for DR

| Gene | Polymorphism | | Relation to DR (significance level) | Population | Number of patients | Author | Year |
|---|---|---|---|---|---|---|---|
| *MnSOD* | rs4880 | VV genotype (V16A) | Positive association ($p = 0.006$) | Slovenian | 426 | Petrovič et al. | 2008 |
| | | AA genotype (V16A) | Positive association ($p = 0.03$) | Finnish | 755 | Kangas-Kontio et al. | 2009 |
| | | C allele (C47T) | No significant association | Different ethnic origins | (17 articles) meta-analysis | Tian et al. | 2011 |
| | | (V16A) | No significant association | North Indian | 758 | Vanita | 2014 |
| | | AV genotype (V16A) | Positive association ($p < 0.0001$) | Northern Iranian | 280 | Haghighi et al. | 2015 |
| *CAT* | rs1001179 | −262C/T | No significant association | Brazilian | 520 | Dos Santos et al. | 2006 |
| *GPx* | rs1050450 | Pro197Leu | No study on DR | / | / | / | / |
| *GSTM1, T1* | Null genotype | GSTT1null | Positive association ($p = 0.01$) | Scottish | 2015 | Doney et al. | 2005 |
| | | GSTT1null GSTM1null | Positive association ($p < 0.0001$) Positive association | Slovenian | 604 | Cilenšek et al. | 2012 |

| Gene | Polymorphism | | Relation to DR (significance level) | Population | Number of patients | Author | Year |
|---|---|---|---|---|---|---|---|
| | | | ($p = 0.01$) | | | | |
| | | GSTM1null | Positive association ($p = 0.04$) | Iranian | 115 | Dadbinpour et al. | 2013 |
| | | GSTM1null GSTT1null | No significant association | Iranian | 404 | Moasser et al. | 2014 |
| | | GSTT1null | Positive association | Caucasian | 3563 (meta-analysis) | Sun et al. | 2015 |
| *GSTP1* | rs947894 | Ile105Val | No significant association | Slovenian | 604 | Cilenšek et al. | 2012 |
| | | A313G | No significant association | Egyptian | 105 | Zaki et al. | 2015 |
| *Trx* | rs4485648 | CT genotype (T9921C) TT genotype (T9921C) | Positive association ($p = 0.028$) Positive association ($p = 0.026$) | Slovenian | 953 | Mankoč Ramuš et al. | 2015 |

**Table 1.** Genes affecting oxidative stress and diabetic retinopathy.

### 5.1. Manganese superoxide dismutase (MnSOD)

SOD catalyzes the breakdown of superoxide into $H_2O_2$ scavenging superoxide, and, because of its mitochondrial localization, MnSOD is considered as the first line of defense against oxidative stress [19]. A number of polymorphisms in the mitochondrial targeting sequence of *MnSOD* have been described, but only the A16V (C47T; rs4880) evokes functional consequences [21–24]. In fact, the alanine variant of MnSOD is thought to have an $\alpha$-helical mitochondrial-targeting domain, whereas the valine variant of MnSOD appears to have a β-pleated sheet conformation. This conformational difference is thought to result in a more efficient transport of the alanine variant of MnSOD into mitochondria than the valine variant [25]. Thus, the valine variant has been associated with a 30–40% lower activity and an increased susceptibility to oxidative stress [22].

There are only a few studies indicating the association of the V16A polymorphism of the MnSOD gene with DR (**Table 1**). A meta-analysis comprising 17 studies, including type 1 and type 2 diabetic patients from different ethnic origins, implied that the C (Ala) allele of the C47T polymorphism in the MnSOD gene had a significant protective effect against microvascular complications (DR an diabetic nephropathy), although the aforementioned C allele had no significant effect on the risk for DR alone [26]. Petrovič et al. have reported that the ValVal genotype of the Val16Ala polymorphism of the MnSOD might be a risk factor for DR [27]. In contrast, Kangas-Kontio et al. [24] could not confirm such association in their study, as they found a significantly higher frequency of the AlaAla genotype in diabetics (type 1 or type 2) with DR [24]. Furthermore, a study of northern Iranian T2DM patients revealed that the heterozygosity in codon 16 of the MnSOD is considered as a risk factor for DR in T2DM [28]. However, another study from north India did not confirm an association between this SNP and DR in T2DM patients [29].

These conflicting results may be due to the ethnical differences, different genetic backgrounds, and sizes of the study populations.

### 5.2. Catalase (CAT)

CAT is a potent scavenger of $H_2O_2$ and provides a powerful antioxidant defense in the retina. It prevents the formation of the more toxic hydroxyl radical ($HO^{\bullet}$) resulting from the reaction of $H_2O_2$ and ferrous ions [30]. In structures like the eye, a significant contribution of CAT to $H_2O_2$ detoxification was reported. The inhibition of catalase activity in the rabbit eyes increased the $H_2O_2$ concentration 2.5-fold, which was not compensated for by GPx activity [31].

It has been shown that genetic variations in the *CAT* gene and its promoter may play a role in a number of diseases associated with oxidative stress (e.g., atherosclerosis, hyperlipidemia, diabetes mellitus, hypertension, and neurodegenerative diseases) [32]. Although catalase is broadly studied, to the best of our knowledge, there is only one report in which no association was observed between the −262C/T polymorphism in the promoter region of the *CAT* gene and DR in Caucasian-Brazilian T2DM patients (**Table 1**) [33].

### 5.3. Glutathione peroxidases (GPxs)

GPxs are selenocysteine-containing enzymes that catalyze the reduction of $H_2O_2$ and lipid hydroperoxides to $H_2O$ and lipid alcohols, respectively, in a reaction that utilizes reduced glutathione (GSH) as a reducing co-substrate. There are five known forms of GPx: cellular (GPx-1), gastrointestinal (GPx-2), plasma (GPx-3), phospholipid (GPx-4), and sperm (snGPx) [34]. The most abundant intracellular isoform is GPx-1; it is known as the classical or cytosolic antioxidant enzyme and is ubiquitously expressed. GPx-1 deficiency has been shown to promote endothelial dysfunction, heart failure, and abnormal structural changes in vasculature and myocardium [2,34].

GPx-1 has four SNPs that change the amino acid produced, but only one has been studied extensively in human disease [35]. This missense polymorphism changes the amino acid from proline (Pro) to leucine (Leu) at position 197 (rs1050450) and was associated with a reduction in transcription and enzyme activity of GPx-1 [36].

The GPx-1 Pro/Leu genotype has been linked to lung cancer, bladder cancer, and complications in T2DM. Studies assessing the association between GPx-1 Pro197Leu SNP genotypes and diabetes, stroke, brain tumors, and prostate cancer are inconclusive [35].

An abundance of GPx has been localized in the rabbit retina through immunohistochemistry [37]. However, to date, there has been no study to show the association between *GPx* gene polymorphisms and DR in T2DM patients (**Table 1**).

### 5.4. Glutathione S-transferases (GSTs)

The human glutathione S-transferases (GSTs) are a family of enzymes known to act in the body as a defense system for neutralizing free radicals. They play an important role in the detoxification of electrophiles by glutathione conjugation [38]. GST enzymes are coded by at least eight distinct loci: $\alpha$ (GSTA), $\mu$ (GSTM), $\theta$ (GSTT), $\pi$ (GSTP), $\sigma$ (GSTS), $k$ (GSTK), o (GSTO), and $\tau$ (GSTZ), each containing one or more homodimeric or heterodimeric isoforms. Three loci in particular, GSTM1, GSTT1, and GSTP1, have received most of the attention. The GSTM1 locus has been mapped on chromosome 1p13.3, while the GSTT1 and GSTP1 loci can be found on chromosomes 22q11.2 and 11q13. Persons with homozygous deletions of either the GSTM1 or GSTT1 loci have no enzymatic functional activity of the respective enzyme [39,40]. A GSTP1 variant with a substitution in the active site of valine for isoleucine at codon 105 (Ile105Val) has a reduced ability to conjugate reactive electrophiles with glutathione and may therefore sensitize cells to free radical-mediated damage. The Val105 variant has been associated with susceptibility to smoking-related cancer and cardiovascular disease [41].

Numerous GST polymorphisms have been associated with an increased or decreased susceptibility to several diseases [39,42–45], but only a few studies examined the association of GST polymorphisms and DR in T2DM patients (**Table 1**). Cilenšek et al. proposed a protective effect for the GSTM1-null genotype against retinopathy [46], explained by an up-regulation of other antioxidant enzymes, such as MnSOD [47]. On the contrary, the result of the aforementioned study is inconsistent with the study that showed a significant correlation between the GSTM1-null genotype and DR [38]. The study carried out by Doney et al. demonstrated that GSTT1-null individuals have a more generalized vasculopathy with an increased risk of progression of both retinopathy and nephropathy [41]. These findings are in agreement with the reports by Cilenšek et al., who recently reported that individuals homozygous for the deletion of GSTT1 are at an ≈ 2-fold-greater risk of DR [46]. There is only one report suggesting that GST allelic variants are not associated with individual susceptibility to DR [48].

Since the results of studies were conflicting and inconclusive, Sun et al. [49] performed a meta-analysis. A total of five studies were included, all of which were conducted in Caucasians; one study used T1DM patients, while other studies used T2DM patients. They reported that an increased risk of DR was associated with the null genotype of GSTT1 and GSTT1 polymorphisms, respectively [49].

As regards the GSTP1 gene polymorphism (rs947894), the domination of the G allele results in the reduction of GSTP1 enzyme activity. Consequently, the cell becomes more susceptible to mutation and damage from exposure to electrophiles and ROS [50]. Despite the significance noted in the G allele in the GSTP1 gene polymorphism among diabetic cases [51,52], two studies failed to demonstrate any significant association between the GSTP1 polymorphism and DR in T2DM patients [46,50].

### 5.5. Trx system

The Trx system is one of the central antioxidant systems in mammalian cells, maintaining a reducing environment by catalyzing electron flux from NADPH through Trx reductase to Trx, which reduces its target proteins using highly conserved thiol groups [53]. In mammals, both Trx and TrxR are expressed as dedicated isoforms for either predominantly cytosolic (Trx1 and TrxR1) or mitochondrial (Trx2 and TrxR2) localization [54].

Up-regulation of thioredoxin-interacting protein (TXNIP), an endogenous inhibitor of Trx, compromises cellular antioxidant and antiapoptotic defenses and stimulates pro-inflammatory cytokines expression [55]. Moreover, it is highly induced in the diabetic retina and plays a critical role in DR pathogenesis [56–59]. Mankoč Ramuš et al. searched for a connection between genetic variants within the mitochondrial Trx antioxidant defense system and DR (**Table 1**). The aforementioned study was the first to explore the association between seven single nucleotide polymorphisms (SNPs), including rs8140110, rs7211, rs7212, rs4755, rs1548357, rs4485648, and rs5748469, in the Trx2/TXNIP and TrxR2 genes, and the risk of DR in a case–control study of Slovenian patients with T2DM. They found an association between the rs4485648 polymorphism of the TrxR2 gene and DR in Caucasians with T2DM [60].

## 6. The role of epigenetics in the pathogenesis of diabetic retinopathy

The heritable, yet reversible changes in the gene expression that are independent of the order of the nucleotides within a gene are called epigenetic modifications. An organism's genome can be modified by naturally occurring ROS which are regularly produced as an inevitable by-product of the normal oxygen metabolism. Oxidative stress is defined as a condition associated with an aberrant increase in ROS generation in a cell.

In diabetes, oxidative stress is increased in the retina and its capillary cells and is considered as one of the major metabolic abnormalities associated with the development of DR [61–63]. Arguably, the resulting hyperglycemia-induced ROS production may also promote epigenetic alterations in DR. Fundamental epigenetic mechanisms include DNA cytosine methylation, histone post-translational modifications (PTMs) in the chromatin, and noncoding RNAs (ncRNAs), all of which can affect gene expression individually or cooperatively and modulate disease states [64].

DNA methylation is considered to be one of the most important modifications leading to disease [65]. In general, DNA methylation at 5′ cytosine of the CpG dinucleotides forms 5-methylated cytosine (5mC). The formation of 5mC in the promoter regions leads to gene

http://dx.doi.org/10.5772/63353

repression, whereas in genes bodies it might regulate transcription elongation and alternative splicing [66]. DNA methylation is brought about by DNA methyltransferases (Dnmts), and these enzymes use S-adenosyl methionine (SAM) as the methyl donor [67,68]. It is noteworthy that some studies have begun to uncover the role of DNA methylation in diabetes and its complications. In animal models, epigenetic silencing due to increased promoter DNA methylation has been linked to islet dysfunction and development of diabetes [69,70]. In a case-controlled study of 168 patients with type 2 DM, the global DNA methylation status was shown to be associated with DR. Additionally, the DNA methylation status exhibited a strong correlation with the progression of DR [71,72]. Apart from the increased activity of Dnmts in the retina and its capillary cells [73], histone-modifying machinery is also affected in diabetes.

In mammalian cells, chromosomal DNA is packed into chromatin, and chromatin is made up of subunits called nucleosomes. Each nucleosome consists of an octamer protein complex, containing two copies each of core histone proteins H2A, H2B, H3, and H4 with 147 bp of chromosomal DNA wrapped around it [74]. Despite such sophisticated DNA packaging, the N-terminal of histones remains vulnerable for PTMs and can be acetylated, methylated, and phosphorylated. Such epigenetic modifications alter the chromatin structure which subsequently affects the binding of transcription factors and can regulate the selective expression of genes in a particular tissue by acting as switches to control gene activity [75–79]. Acetylation, the most common histone modification, which is generally associated with gene activation, is regulated [80] by fine-tune between histone-acetylating and histone-deacetylating enzymes; histone acetyltransferases (HATs) add the acetyl group, while histone deacetylase (HDAC) removes the acetyl group. Histone K acetylation (Kac) is enzymatically mediated by HATs, such as p300, the CREB-binding protein (CBP), and the Tat-interactive protein 60 kDa (Tip60). In general, histone Kac (such as H3K9ac, H3K14ac, and H4K5ac) at gene promoters correlates with transcriptional activation, whereas its removal is associated with gene repression [81]. Experimental evidence using *in vitro* and *in vivo* models of DR has shown increased HDACs and decreased HAT activities and global acetylation [82]. However, Kadiyala et al. have discovered an increased histone acetylation [83]. The reason for the divergence of the published data is not yet known.

Histone methylation is the most complex modification, since its function depends on the precise methylation site and the degree of modification. Lysine residues can have up to three methylation sites, whereas arginines (R) can have up to two methylation sites [84]. Lysine methylation (Kme) is mediated by histone K methyltransferases (HMTs) and removed by K demethylases (KDMs) [85,86]. H3K4me1/2/3 and H3K36me2/3 are generally associated with transcriptionally active genome regions, whereas H3K9me3, H3K27me3, and H4K20me3 are related with repressed domains [81]. In the development of DR, superoxide levels are elevated in the retina, antioxidant defense system is compromised, MnSOD is inhibited, and mitochondria are swollen and dysfunctional [77,87–90]. Overexpression of MnSOD protects diabetes-induced mitochondrial damage and the development of DR [19,91]. Furthermore, *SOD2* is epigenetically modified with increased H4K20me3, H3K9ac, and p65 subunit of NF-kB at its promoter/enhancer [77]. Besides, Zhong and Kowluru revealed that the exposure of retinal capillary cells to high glucose decreases H3K4me at *SOD2* promoter and enhancer regions, suggesting the role of H3K4 methylation in *SOD2* repression [78]. The possible mechanism for such decrease of methylation is the activation of lysine-specific demethylase-1 (LSD1).

Apart from histone epigenetic modifications, the role of ncRNA has evoked great interest because gene expression can vary due to the function of RNA molecules themselves as well as their interactions with DNA and/or proteins [92]. NcRNAs with less than 200 nucleotides are generally classified as short (i.e., microRNAs), while all larger transcripts are regarded as long ncRNA (lncRNA). There are several subtypes of long and short ncRNA species, many of which are involved in the regulation of gene expression, and these can be further grouped according to their genomic origins and biogenic processes [92]. Specifically, increasing emphasis is being placed on the ability of miRNAs and lncRNAs to regulate gene expression and modulate the actions of growth and inflammatory factors related to diabetic complications [64]. MicroRNAs are a class of highly conserved 19–25 nucleotide single-stranded ncRNAs that regulate gene expression at the posttranscriptional level [93,94]. They block gene translation via binding to complementary regions of the mRNA. Micro-RNAs are also able to initiate the degradation of mRNA strands to which they are bound [95]. Various recent reports have demonstrated alterations in miRNA expression in diabetic eyes. Subjects with proliferative and nonproliferative DR have different serum levels of miR-21, miR-181c, and miR-1179 [96]. Downregulation of miR-200b was observed in the retina in diabetes. In parallel, VEGF (target of miR-200b) mRNA and protein were elevated [97]. It is now becoming clear that oxidative stress causes the activation of the redox-sensitive transcription factors and altered expression of a number of genes, including *VEGF*. Under diabetic conditions, it acts to increase vascular permeability in the early stages of DR and fluid accumulates in the retinal tissue, causing macular oedema and exudate [98]. Up-regulation of miR-195 is shown to downregulate deacetylase Sirtuin 1(Sirt 1) [99], and in DR, the inhibition of Sirt 1 in the retina activates NF-kB, a redox-sensitive proapoptotic factor [100]. On the other hand, up-regulation of miR-29b exerted an antiapoptotic function in the retinal ganglion cells [101]. In addition, miRNAs are stable in biological fluids, such as urine and serum [64], in this view; miRNAs appear to represent valuable noninvasive biomarkers and a promising tool of new approaches for the treatment of DR.

LncRNAs participate in a variety of biological processes, such as chromosome imprinting, epigenetic regulation, cell-cycle control, cell apoptosis, and reprogramming of induced pluripotent stem cells [102,103]. Recently, a human β-cell transcriptome analysis had indicated that lncRNAs are dynamically regulated and abnormally expressed in type 2 diabetes [104]. The field of lncRNA research in ocular diseases is expanding rapidly. Notably, lncRNAs are involved in the pathogenesis of DR through the modulation of multiple pathogenetic pathways. Metastasis-associated lung adenocarcinoma transcript 1, a conserved lncRNA, may become a potential therapeutic target for the prognosis, diagnosis, and treatment of DR [105]. The following year, Yan et al. revealed a regulatory role of the lncRNA myocardial infarction-associated transcript (MIAT) in diabetes mellitus-induced microvascular dysfunction [106].

In the pathogenesis of DR, retinal mitochondria become dysfunctional, and capillary cell apoptosis precedes the development of retinal histopathology associated with DR [107–109]. Mitochondrial homeostasis is maintained by a close cooperation between nuclear DNA and mitochondrial DNA (mtDNA) [110]. Due to the lack of supporting histones, and the close proximity to the superoxide-generating electron transport chain, mtDNA is prone to oxidative damage [111,112]. In diabetes, the activity of retinal Dnmts is increased, and the mtDNA replication enzyme, the polymerase $\gamma$-1 (*POLG1*) gene, is hypermethylated and its binding at the *D-loop* is impaired, resulting in decreased mtDNA biogenesis [73].

Lately, it is becoming apparent that small interfering RNAs ameliorated the hyperglycemia-induced decrease in mtDNA transcription and the increase in apoptosis. In fact, Mishra and Kowluru have recently discovered that modulation of Dnmt1 by pharmaceutical or molecular means could help maintain mitochondrial integrity and serve as a potential strategy to inhibit/halt the development of DR [113].

The "new antioxidant" concept represents the benefit of the consumption of fresh fruit and vegetables in diabetic patients. Research on foods of plant origin shows that they contain many non-nutritional compounds with an oxidative stress-protective effect (green tea, $\alpha$-lipoic acid, carnitine, glucosinolates, carotenoids, epigallocatechin, flavonoids, resveratrol, etc.) [100,114–118]. It has been suggested that these compounds regulate free radical over-generation at the mitochondrial level, increase intracellular defenses, and secrete and activate detoxifying enzymes [100,118]. The same principles work for the aforementioned novel compounds.

## 7. Antioxidants and diabetic retinopathy

So far, oxidative stress has been demonstrated to play an important role in the development and progression of DR; therefore antioxidants are expected to be helpful in preventing DR and its progression [100,114–118]. Lipid peroxidation (LPO) is considered to be a major harmful consequence of ROS formation, as it reflects irreversible oxidative changes of membranes. Moreover, it must be emphasized that retinal cells are highly sensitive to oxidative damage caused by the constant photochemical reactions, and the high concentrations of polyunsaturated fatty acids that constitute their membranes are directly affected by LPO.

Several antioxidants have so far been considered helpful in terms of prevention of DR and its progression; however, only a few research groups demonstrated an important effect of antioxidants in a few ocular disorders, such as in macular degeneration and in DR [119,120].

The administration of combined antioxidant therapy is helpful by improving antioxidant capacity against ROS and protecting photoreceptors against radiation. Vitamins C and E act by normalizing numerous chemical reactions to diminish aging and degeneration caused by ROS. CAT is recommended in macular degeneration [119]. Just recently an interesting study has been reported to demonstrate the effect of an adjunctive antioxidant treatment in subjects with DR [120]. Either coenzyme Q10 (400 mg/day) or combined antioxidant therapy (composed of 10 mg of lutein, 4 mg of astaxanthin, 1 mg of zeaxanthin, 180 mg of vitamin C, 30 mg of vitamin E, 20 mg of zinc, and 1 mg of copper) proved to be effective and safe for improving the oxidative stress in DR [120]. Moreover, ingestion of coenzyme Q10 and combined antioxidant therapy was significantly superior for decreasing the LPO levels, to values closer to normal, an outcome similar to that reported recently in vitreous humor [120,121].

## 8. Pespectives

Changes in dietary habits and lifestyles associated with rapid economic growth have dramatically increased the incidence of diabetes and related chronic microvascular complications, i.e., DR. So far, several studies have demonstrated the importance of several environmental, genetic, and epigenetic factors. Modulation of epigenetic changes by pharmaceutical means may provide a potential strategy to retard the progression of DR. Besides intense medical management, these strategies include dietary measures and the introduction of epigenetic drugs, such as inhibitors of DNA methylation and histone demethylases. We presume that intense medical management may be especially helpful with subjects having increased genetic risk according to the findings of genetic studies.

To conclude, the impact of nutritional factors is still insufficiently understood for patients with DR and well-designed prospective randomized clinical trials are needed to address the role of nutritional factors, including antioxidants. Genetic biomarkers (DNA and RNA gene polymorphisms) may be especially helpful in risk prediction, prognosis, or prediction of response of DR on drugs or nutritional factors. Finally, personalized medicine will most probably have an important part in managing subjects at increased risk for DR according to clinical, genetic, and epigenetic information providing that genetic tests (i.e., cost) become more widely available and that the genetic markers will be confirmed in prospective studies.

## Acknowledgements

The authors thank Mrs. Brina Beškovnik, BA, for revising the English.

## Author details

Ines Cilenšek[1], Sara Mankoč Ramuš[1], Mojca Globočnik Petrovič[2] and Daniel Petrovič[1*]

*Address all correspondence to: daniel.petrovic@mf.uni-lj.si

1 Institute of Histology and Embryology, Faculty of Medicine, University of Ljubljana, Ljubljana, Slovenia

2 University Medical Centre, Eye Clinic, Ljubljana, Slovenia

# References

[1] American Diabetes Association. Diagnosis and classification of diabetes mellitus. Diabetes Care. 2012;35(Suppl 1):S64–S71.

[2] Chen L, Magliano DJ, Zimmet PZ. The worldwide epidemiology of type 2 diabetes mellitus—present and future perspectives. Nat Rev Endocrinol. 2011; 8(4):228–36.

[3] Kowluru RA, Kowluru A, Mishra M, Kumar B. Oxidative stress and epigenetic modifications in the pathogenesis of diabetic retinopathy. Prog Retin Eye Res. 2015; 48:40–61

[4] Fong DS, Aiello L, Gardner TW, King GL, Blankenship G, Cavallerano JD, Ferris FL 3rd, Klein R; American Diabetes Association. Diabetic retinopathy. Diabetes Care. 2003; 26(1):226–9.

[5] Nwanyanwu KH, Newman-Casey PA, Gardner TW, Lim JI. Beyond HbA1c: environmental risk factors for diabetic retinopathy. J Clin Exp Ophthalmol. 2015; 6:2.

[6] Madsen-Bouterse SA, Kowluru RA. Oxidative stress and diabetic retinopathy: pathophysiological mechanisms and treatment perspectives. Rev Endocr Metab Disord. 2008; 9(4):315–27.

[7] The Diabetes Control and Complications Trial Research Group. The effect of intensive treatment of diabetes on the development and progression of long-term complications in insulin-dependent diabetes mellitus. N Engl J Med. 1993; 329:977–86.

[8] UK Prospective Diabetes Study (UKPDS) Group. Intensive blood-glucose control with sulphonylureas or insulin compared with conventional treatment and risk of complications in patients with type 2 diabetes (UKPDS 33). Lancet. 1998; 352:837–53.

[9] Brownlee M. The pathobiology of diabetic complications: a unifying mechanism. Diabetes. 2005; 54(6):1615–25.

[10] Tarr JM, Kaul K, Chopra M, Kohner EM, Chibber R. Pathophysiology of diabetic retinopathy. ISRN Ophthalmol. 2013; 2013:343560.

[11] Petrovič D. Candidate genes for proliferative diabetic retinopathy. Biomed Res Int. 2013; 2013:540416.

[12] https://www.broadinstitute.org/scientificcommunity/science/platforms/proteomics/biomarkers/.

[13] Rahal A, Kumar A, Singh V, Yadav B, Tiwari R, Chakraborty S, Dhama K. Oxidative stress, prooxidants, and antioxidants: the interplay. Biomed Res Int. 2014; 2014:761264.

[14] Gürler B, Vural H, Yilmaz N, Oguz H, Satici A, Aksoy N. The role of oxidative stress in diabetic retinopathy. Eye (Lond). 2000; 14 Pt 5:730–5.

[15] Lu J, Holmgren A. The thioredoxin antioxidant system. Free Radic Biol Med. 2014; 66:75–87.

[16] Allen RG, Tresini M. Oxidative stress and gene regulation. Free Radic Biol Med. 2000; 28(3):463–99.

[17] Du Y, Miller CM, Kern TS. Hyperglycemia increases mitochondrial superoxide in retina and retinal cells. Free Radic Biol Med. 2003; 35(11):1491–9.

[18] Jain SK, McVie R, Duett J, Herbst JJ. Erythrocyte membrane lipid peroxidation and glycosylated hemoglobin in diabetes. Diabetes. 1989; 38(12):1539–43.

[19] Kowluru RA, Atasi L, Ho YS. Role of mitochondrial superoxide dismutase in the development of diabetic retinopathy. Invest Ophthalmol Vis Sci. 2006; 47(4):1594–9.

[20] Anderson RE, Rapp LM, Wiegand RD. Lipid peroxidation and retinal degeneration. Curr Eye Res. 1984; 3:223–7.

[21] Degoul F, Sutton A, Mansouri A, Cepanec C, Degott C, Fromenty B, Beaugrand M, Valla D. Homozygosity for alanine in the mitochondrial targeting sequence of superoxide dismutase and risk for severe alcoholic liver disease. Gastroenterology. 2001;120:1468–74.

[22] AQ: Please provide volume number for Ref. [22].Shimoda-Matsubayashi S, Matsumine H, Kobayashi T, Nakagawa-Hattori Y, Shimizu Y, Mizuno Y. Structural dimorphism in the mitochondrial targeting sequence in the human manganese superoxide dismutase gene. A predictive evidence for conformational change to influence mitochondrial transport and a study of allelic association in Parkinsons disease. Biochem Biophys Res Commun. 1996; 561–5.

[23] Sutton A, Imbert A, Igoudjil A, Descatoire V, Cazanave S, Pessayre D, Degoul F. The manganese superoxide dismutase Ala16Val dimorphism modulates both mitochondrial import and mRNA stability. Pharmacogenet Genomics. 2005; 15:311–19.

[24] Kangas-Kontio T, Vavuli S, Kakko SJ, Penna J, Savolainen ER, Savolainen MJ, Liinamaa MJ. Polymorphism of the manganese superoxide dismutase gene but not of vascular endothelial growth factor gene is a risk factor for diabetic retinopathy. Br J Ophthalmol. 2009; 93(10):1401–6.

[25] Fujimoto H, Taguchi J, Imai Y, Ayabe S, Hashimoto H, Kobayashi H, Ogasawara K, Aizawa T, Yamakado M, Nagai R, Ohno M. Manganese superoxide dismutase polymorphism affects the oxidized low-density lipoprotein-induced apoptosis of macrophages and coronary artery disease. Eur Heart J. 2008; (10):1267–74.

[26] Tian C, Liu T, Fang S, Du X, Jia C. Association of C47T polymorphism in SOD2 gene with coronary artery disease: a case–control study and a meta-analysis. Mol Biol Rep. 2012; 39(5):5269–76.

[27] Petrovic MG, Cilensek I, Petrovic D. Manganese superoxide dismutase gene polymorphism (V16A) is associated with diabetic retinopathy in Slovene (Caucasians) type 2 diabetes patients. Dis Markers. 2008; 24(1):59–64.

[28] Haghighi SF, Salehi Z, Sabouri MR, Abbasi N. Polymorphic variant of MnSOD A16V and risk of diabetic retinopathy. Mol Biol (Mosk). 2015; 49(1):114–8.

[29] Vanita V. Association of RAGE (p.Gly82Ser) and MnSOD (p.Val16Ala) polymorphisms with diabetic retinopathy in T2DM patients from north India. Diabetes Res Clin Pract. 2014; 104(1):155–62.

[30] Chen B, Tang L. Protective effects of catalase on retinal ischemia/reperfusion injury in rats. Exp Eye Res. 2011; 93(5):599–606.

[31] Ohta Y, Yamasaki T, Niwa T, Niimi K, Majima Y, Ishiguro I. Role of catalase in retinal antioxidant defence system: its comparative study among rabbits, guinea pigs, and rats. Ophthalmic Res. 1996; 28(6):336–42.

[32] Kodydková J, Vávrová L, Kocík M, Žák A. Human catalase, its polymorphisms, regulation and changes of its activity in different diseases. Folia Biol (Praha). 2014; 60(4): 153–67.

[33] dos Santos KG, Canani LH, Gross JL, Tschiedel B, Souto KE, Roisenberg I. The catalase −262C/T promoter polymorphism and diabetic complications in Caucasians with type 2 diabetes. Dis Markers. 2006; 22(5–6):355–9.

[34] Banerjee M, Vats P. Reactive metabolites and antioxidant gene polymorphisms in Type 2 diabetes mellitus. Indian J Hum Genet. 2014; 20(1):10–9.

[35] Crawford A, Fassett RG, Geraghty DP, Kunde DA, Ball MJ, Robertson IK, Coombes JS. Relationships between single nucleotide polymorphisms of antioxidant enzymes and disease. Gene. 2012; 501(2):89–103.

[36] Matsuno S, Sasaki H, Yamasaki, Yamaoka H, Ogawa K, Nakatani M, Hamanishi T, Doi A, Nakano Y, Wakasaki H, Furuta H, Nishi M, Akamizu T, Nanjo K. Pro198Leu missense polymorphism of the glutathione peroxidase 1 gene might be a common genetic predisposition of distal symmetric polyneuropathy and macrovascular disease in Japanese type 2 diabetic patients. J Diabetes Investig. 2011; 2(6):474-82.

[37] Atalla LR, Sevanian A, Rao NA. Immunohistochemical localization of peroxidative enzymes in ocular tissue. CLAO J. 1990; 16(1 Suppl):S30–3.

[38] Dadbinpour A, Sheikhha MH, Darbouy M, Afkhami-Ardekani M. Investigating GSTT1 and GSTM1 null genotype as the risk factor of diabetes type 2 retinopathy. J Diabetes Metab Disord. 2013; 12(1):48.

[39] Mo Z, Gao Y, Cao Y, Gao F, Jian L. An updating meta-analysis of the GSTM1, GSTT1, and GSTP1 polymorphisms and prostate cancer: a HuGE review. Prostate. 2009; 69(6): 662–88.

[40] Pemble S, Schroeder KR, Spencer SR, Meyer DJ, Hallier E, Bolt HM, Ketterer B, Taylor JB. Human glutathione S-transferase theta (GSTT1): cDNA cloning and the characterization of a genetic polymorphism. Biochem J. 1994; 300 (Pt 1):271–6.

[41] Doney AS, Lee S, Leese GP, Morris AD, Palmer CN. Increased cardiovascular morbidity and mortality in type 2 diabetes is associated with the glutathione S transferase theta-null genotype: a Go-DARTS study. Circulation. 2005; 111(22):2927–34.

[42] Stoian A, Bănescu C, Bălaşa RI, Moţăţăianu A, Stoian M, Moldovan VG, Voidăzan S, Dobreanu M. Influence of GSTM1, GSTT1, and GSTP1 polymorphisms on type 2 diabetes mellitus and diabetic sensorimotor peripheral neuropathy risk. Dis Markers. 2015; 2015:638693.

[43] Petrovič D, Peterlin B. GSTM1-null and GSTT1-null genotypes are associated with essential arterial hypertension in patients with type 2 diabetes. Clin Biochem. 2014; 47(7–8):574–7.

[44] Safarinejad MR, Safarinejad S, Shafiei N, Safarinejad S. Association of genetic polymorphism of glutathione S-transferase (GSTM1, GSTT1, GSTP1) with bladder cancer susceptibility. Urol Oncol. 2013; 31(7):1193–203.

[45] Boccia S, La Torre G, Gianfagna F, Mannocci A, Ricciardi G. Glutathione S-transferase T1 status and gastric cancer risk: a meta-analysis of the literature. Mutagenesis. 2006; 21(2):115–23.

[46] Cilenšek I, Mankoč S, Petrovič MG, Petrovič D. GSTT1 null genotype is a risk factor for diabetic retinopathy in Caucasians with type 2 diabetes, whereas GSTM1 null genotype might confer protection against retinopathy. Dis Markers. 2012; 32(2):93–9.

[47] Otto-Knapp R, Jurgovsky K, Schierhorn K, Kunkel G. Antioxidative enzymes in human nasal mucosa after exposure to ozone. Possible role of GSTM1 deficiency. Inflamm Res. 2003; 52(2):51–5.

[48] Moasser E, Azarpira N, Shirazi B, Saadat M, Geramizadeh B. Genetic polymorphisms of glutathione-S-transferase M1 and T1 genes with risk of diabetic retinopathy in Iranian population. Iran J Basic Med Sci. 2014; 17(5):351–6.

[49] Sun L, Zhang Y, Xiong Y. GSTM1 and GSTT1 null genotype and diabetic retinopathy: a meta-analysis. Int J Clin Exp Med. 2015; 8(2):1677–83.

[50] Zaki MA, Moghazy TF, El-Deeb MMK, Mohamed AH, Mohamed NAA. Glutathione S-transferase M1, T1 and P1 gene polymorphisms and the risk of developing type 2 diabetes mellitus in Egyptian diabetic patients with and without diabetic vascular complications. Alexandria J Med. 2015; 51(1):73–82.

[51] Bid HK, Konwar R, Saxena M, Chaudhari P, Agrawal CG, Banerjee M. Association of glutathione S-transferase (GSTM1, T1 and P1) gene polymorphisms with type 2 diabetes mellitus in north Indian population. J Postgrad Med. 2010; 56(3):176–81.

[52] Amer MA, Ghattas MH, Abo-Elmatty DM, Abou-El-Ela SH. Evaluation of glutathione S-transferase P1 genetic variants affecting type-2 diabetes susceptibility and glycemic control. Arch Med Sci. 2012; 8(4):631–6.

[53] Lee S, Kim SM, Lee RT. Thioredoxin and thioredoxin target proteins: from molecular mechanisms to functional significance. Antioxid Redox Signal. 2013; 18(10):1165–207.

[54] Arnér ES, Holmgren A. The thioredoxin system in cancer. Semin Cancer Biol. 2006; 16(6):420–6.

[55] Al-Gayyar MM, Abdelsaid MA, Matragoon S, Pillai BA, El-Remessy AB. Thioredoxin interacting protein is a novel mediator of retinal inflammation and neurotoxicity. Br J Pharmacol. 2011; 164(1):170–80.

[56] Devi TS, Lee I, Hüttemann M, Kumar A, Nantwi KD, Singh LP. TXNIP links innate host defense mechanisms to oxidative stress and inflammation in retinal Muller glia under chronic hyperglycemia: implications for diabetic retinopathy. Exp Diabetes Res. 2012; 2012:438238.

[57] Devi TS, Hosoya K, Terasaki T, Singh LP. Critical role of TXNIP in oxidative stress, DNA damage and retinal pericyte apoptosis under high glucose: implications for diabetic retinopathy. Exp Cell Res. 2013; 319(7):1001–12.

[58] Perrone L, Devi TS, Hosoya K, Terasaki T, Singh LP. Thioredoxin interacting protein (TXNIP) induces inflammation through chromatin modification in retinal capillary endothelial cells under diabetic conditions. J Cell Physiol. 2009; 221(1):262–72.

[59] Perrone L, Devi TS, Hosoya KI, Terasaki T, Singh LP. Inhibition of TXNIP expression in vivo blocks early pathologies of diabetic retinopathy. Cell Death Dis. 2010; 1:e65.

[60] Ramus SM, Cilensek I, Petrovic MG, Soucek M, Kruzliak P, Petrovic D. Single nucleotide polymorphisms in the Trx2/TXNIP and TrxR2 genes of the mitochondrial thioredoxin antioxidant system and the risk of diabetic retinopathy in patients with Type 2 diabetes mellitus. J Diabetes Complications. 2015; pii: S1056-8727(15)00459-6.

[61] Kowluru RA. Effect of reinstitution of good glycemic control on retinal oxidative stress and nitrative stress in diabetic rats. Diabetes. 2003; 52(3):818–23.

[62] Kowluru RA, Engerman RL, Kern TS. Abnormalities of retinal metabolism in diabetes or experimental galactosemia. VI. Comparison of retinal and cerebral cortex metabolism, and effects of antioxidant therapy. Free Radic Biol Med. 1999; 26(3–4):371–8.

[63] Kowluru RA, Tang J, Kern TS. Abnormalities of retinal metabolism in diabetes and experimental galactosemia. VII. Effect of long-term administration of antioxidants on the development of retinopathy. Diabetes. 2001; 50(8):1938–42.

[64] Kato M, Natarajan R. Diabetic nephropathy—emerging epigenetic mechanisms. Nat Rev Nephrol. 2014; 10(9):517–30.

[65] Rasool M, Malik A, Naseer MI, Manan A, Ansari S, Begum I, Qazi MH, Pushparaj P, Abuzenadah AM, Al-Qahtani MH, Kamal MA, Gan S. The role of epigenetics in

personalized medicine: challenges and opportunities. BMC Med Genomics. 2015; 8 (Suppl 1):S5.

[66] Jones PA. Functions of DNA methylation: islands, start sites, gene bodies and beyond. Nat Rev Genet. 2012; 13(7):484–92.

[67] Deaton AM, Bird A. CpG islands and the regulation of transcription. Genes Dev. 2011; 25(10):1010–22.

[68] Majumdar S, Buckles E, Estrada J, Koochekpour S. Aberrant DNA methylation and prostate cancer. Curr Genomics. 2011; 12(7):486–505.

[69] Ling C, Del Guerra S, Lupi R, Rönn T, Granhall C, Luthman H, Masiello P,Marchetti P, Groop L, Del Prato S. Epigenetic regulation of PPARGC1A in human type 2 diabetic islets and effect on insulin secretion. Diabetologia. 2008; 51(4):615–22.

[70] Park JH, Stoffers DA, Nicholls RD, Simmons RA. Development of type 2 diabetes following intrauterine growth retardation in rats is associated with progressive epigenetic silencing of Pdx1. J Clin Invest. 2008; 118(6):2316–24.

[71] Maghbooli Z, Larijani B, Emamgholipour S, Amini M, Keshtkar A, Pasalar P. Aberrant DNA methylation patterns in diabetic nephropathy. J Diabetes Metab Disord. 2014; 13:69.

[72] Maghbooli Z, Hossein-nezhad A, Larijani B, Amini M, Keshtkar A. Global DNA methylation as a possible biomarker for diabetic retinopathy. Diabetes Metab Res Rev. 2015; 31(2):183–9.

[73] Tewari S, Zhong Q, Santos JM, Kowluru RA. Mitochondria DNA replication and DNA methylation in the metabolic memory associated with continued progression of diabetic retinopathy. Invest Ophthalmol Vis Sci. 2012; 53(8):4881–8.

[74] Luger K, Mäder AW, Richmond RK, Sargent DF, Richmond TJ. Crystal structure of the nucleosome core particle at 2.8 A resolution. Nature. 1997; 389(6648):251–60.

[75] Berger SL. The complex language of chromatin regulation during transcription. Nature. 2007; 447(7143):407–12.

[76] Vaissière T, Sawan C, Herceg Z. Epigenetic interplay between histone modifications and DNA methylation in gene silencing. Mutat Res. 2008; 659(1–2):40–8.

[77] Zhong Q, Kowluru RA. Epigenetic changes in mitochondrial superoxide dismutase in the retina and the development of diabetic retinopathy. Diabetes. 2011; 60(4):1304–13.

[78] Zhong Q, Kowluru RA. Epigenetic modification of Sod2 in the development of diabetic retinopathy and in the metabolic memory: role of histone methylation. Invest Ophthalmol Vis Sci. 2013; 54(1):244–50.

[79] Zhong Q, Kowluru RA. Regulation of matrix metalloproteinase-9 by epigenetic modifications and the development of diabetic retinopathy. Diabetes. 2013; 62(7):2559–68.

[80] Glozak MA, Seto E. Histone deacetylases and cancer. Oncogene. 2007; 26(37):5420–32.

[81] Kouzarides T. Chromatin modifications and their function. Cell. 2007; 128(4):693–705.

[82] Zhong Q, Kowluru RA. Role of histone acetylation in the development of diabetic retinopathy and the metabolic memory phenomenon. J Cell Biochem. 2010; 110(6): 1306–13.

[83] Kadiyala CS, Zheng L, Du Y, Yohannes E, Kao HY, Miyagi M, Kern TS. Acetylation of retinal histones in diabetes increases inflammatory proteins: effects of minocycline and manipulation of histone acetyltransferase (HAT) and histone deacetylase (HDAC). J Biol Chem. 2012; 287(31):25869–80.

[84] Izzo A, Schneider R. Chatting histone modifications in mammals. Brief Funct Genomics. 2010; 9(5–6):429–43.

[85] Klose RJ, Zhang Y. Regulation of histone methylation by demethylimination and demethylation. Nat Rev Mol Cell Biol. 2007; 8(4):307–18.

[86] Zhou VW, Goren A, Bernstein BE. Charting histone modifications and the functional organization of mammalian genomes. Nat Rev Genet. 2011; 12(1):7–18.

[87] Kowluru RA, Abbas SN. Diabetes-induced mitochondrial dysfunction in the retina. Invest Ophthalmol Vis Sci. 2003; 44(12):5327–34.

[88] Kowluru RA, Kowluru V, Xiong Y, Ho YS. Overexpression of mitochondrial superoxide dismutase in mice protects the retina from diabetes-induced oxidative stress. Free Radic Biol Med. 2006; 41(8):1191–6.

[89] Madsen-Bouterse SA, Mohammad G, Kanwar M, Kowluru RA. Role of mitochondrial DNA damage in the development of diabetic retinopathy, and the metabolic memory phenomenon associated with its progression. Antioxid Redox Signal. 2010; 13(6):797–805.

[90] Zhong Q, Kowluru RA. Diabetic retinopathy and damage to mitochondrial structure and transport machinery. Invest Ophthalmol Vis Sci. 2011; 52(12):8739–46.

[91] Kanwar M, Chan PS, Kern TS, Kowluru RA. Oxidative damage in the retinal mitochondria of diabetic mice: possible protection by superoxide dismutase. Invest Ophthalmol Vis Sci. 2007; 48(8):3805–11.

[92] Peschansky VJ, Wahlestedt C. Non-coding RNAs as direct and indirect modulators of epigenetic regulation. Epigenetics. 2014; 9(1):3–12.

[93] Bartel DP. MicroRNAs: genomics, biogenesis, mechanism, and function. Cell. 2004; 116(2):281–97.

[94] Plasterk RH. Micro RNAs in animal development. Cell. 2006; 124(5):877–81.

[95] Wutz A. RNA-mediated silencing mechanisms in mammalian cells. Prog Mol Biol Transl Sci. 2011; 101:351–76.

[96] Qing S, Yuan S, Yun C, Hui H, Mao P, Wen F, Ding Y, Liu Q. Serum miRNA biomarkers serve as a fingerprint for proliferative diabetic retinopathy. Cell Physiol Biochem. 2014; 34(5):1733–40.

[97] McArthur K, Feng B, Wu Y, Chen S, Chakrabarti S. MicroRNA-200b regulates vascular endothelial growth factor-mediated alterations in diabetic retinopathy. Diabetes. 2011; 60(4):1314–23.

[98] Cukiernik M, Hileeto D, Evans T, Mukherjee S, Downey D, Chakrabarti S. Vascular endothelial growth factor in diabetes induced early retinal abnormalities. Diabetes Res Clin Pract. 2004; 65(3):197–208.

[99] Chen Z, Shentu TP, Wen L, Johnson DA, Shyy JY. Regulation of SIRT1 by oxidative stress-responsive miRNAs and a systematic approach to identify its role in the endothelium. Antioxid Redox Signal. 2013; 19(13):1522–38.

[100] Kowluru RA, Santos JM, Zhong Q. Sirt1, a negative regulator of matrix metalloproteinase-9 in diabetic retinopathy. Invest Ophthalmol Vis Sci. 2014; 55(9):5653–60.

[101] Silva VA, Polesskaya A, Sousa TA, Corrêa VM, André ND, Reis RI, Kettelhut IC, Harel-Bellan A, De Lucca FL. Expression and cellular localization of microRNA-29b and RAX, an activator of the RNA-dependent protein kinase (PKR), in the retina of streptozotocin-induced diabetic rats. Mol Vis. 2011; 17:2228–40.

[102] Mercer TR, Dinger ME, Mattick JS. Long non-coding RNAs: insights into functions. Nat Rev Genet. 2009; 10(3):155–9.

[103] Wapinski O, Chang HY. Long noncoding RNAs and human disease. Trends Cell Biol. 2011; 21(6):354–61.

[104] Morán I, Akerman I, van de Bunt M, Xie R, Benazra M, Nammo T, Arnes L, Nakić N, García-Hurtado J, Rodríguez-Seguí S, Pasquali L, Sauty-Colace C, Beucher A, Scharfmann R, van Arensbergen J, Johnson PR, Berry A, Lee C, Harkins T, Gmyr V, Pattou F, Kerr-Conte J, Piemonti L, Berney T, Hanley N, Gloyn AL, Sussel L, Langman L, Brayman KL, Sander M, McCarthy MI, Ravassard P, Ferrer J. Human β cell transcriptome analysis uncovers lncRNAs that are tissue-specific, dynamically regulated, and abnormally expressed in type 2 diabetes. Cell Metab. 2012; 16(4):435–48.

[105] Yan B, Tao ZF, Li XM, Zhang H, Yao J, Jiang Q. Aberrant expression of long noncoding RNAs in early diabetic retinopathy. Invest Ophthalmol Vis Sci. 2014; 55(2):941–51.

[106] Yan B, Yao J, Liu JY, Li XM, Wang XQ, Li YJ, Tao ZF, Song YC, Chen Q, Jiang Q. lncRNA-MIAT regulates microvascular dysfunction by functioning as a competing endogenous RNA. Circ Res. 2015; 116(7):1143–56.

[107] Kern TS, Tang J, Mizutani M, Kowluru RA, Nagaraj RH, Romeo G, Podesta F, Lorenzi M. Response of capillary cell death to aminoguanidine predicts the development of retinopathy: comparison of diabetes and galactosemia. Invest Ophthalmol Vis Sci. 2000; 41(12):3972–8.

[108] Kowluru RA. Mitochondria damage in the pathogenesis of diabetic retinopathy and in the metabolic memory associated with its continued progression. Curr Med Chem. 2013; 20(26):3226–33.

[109] Kowluru RA, Chan PS. Metabolic memory in diabetes—from in vitro oddity to in vivo problem: role of apoptosis. Brain Res Bull. 2010; 81(2–3):297–302.

[110] Scarpulla RC. Nucleus-encoded regulators of mitochondrial function: integration of respiratory chain expression, nutrient sensing and metabolic stress. Biochim Biophys Acta. 2012; 1819(9–10):1088–97.

[111] Alexeyev M, Shokolenko I, Wilson G, LeDoux S. The maintenance of mitochondrial DNA integrity—critical analysis and update. Cold Spring Harb Perspect Biol. 2013; 5(5):a012641.

[112] Shokolenko I, Venediktova N, Bochkareva A, Wilson GL, Alexeyev MF. Oxidative stress induces degradation of mitochondrial DNA. Nucleic Acids Res. 2009; 37(8):2539–48.

[113] Mishra M, Kowluru RA. Epigenetic modification of mitochondrial DNA in the development of diabetic retinopathy. Invest Ophthalmol Vis Sci. 2015; 56(9):5133–42.

[114] Cao Y, Cao R. Angiogenesis inhibited by drinking tea. Nature. 1999;398(6726):381.

[115] Chan CM, Chang HH, Wang VC, Huang CL, Hung CF. Inhibitory effects of resveratrol on PDGF-BB-induced retinal pigment epithelial cell migration via PDGFRβ, PI3K/Akt and MAPK pathways. PLoS One. 2013; 8(2):e56819.

[116] Alqahtani A, Hamid K, Kam A, Wong KH, Abdelhak Z, Razmovski-Naumovski V, Chan K, Li KM, Groundwater PW, Li GQ. The pentacyclic triterpenoids in herbal medicines and their pharmacological activities in diabetes and diabetic complications. Curr Med Chem. 2013; 20(7):908–31.

[117] Please provide the volume number and page range for Ref. [117].Zeng K, Yang N, Wang D, Li S, Ming J, Wang J, Yu X, Song Y, Zhou X, Yang Y. Resveratrol prevents retinal dysfunction by regulating glutamate transporters, glutamine synthetase expression and activity in diabetic retina. Neurochem Res. 2015 Dec 16 [Epub ahead of print].

[118] Ulker E, Parker WH, Raj A, Qu ZC, May JM. Ascorbic acid prevents VEGF-induced increases in endothelial barrier permeability. Mol Cell Biochem. 2016; 412(1–2):73–9.

[119] Parisi V, Tedeschi M, Gallinaro G, Varano M, Saviano S, Piermarocchi S, CARMIS Study Group. Carotenoids and anti- oxidants in age-related maculopathy Italian study:

multifocal electroretinogram modifications after 1 year. Ophthalmology. 2008; 115(2): 324–33.

[120] Rodríguez-Carrizalez AD, Castellanos-González JA, Martínez-Romero EC, Miller-Arrevillaga G, Pacheco-Moisés FP, Román-Pintos LM, Miranda-Díaz AG. The effect of ubiquinone and combined antioxidant therapy on oxidative stress markers in non-proliferative diabetic retinopathy: a phase IIa, randomized, double-blind, and placebo-controlled study. Redox Rep. 2015 Aug 31 [Epub ahead of print].

[121] Mancino R, Di Pierro D, Varesi C, Cerulli A, Feraco A, Cedrone C, et al. Lipid peroxidation and total antioxidant capacity in vitreous, aqueous humor, and blood samples from patients with diabetic retinopathy. Mol Vis. 2011; 17:1298–304.

Chapter 5

# Novel Biomarkers to Understand Cardiovascular Complications in Diabetes

Ramu Adela and Sanjay K. Banerjee

Additional information is available at the end of the chapter

http://dx.doi.org/10.5772/62595

**Abstract**

Diabetic subjects have shown two- to fourfold increased risk of cardiovascular diseases (CVDs) than without diabetes. Diabetes can be prevented if detected early at prediabetes stage. Progression of diabetes not only causes hyperglycaemia; it also increased the risk of macrovascular and microvascular complications. Different mechanisms, i.e. inflammation, abnormal adipocyte signalling, insulin resistance, endothelial dysfunction, and oxidative stress, are involved in the progression of diabetes and associated cardiovascular complication. These mechanisms alter different signalling molecules in blood and other body fluids. These altered molecules offer potential biomarkers for the identification and early detection of the disease progression. If we are able to detect the early biomarkers based on the alteration of different mediators responsible for cardiac complications in diabetes, we can prevent the cardiac diseases in diabetes by selective therapy. Different kinds of biomarkers, i.e. miRNA, protein, metabolites, cytokines, and adipokines, can be used together to detect the different stages of the disease. In the present book chapter, we are explaining briefly about characteristics of biomarkers and their applications and different approaches that were used to identify biomarkers. Different existing and novel biomarkers and their scope to detect patients with prediabetes, diabetes and cardiovascular complication in diabetes have been discussed.

**Keywords:** type 2 diabetes, biomarkers, cardiovascular diseases, metabolic syndrome, coronary artery diseases

## 1. Introduction

A biomarker is defined as "any substance, structure, or process that can be measured in the body or its products and influence or predict the incidence of outcome or disease" [1]. Research interest on biomarkers has increased in recent years. In MedLine search in 1990, there were only 21 hits on cardiovascular risk markers, while by 2010, it is increased to 2032 hits, thus indicating huge increase in number of publications in biomarkers in the last decade [2]. There were 37% more biomarker studies in 2014 as compared to 2013 [3]. However, only few biomarkers are routinely used in clinical practice. For example, fasting blood sugar, glycated haemoglobin, cardiac troponin T (cTnT), cardiac troponin I (cTnI), and B-type natriuretic peptide (BNP) are used regularly for diabetes, myocardial infarction, and heart failure. Biomarkers should have specific characteristics, i.e. specific to the particular diseases and easily detectable. Biomarker can be predictive to identify disease progression after treatment. The detection method should be fast, simple, and low cost. It should be stable at any time of the day and samples should be available easily by invasive method (blood and urine). Identified biomarker should be proven of its importance preclinically and clinically. Biomarker can be used for different purposes such as the early detection of disease, evaluation of acute and chronic clinical condition, risk stratification of patients to suspect or confirm the diagnosis, selection of appropriate therapeutic treatment, and observation of patient response for the treatment (**Figure 1**) [4]. Identification of early biomarkers for noncommunicable chronic diseases such as diabetes is very important for finding appropriate therapeutic strategy.

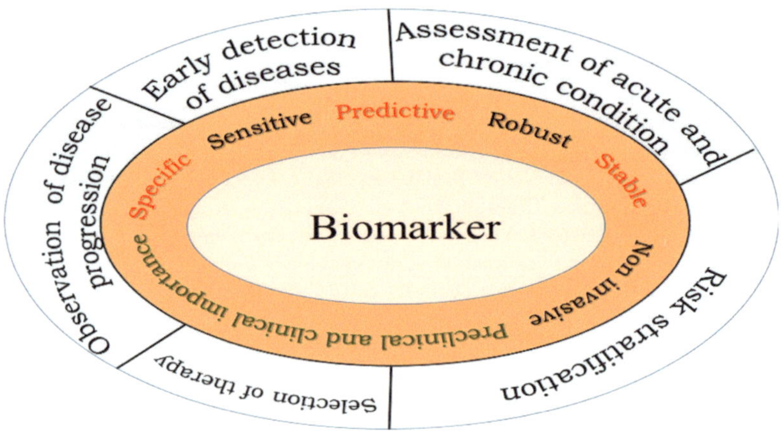


**Figure 1.** Biomarker characteristics (inner circle) and applications (outer circle).

Prevalence of diabetes is reaching epidemic proportions in developed and developing nations due to increase in life expectancy, sedentary lifestyle, and obesity. As per the International Diabetic Federation (IDF) Diabetes Atlas (Sixth Edition 2013), the number of people with diabetes is 382 million and it is going to rise to 592 million by 2035. Global burden of diabetes is huge and 548 billion dollars was spent in 2013. In India, approximately 65.1 million people are with diabetes. Cardiovascular diseases (CVDs) are the major complications of diabetes. The prevalence, incidence, and mortality of cardiovascular diseases are two- to fourfold higher in persons having diabetes than those without diabetes [5]. Prediction of cardiovascular disease (CVD) risk among people with diabetes is important not only to give better clinical therapy but also to distinguish higher risk patients for extra care. Biomarkers may help in early detection of diseases, distinguishing patients based on disease severity, and find the cardiovascular risk among diabetic patients.

### 1.1. Diabetes and its cardiovascular complications

Diabetes is characterised by high glucose level in blood due to either less insulin secretion from pancreas or developing insulin resistance in skeletal muscle. Type 2 diabetes (T2DM) is the commonest form and it is characterised by insulin resistance mostly in skeletal muscle and deficiency of insulin release at end stage. In general, T2DM causes elevation of blood glucose level and other components of metabolic syndrome. Parameters of metabolic syndrome are elevated blood pressure, increased triglycerides, reduced high density lipoprotein levels, and abdominal obesity [5]. In obese condition, increased adipocytes secrete adipocytokines. Released adipocytokines integrate the endocrine, autocrine, and paracrine signals to mediate the insulin sensitivity, oxidative stress, energy metabolism, blood coagulation, and inflammatory responses. Elevated levels of free fatty acids (FFAs) induce insulin resistance and increase fibrinogen and plasminogen activator inhibitor-1 (PAI-1). In the long run, high FFA and glucose together impair beta-cell function through lipotoxicity and glucotoxicity and develop macro- and microvascular complications [6,7].

Diabetes and cardiovascular diseases are involved in different abnormalities in genes, proteins, metabolites, and lipids by different mechanisms such as oxidative stress, inflammation, and endothelial dysfunction. Identification of highly sensitive and specific potential biomarkers would be beneficial for the detection of cardiovascular diseases risk among diabetic patients with different advanced omics approaches such as genomics (genes), metabolomics (metabolites), proteomics (proteins), transcriptomics (mRNA), and lipidomics (lipids) (**Figure 2**). These

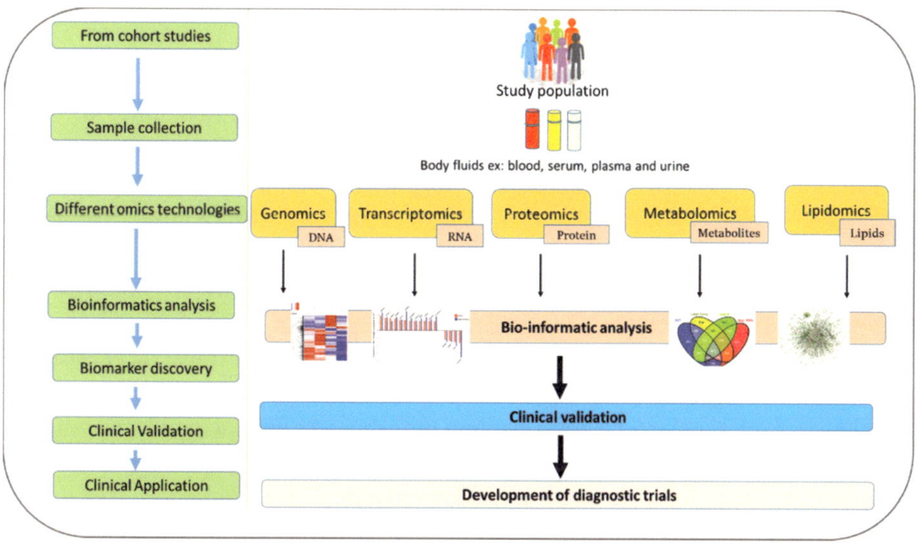


**Figure 2.** Development of biomarkers with the help of different omics approaches.

new techniques are useful for simultaneous investigation of multiple molecules and to identify different kinds of biomarkers (**Table 1**).

| Different omics approaches | Study of different molecules | Technology used |
|---|---|---|
| Genomics | DNA | DNA microarray<br>Single nucleotide polymorphism<br>Hot spot mutation<br>Epigenomics |
| Transcriptomics | mRNA<br>tRNA<br>rRNA<br>Noncoding RNA | RNA microarray<br>New-generation sequencing (NGS)<br>Exome sequencing |
| Proteomics | Proteins and their abundance, variation, modific ations, and interactions | 2D-PAGE<br>Protein microarray<br>Mass spectrometry<br>MALDI-TOF-MS<br>ESI-MS |
| Metabo lomics | Metabolites | NMR<br>Mass spectrometry–LC–MS |
| Lipi domics | Lipids | Mass spectrometry–LC–MS/MS |

**Table 1.** Omics approaches target for different molecules.

## 2. Different omics approaches used for the identification of biomarkers

(*i*) *Genomics* is a systematic study of structure, function, and expression of organism's genome. This involves DNA sequencing, assembly, as well as analysis of an annotation of structure and function of the gene. The single nucleotide polymorphism array (SNP array) is a type of DNA microarray that can be used to detect polymorphisms within the whole genome. Next-generation sequencing (NGS) has gained considerable attention for investigations at the nucleotide levels including both DNA and RNA sequences. (*ii*) *Transcriptomics* is a study of total set of RNA including mRNA, tRNA, rRNA, and microRNA. Single gene was analysed by single-gene detection method individually, and thousands of gene expression are analysed simultaneously by high-throughput analysis such as DNA microarrays. (*iii*) *Proteomics* is a study of all expressed proteins and it gives information about protein abundance, variation, modification, and interaction through signalling pathway and network analysis. Initially two-dimensional polyacrylamide gel electrophoresis (2D-PAGE) technique was used to determine whole protein expression. In this method we can separate a large number of protein mixture based on molecular weight and isoelectric point. This technique has initially been used to find global changes of protein expression. However, recently mass spectrophotometer has been used to identify protein alterations. Mass spectrometry has been utilised to separate ions from proteins, peptides, or metabolites according to their mass-to-charge ratio (*m/z*) and to provide data as mass spectrum that can be further analysed to determine characteristics of molecular mass and structure. However, proteomics studies are more complicated due to presence of high-abundant proteins such as albumin and immunoglobulins (serum) that may mask the important biomarker candidates. To overcome this problem, different depletion columns are available for removing high-abundant proteins and immunoglobulins. With mass spectrometry the two types of approaches were targeted (preselected panel of proteins) and untargeted (without any assumptions total proteins are captured). Protein microarray has also been developed to detect thousands of proteins based on specific antibody detection. (*iv*) *Metabolomics* is a systemic approach to evaluate the metabolic profile, which can be useful in biomarker discovery. Metabolites are usually considered as good biomarkers due their stability. Metabolome analysis can be performed using a variety of techniques such as nuclear magnetic resonance (NMR) as well as mass spectrometry. Metabolites were also studied in two ways as same as proteomics, i.e. targeted and untargeted [8]. (*v*) *Lipidomics* is systemic approach to study large-scale changes in lipids and understand the regulation of lipid metabolism. This will be analysed with the help of LC–MS/MS. These omics approaches offer simultaneous estimation of different molecules through high-throughput screening. After identification of set of proteins/genes/metabolites/lipids by omics approach, there is a need for validation of each marker by other methods. **Table 2** shows a list of biomarkers identified by different omics approaches.

| Diseases | Study name | Approach | Sample type | No. of patients | Biomarkers identified | Reference |
|---|---|---|---|---|---|---|
| Prediabetes | KORA | Metabo lomics | Serum | 4297 | Three metabolites (glycine, lysoph osphatid', and acetylcarnitine) that altered significant levels in impaired glucose tolerance (IGT) as compared with normal glucose tolerance | [98] |
| Type 2 diabetes | – | Prote omics (2D-LC–MS/MS) | Saliva | 40 (10 control, 10 I FG, 10 IGT, 10 T2DM patients) | 487 biomarkers identified | [99] |
| T2DM | Frami ngham Off spring | Metabo lomics | Plasma | Rando mly se lected | Out of 70 metabolites 2-AAA (2-amino adipic acid) had the | [100] |

| Diseases | Study name | Approach | Sample type | No. of patients | Biomarkers identified | Reference |
|---|---|---|---|---|---|---|
| | Study | | | 1561 ind ividuals | strongest association with risk of future diabetes mellitus | |
| Cardio vascular diseases | Bruneck study | Lipi domics | Plasma | 685 subj ects with 10-year observ ation period | Cholesterol esters (CEs) , lysophosphatidylcholines, phosphatidylcholines, phosphatidylethanolamines (PEs), sphingomyelins, and triacylglycerols (TAGs) were associated with cardiovascular disease | [101] |
| Obesity and insulin resistance | The Western Australian Pregnancy Cohort (Raine) Study | Lipi domics | Plasma | 1126 patients with 20-year follow-up | Sphingomyelins, particularly those with two double bonds, and lysophosphatidylcholines were identified between subjects with normal weight and obesity independent of LDL-C and HDL-C concentrations | [102] |
| Cardiov ascular diseases | National Finnish FINRISK study, SABRE study, and BWHH Study | Metabo lomics | Serum | FINRISK ($n$ = 7256; 800 events), SABRE ($n$ = 2622; 573 events), and British Women's ($n$ = 3563; 368 events) | Higher phenylalanine and monounsaturated fatty acid levels were associated with increased cardiovascular risk, while higher omega-6 fatty acids and docos ahexaenoic acid levels were associated with lower risk | [103] |
| Cardiova scular dis eases | – | Metabo lomics | Plasma | 2023 consecutive patients undergoing cardiac catheter isation | Five metabolite factors were independently associated with mortality: factor 1 (medium-chain acylcarnitines, short-chain dic arboxylacylcarnitines, | [104] |

http://dx.doi.org/10.5772/62595

| Diseases | Study name | Approach | Sample type | No. of patients | Biomarkers identified | Reference |
|---|---|---|---|---|---|---|
| | | | | | long-chain dicarboxylacyl carnitines), factor 6 (branched-cha in amino acids) | |
| Type 2 diabetes | – | Lipidomics | Plasma | 104 wo men with previ ous ges tational diabetes; 21 (20%) developed diabetes during the median follow-up period of 8.5 years | Cholesteryl ester species CE 20:4 , alkenylphosphatidylethan olamine species PE (P-36:2), and the phosphatidyls erine species PS 38:4 were independently and positively associated with the development of type 2 diabetes | [105] |

**Table 2.** Biomarkers identified by different omics approaches in diabetes and cardiovascular diseases.

Although there are a high number of research articles describing existing and promising biomarkers for diabetes and cardiovascular disease, here we are providing an overview of a few standard and exciting biomarkers that regularly used in clinic.

# 3. Existing and standard biomarkers in diabetes and cardiovascular diseases

Glycated haemoglobin (HbA1c) and glucose levels are mostly used for the diagnosis of diabetes. These two tests give idea about sugar levels in the body in the presence and absence of medication. However, these tests can be used to predict the disease in the later stages not in the early stages. So, there is an urgent need to identify novel biomarkers to detect the early stage of diabetes, i.e. prediabetic stage.

Troponin T (cTnT), troponin I (cTnI), and creatinine kinase-MB (CK-MB) are the common markers for the diagnosis of myocardial injury and stratification of the risk in acute coronary syndrome. cTnI is as effective as cTnT in diagnosing myocardial necrosis in the setting of trauma and coronary bypass grafting [9]. Increased hs-cTnT concentrations are associated with extent and complexity of CAD as well as diabetic patients with stable CAD [10]. Recently, Brendan et al. reported that cardiac troponin T concentration was an independent predictor of death from cardiovascular causes, myocardial infarction, or stroke in patients who had both type 2 diabetes and stable ischemic heart disease [11]. European Society of Cardiology (ESC) and the American College of Cardiology (ACC) guidelines have recommended cardiac troponins are markers for the acute myocardial infarction. These sensitive markers (cTnT and cTnI) begin to rise in the first 4–8 h following injury and peak at 12–24 h. However, cTnT may remain raised for more than two weeks while cTnI for more than 5–7 days. These two detect myocardial injury below the detection limit of CK-MB. Some of the clinicians measured CK-MB to rule out myocardial infarction and to monitor for additional cardiac muscle injury over time [9].

Natriuretic peptides [brain natriuretic peptide (BNP), atrial natriuretic peptide (ANP)] and their N-terminal pro-hormones [N-terminal pro-atrial natriuretic peptide (NT-pro-ANP) and N-terminal pro-brain natriuretic peptide (NT-pro-BNP)] were increased in patients with heart failure, i.e. left ventricular dysfunction. In general, these markers are produced initially within the heart and released into the circulation in response to increased wall tension. BNP and ANP are secreted not only from the atria but also from the ventricles, especially in patients with heart failure. BNP and NT-pro-BNP may be superior to ANP and NT-pro-ANP in the detection of left ventricular dysfunction [12].

C-reactive protein (CRP) is a liver-derived pattern recognition molecule and systemic inflammatory marker that is increased in inflammatory states. It releases rapidly after immediate tissue injury and work as host defence [13]. Interleukin-6 (IL-6) is the most potent inducer of CRP production, and hsCRP (high-sensitivity C-reactive protein) is released from activated leukocytes in response to infection or trauma and from vascular smooth muscle cells in response to atherosclerosis [14]. Inflammation plays a major role in type 2 diabetes and cardiovascular diseases. Inflammation is the one of the risk factors for the development of T2DM and CVD. Researchers have identified that increased hsCRP levels were associated with obesity, metabolic syndrome, type 1 diabetes, type 2 diabetes, atherosclerosis, and coronary artery diseases (CADs) [15]. Increased blood hsCRP levels indicate the coexistence of subclinical systemic inflammation and insulin resistance and correlated with elevated insulin, C-peptide, and HOMA-IR (Homeostatic Model Assessment-insulin resistance) [16]. Treatment with aspirin, statins, cyclooxygenase-2 inhibitors, and fibrates are able to reduce hsCRP levels [13]. Treatment with peroxisome proliferator-activated receptor gamma (PPAR-$\gamma$) agonist pioglitazone also decreased hsCRP along with other cardiovascular risk markers [17].

Pro-inflammatory cytokines, i.e. tumour necrosis factor-alpha (TNF-$\alpha$), interleukin-6 (IL-6), IL-1-beta, and IL-8 and monocyte chemoattractant protein (MCP-1); cell adhesion molecules, i.e. intra-cell adhesion molecule-1 (ICAM-1) and vascular cell adhesion molecule-1 (VCAM-1); and markers of cardiovascular risk, i.e. C-reactive protein (CRP), homocysteine, and plasminogen activator inhibitor-1 (PAI-1) and reactive oxygen species (ROS) are the common markers for inflammation and oxidative stress. Metabolic hormones such as resistin, leptin, adiponectin, ghrelin, and visfatin were also altered in diabetes and metabolic disorder and considered as important biomarkers for understanding the diabetic complication.

All these above markers are used to predict diabetes and cardiovascular diseases independently but not in a combination to understand the disease complexity. Even these biomarkers

http://dx.doi.org/10.5772/62595

are not able to predict the disease in the early stages. Thus, there is an urgent need to identify novel biomarkers to predict the early detection of the disease and disease progression.

## 4. Exploring novel biomarkers for diagnostic and prognostic biomarkers for diabetes and its cardiovascular complications

### 4.1. Galectin-3

Galectin-3 (Gal-3) a 30-kDa β-galactoside-binding lectin mainly present in the cytoplasm, and also in the nucleus, is expressed by different types of cells and regulates various T-cell functions and innate immune responses. Expression of galectin-3 increased in activated macrophages and involved in inflammation, tumour growth, and fibrosis [18,19]. Gal-3 protects β-cells from the cytotoxic effect of IL-1β [20] and advanced glycation end product (AGE)-induced tissue injury. Removal of Gal-3 accelerates AGE-induced kidney injury in diabetes [21], enhances atherogenesis [22], accelerates high-fat diet-induced obesity, and increases inflammation in adipose tissue and pancreatic islets. Gal-3 shows protective effect in obesity-induced inflammation and diabetes [18]. Ohkura et al. reported that low levels of Gal-3 were associated with insulin resistance in T2DM patients [23]. On the contrary, elevated levels of Gal-3 are associated with increased risk of heart failure and mortality [24]. Recently, Ozturk et al. identified that Gal-3 concentrations were significantly higher in the coronary artery disease (CAD) group than in the non-CAD group. Gal-3 levels were correlated positively with BMI (Body mass index), high-sensitivity C-reactive protein, the total number of diseased vessels, the number of plaques, and the calcified plaque type. In addition, galectin-3 levels were found to be independent predictor of coronary atherosclerosis in type 2 diabetic patients. Gal-3 is a novel and promising biomarker that may help to identify type 2 diabetic patients who may require early CAD intervention because of the potential risk of coronary atherosclerosis [25]. Jin et al. reported that elevated galectin levels were associated with increase in vascular complications, i.e. the heart failure, nephropathy, and peripheral artery diseases. Several research articles have shown association of Gal-3 with diabetes and cardiovascular diseases. However, many questions still need to be answered before considering Gal-3 as a biomarker in diabetes and cardiovascular diseases: Can Gal-3 specifically be used as a biomarker for diabetes-associated cardiovascular diseases (Gal-3 is usually expressed in the inflammatory and fibrinolytic conditions in the liver, kidney, and lungs; this shows lack of tissue specificity)? Can Gal-3 alone predict the disease prevention strategy? Can it be used with any other established marker to predict diabetes-associated cardiovascular complications?

### 4.2. Irisin

Irisin is a newly discovered hormone which is mainly secreted by the heart, skeletal muscle, liver, and kidneys. Bostrom et al. reported that cardiac muscle produces more irisin than skeletal muscle. Irisin is mainly produced within heart and skeletal muscle [26]. Irisin is essential to convert white adipose tissue to brown adipose tissue. He et al. found that irisin levels were decreased and urotensin II (UII) levels were increased in type 2 diabetic subjects.

Circulating urotensin II levels were increased in diabetes and could inhibit the glucose transport in skeletal muscle in diabetic mouse and aggravated the insulin resistant [27]. The study found the association between both irisin and urotensin II and concluded that urotensin II and high glucose may inhibit the release of irisin from skeletal muscle in diabetic patients [28]. Increased circulating irisin predicts the insulin resistance onset in association with weight regain and authors concluded that irisin could be secreted as an adaptive response to counteract the deleterious effect of excess adiposity on glucose homeostasis [29]. Two-week treatment with simvastatin increased circulating irisin concentrations in healthy individuals and also in primary human skeletal muscle cells. Simvastatin induces both cellular stress markers as well as protective response markers. Simvastatin-induced irisin secretion can block mitochondrial oxidative stress and thus play an important role in the regulation of oxidative stress in human skeletal muscle [30]. Irisin is also secreted in response to the activation of PGC-1$\alpha$. Previous studies have explained well regarding the regulation of PGC-1$\alpha$ in mitochondrial biogenesis, oxidative metabolism, mitochondrial function, and modulation of insulin resistance. Decreased PGC-1$\alpha$ levels in type 2 diabetic subjects as reported earlier [31–33] might be responsible for reduced irisin levels. There is a controversy regarding irisin levels in obesity, insulin resistance, and metabolic syndrome in type 2 diabetic patients. While some reported higher irisin levels in diabetic patients, others reported the opposite [34–36]. These discrepancies were due to the data analysed from different stages of diseases and the presence of other complications [26]. Researchers have reported that serum irisin levels were decreased in type 2 diabetes and myocardial infarction patients [37,38]. Aronis et al. reported that increased irisin levels predict the development of major cardiovascular events, especially unstable angina, in patients with CAD after percutaneous intervention (PCI) [39]. Hanatani et al. also reported that irisin is a novel biomarker providing prognostic information in patients with heart failure with reduced ejection fraction. However, further clinical studies are needed to find whether irisin is associated with cardiometabolic disease and evaluate whether circulatory irisin levels could serve as an independent prognostic marker in diabetic patients with cardiovascular complications and also elucidate beneficial effects by finding molecular mechanism and intervention studies in different animal models.

### 4.3. Apelin

Apelin is identified as a 36-amino acid peptide and is an endogenous ligand of G-protein-coupled receptors (GPCRs) of apelin receptor. Recently, apelin was recognised as adipokine and secreted from white adipose tissue. Apelin receptor is present in ventricular cardiomyocytes, vascular smooth muscle cells (VSMCs), and intra-myocardial endothelial cells (ECs) [40]. Apelin stimulates endothelium-dependent nitric oxide-mediated vasorelaxation and reduces arterial blood pressure. Apelin synthesis in adipocytes is stimulated by insulin, and apelin plasma levels are markedly increased in obesity associated with insulin resistance [41]. Apelin shows antioxidant effects and attenuates reactive oxygen species (ROS)-induced adipogenesis, lipogenesis, lipolysis, and release of free fatty acids [42]. Apelin knockout mice show diminished insulin sensitivity [43]. Tumour necrosis factor-$\alpha$ (TNF-$\alpha$) induces the expression of apelin via phosphatidylinositol 3-kinase (PI3K), c-Jun N-terminal kinase (JNK) and MEK1/2 signalling pathways in adipocytes [44]. Chronic treatment with apelin ameliorates both glucose and lipid metabolism and also increases muscle mitochondrial performance through increased mitochondrial biogenesis and a tighter matching between fatty acid oxidation and the tricarboxylic acid cycle. Therefore, chronic apelin treatment can be a targeted therapy for type 2 diabetes and its complications [45]. Furthermore, in studies using lipopolysaccharide (LPS) and cytokines to elicit an immune response in rodents, the expression of apelin mRNA has been reported to be upregulated, involving the JAK/STAT pathway [40]. Ma et al. reported that plasma apelin is a novel biomarker for predicting type 2 diabetes in men [46]. It was reported that suppressed apelin levels were associated with increased cardiovascular risk in women with previous history of gestational diabetes [47]. Recently, Abd-Elbaky et al. reported that omentin levels were significantly lower and serum apelin and IL-1β concentrations were significantly higher in obese diabetic groups compared to nonobese controls. This study concluded that abnormal production of omentin and apelin can contribute to the pathogenesis of obesity-related complications including T2DM and cardiovascular disease [48]. However, further research is needed to confirm whether apelin can be used as biomarker in diabetes and cardiovascular diseases.

### 4.4. Growth differentiation factor-15

Growth differentiation factor-15 (GDF-15) is a stress-responsive cytokine produced as a ≈40 kDa propeptide form and N-terminal cleaved to release as a ≈30 kDa disulphide-linked dimeric active protein form. It is highly expressed in cardiomyocytes, adipocytes, macrophages, endothelial cells, and vascular smooth muscle cells in normal and pathological condition. GDF-15 increases during tissue injury and inflammatory states and is associated with cardiometabolic risk. Increased GDF-15 levels are associated with cardiovascular diseases such as hypertrophy, heart failure, atherosclerosis, endothelial dysfunction, obesity, insulin resistance, diabetes, and chronic kidney diseases in diabetes. Researchers have reported that GDF-15 shows cardioprotective effect through activation of ALK (Activin receptor-like kinase) type 1 receptor (ALK 1–7) and GDF-15 phosphorylates Smad2/3 and Smad1/5/8 which translocate to the nucleus in the form of heteromeric complex with Smad4 and activates PI3K/AKT/eNOS/NO pathway. It also inhibits epidermal growth factor receptor (EGFR) transactivation and NF-kB/JNK/caspase-3 pathway. Many patents have been filed reporting GDF-15 as a marker for the diabetes and cardiovascular diseases. Patent no. EP2439535A1 claimed that GDF-15 can be distinguished between diabetes and diabetes with coronary artery diseases subjects. Recently, we have also shown that GDF-15 levels can be useful to distinguish diabetic patients from cardiovascular complications [5]. However, a large multinational study has to be conducted to validate GDF-15 as a biomarker to detect specific cardiovascular complication in diabetes.

### 4.5. Growth differentiation factor-11

Growth differentiation factor-11 (GDF-11) is a cytokine that belongs to TGF-β super family and also known as bone morphogenetic protein-11 (BMP-11). GDF-11 works like myostatin to modulate metabolic function [49]. Previous scientific literature claimed that GDF-11 is an anti-ageing factor. Fadini et al. showed that circulating GDF-11 levels were decreased with age [50].

Peripheral supplementation of GDF-11 protein in mice attenuated the age-related dysfunction of skeletal muscle [51]. In recent years, researchers are focusing their interest on circulatory GDF-11 levels in heart diseases. GDF-11 levels reversed the age-related hypertrophied heart into a young heart [52]. GDF-11 is also an essential factor for the regeneration of pancreatic islets in diabetic patients [53]. The plasma GDF-11 levels with age and disease condition remain controversial. Egerman et al. in his study showed that an increased GDF-11 protein level was observed with age in rat skeletal muscle. However, serum GDF-11 levels in rat and human were not significantly increased [54]. In contrast, Poggioli et al. explained age-dependent decline in GDF-11 levels in multiple mammalian species such as mice, rats, horses, and sheep. They also showed that exogenous GDF-11 administration rapidly activates SMAD signalling to reduce cardiomyocyte size [55]. This property of reducing cardiomyocytes can be useful against cardiac hypertrophy. Two more recent studies supported the above statement. Heidecker et al. showed that low levels of GDF-11 and high levels of its inhibitor follistatin-like 3 are associated with adverse cardiovascular outcomes in humans [56]. Similarly Olson et al. reported that high levels of GDF-11 are associated with lower prevalence of left ventricular hypertrophy [57]. Recently, Adela et al. reported that plasma GDF-11 levels were decreased in diabetes and diabetes with cardiovascular complications as compared with control subjects [58]. To use GDF-11 as a biomarker for diabetes and diabetes associated with cardiovascular diseases, more research needs to be carried out with a different population. GDF-11 could be used as a biomarker or as an intervention therapy to reduce the disease progression.

### 4.6. Cyclophilin A

Cyclophilin A (CyPA) was discovered three decades ago as the intracellular receptor of the immunosuppressive drug cyclosporine. CyPA is secreted from vascular cell components of endothelial cells and vascular smooth muscle cells in response to the reactive oxygen species (ROS) and also expressed in T cells, neutrophils, monocytes, macrophages, and foam cells and shows cellular effects such as proliferation, migration, activation of NF-kB, induction of matrix metalloproteinases, adhesion of molecules, and induction of ROS [59]. Extracellular CyPA initiates expression of adhesion molecules in endothelial cells (EC), induces apoptosis, and works as a chemoattractant for inflammatory cells. Intracellular and extracellular CyPA promotes intimal thickening, abdominal aortic aneurysms, atherosclerosis, and cardiac hypertrophy in mice [60]. Recently Tsai et al. reported that hyperglycaemia causes release of CyPA in mesangial (MES-13) and tubular (HK-2) cells. Urinary CyPA correlated with the progression of renal function. Significant increase in urinary CyPA was noted in stage 2 diabetic nephropathy and persisted in later stages of the disease. This study concluded that CyPA is a new biomarker for diabetic nephropathy and can be used as an early maker [61]. Type 2 diabetes subjects have increased circulating levels of CyPA than the healthy subjects. CyPA is secreted by monocytes in response to high glucose treatment and responsible for the progression of atherosclerosis in type 2 diabetes [62]. Further authors found that plasma CyPA levels were increased in diabetes subjects with coronary artery disease. This study concluded that CyPA play important role to progress vascular disease in type 2 diabetes subjects. The scientific literature thus provides strong evidence that CyPA work as inflammatory mediator in the progression of atherogenesis [63]. Therefore, all data indicate that CyPA is a promising and potential biomarker for the detection of vascular diseases in type 2 diabetes [64].

### 4.7. Prolactin

Prolactin is a polypeptide released as a pituitary hormone. Prolactin is named so for its ability to promote lactation in post pregnancy in female mammals. Other than lactogenic property, prolactin plays important role in the regulation of reproduction, growth and development, metabolism, immune regulation, brain function, and behaviour [65]. Prevalence of obesity was increased in hyperprolactinaemic patients [66]. Circulating levels of prolactin increase in diabetic patients. Increased prolactin levels were associated with lower prevalence of diabetes and impaired glucose regulation [65,67]. However, Balbach et al. reported that low circulatory prolactin concentration is associated with increased T2DM risk. However, this study did not show any evidence to prove prolactin as a cardiometabolic risk factor [68]. Prolactin levels were increased in essential hypertension, acute coronary syndromes, ischemic strokes, transient ischemic attacks, pre-eclampsia, and heart failure. Carrero et al. also reported that increased prolactin levels were associated with endothelial dysfunction, increased risk of cardiovascular events, and increased mortality in chronic kidney disease (CKD) patients [69]. In vitro studies show that prolactin stimulates integrin-mediated adhesion of circulating mononuclear cells to endothelium and induces vascular smooth muscle cell proliferation. Reuwer et al. study did not predict the prolactin as predictor for the coronary artery diseases in spite of presence of prolactin receptors in human coronary artery plaques [70]. On the other hand, increased plasma prolactin can protect rat cardiomyocytes against hypoxia through the p-JAK2 and p-STAT5 pathways and the PI3K$\alpha$/AKT and MAPK survival pathways [71]. Landberg et al. reported that prolactin concentrations were not associated with cardiovascular mortality and thus not a marker of heart failure [72]. However, a cathepsin D-cleaved 16 kDa form of prolactin mediates postpartum cardiomyopathy and authors claimed that inhibition of prolactin may be a new therapeutic strategy for the paripartum cardiomyopathy [73].

### 4.8. Vitamin D

Vitamin D is a secosteroid that exists in two forms, i.e. ergocalciferol (D2) and cholecalciferol (D3). Ergocalciferol (D2) is synthesised from the vegetable sources. Unlike D2, cholecalciferol (D3) is synthesised by the epidermis on exposure to the UV radiation (sunlight) and also from oily fish supplementation. Vitamin D (D2 and D3) is converted into active metabolite 1, 25(OH)2 D by the two hydroxylation steps. These active metabolites bind with the vitamin D receptor and exert its biological action [74]. Vitamin D receptors are present in many cells such as pancreatic $\beta$ cells, cardiomyocytes, endothelial cells, and vascular smooth muscle cells. Vitamin D plays a pivotal role in the bone and mineral metabolism. Vitamin D deficiency is a common health problem worldwide and is the cause for osteoporosis and osteomalacia, rickets, and other bone-related disorders. In the recent decades, researchers have also identified that lower vitamin D levels were associated with metabolic diseases such as type 1 diabetes, obesity, insulin resistance, hypertension, cardiovascular diseases, and cancer [75,76]. Many epidemiological studies have reported that people from different countries are more prevalence to vitamin D deficiency [77–82]. Eight-week vitamin D replacement therapy in type 2 diabetic patients potentially has beneficial effects on cardiovascular disease risk factors such as HbA1c, total cholesterol, LDL-C, and diastolic blood pressure [83]. Tarcin et al. reported that 25(OH)D-deficient subjects has lower flow-mediated dilatation (FMD) which is useful to measure endothelial dysfunction and was improved after acute treatment with calcitriol [84]. Vitamin D is a negative regulator of renin–angiotensin system and blood pressure [85]. Recently Jisu et al. reported that deletion of macrophage vitamin D receptor promotes insulin resistance and monocyte cholesterol transport to accelerate atherosclerosis in mice. This study suggested that vitamin D plays an important role in inflammation and thus responsible for the development of type 2 diabetes and atherosclerosis [86]. Vitamin D can be used as a biomarker to predict the disease severity of diabetes and cardiovascular complications. However, for better understanding the role of vitamin D in pathophysiology of diabetes and cardiovascular diseases, more intervention studies with long-term follow-up are required.

### 4.9. Pregnancy-associated plasma protein-A (PAPP-A)

PAPP-A is a zinc-binding matrix metalloproteinase that regulates extracellular matrix remodelling. PAPP-A degrades IGFBP-4 and increases the levels of local IGF-1 in response to injury and involved in the pathogenesis of atherosclerosis. Two inflammatory cytokines, i.e. TNF-$\alpha$ and IL-1, are involved in insulin resistance development and most potent stimulators of PAPP-A [95]. Many researchers reported that elevated levels of PAPP-A were associated 36 with coronary artery diseases, e.g. acute coronary syndrome [[88]-[93]]. On this contrary, Pellitero et al. reported in their study that serum PAPP-A concentrations were significantly lower in diabetic subjects and correlated negatively with HbA1C. PAPP-A concentration was lower in patients with HbA1C > 8.2% (0.35 mUI/l [0.07–0.43]) compared with that in patients with HbA1C < 5.9% (0.72 mUI/l [0.2–0.92], $P < 0.03$). However, PAPP-A levels were not changed in hypercholesteraemic subjects when compared with normal cholesterolaemia subjects. It is also reported that genetic deletion of PAPP-A is associated with resistance to atherosclerotic lesion development in apolipoprotein E-deficient mice fed with a high-fat diet by decreasing bioavailability of IGF-1. This study indicates that PAPP-A is essential to promote lesion formation through regulation of IGF-1 action [94]. Serum PAPP-A and IGF-1 do not appear to be useful serum biomarkers for carotid atherosclerosis in type 2 diabetic patients with stable glycemic control, despite scientific evidence of their local role in atherosclerosis. [87]. However, Hjortebjerg et al. have reported that PAPP-A is a prognostic marker for acute coronary syndrome [96]. Recently Conover et al. reported that targeted inhibition of PAPP-A reduces atherosclerotic plaque burden in mice. This study is giving evidence that inhibition of PAPP-A can be used as therapeutic strategy in atherosclerosis [97]. However, further studies need to be conducted to find its role in diabetes and associated cardiovascular complication.

http://dx.doi.org/10.5772/62595

## 5. Conclusion

Cardiovascular complication is the major cause of the death of diabetes worldwide. At present, all standard available markers are useful to detect diabetes and cardiovascular disease separately but not suitable for identifying the cardiovascular complication at early and late stages of the diseases progression. There is an urgent need to identify novel biomarkers by using different omics approaches using large number of patients having desired phenotype. Identified markers can also able to assist in clinical decision making such as interventions and medications. Recently all new markers such as vitamin D, GDF-15, galectin-3, and cyclophilin-A identified have a strong association with type 2 diabetes and cardiovascular disease. However, these yet have not been implemented in the clinical practice. Before accepting any new markers as clinical biomarkers, the following questions need to be answered: whether new identified biomarkers can be used to take clinical decision for any particular diseases, whether it can be useful in therapeutic management and provide any diagnostic and prognostic information, and whether identified biomarkers can be used as a single marker or in a combination with other biomarkers. Identifying new biomarker may also help to understand the affected signalling pathways related to the disease and discover novel therapy against diabetes and cardiovascular complications.

Future biomarker discovery is showing excitement and raising many challenges. One of the major challenges in biomarker discovery is to develop biomarkers for personalised medicine. Biomarkers can play a critical role in classifying patients into subpopulations. In the present days, predicting the therapeutic strategy through personalised medicine is more familiar. However, more research needs to be done to develop specific biomarker to make personalised medicine successful. Personalised medicine is developing tremendously in cancer treatment. However, researchers should focus more on diabetes and cardiovascular disease to initiate personalised medicine in metabolic diseases. Other challenges in biomarker discovery include active collaboration between basic scientists and clinicians. Formation of different societies and organisations need to be established like HUPO (Human Proteome Organization) organisation for the proteomics and to prepare biomarkers databases for free access. Scientific communities need to debate with the issue whether individual diagnostic and prognostic biomarker or combined panel of biomarkers are more useful to predict the cardiovascular outcome among diabetic patients.

## Author details

Ramu Adela and Sanjay K. Banerjee*

*Address all correspondence to: skbanerjee@thsti.res.in; banerjees74@hotmail.com

Drug Discovery Research Centre (DDRC), Translational Health Science and Technology Institute (THSTI), Faridabad, Haryana, India

## References

[1] Prentice RL. Surrogate endpoints in clinical trials: definition and operational criteria. Stat Med. 1989; 8:431–440.

[2] Lindahl B. The story of growth differentiation factor 15: another piece of the puzzle. Clin Chem. 2013; 59(11):1550–2. DOI: 10.1373/clinchem.2013.212811.

[3] Audette J. Chart of the week: clinical trials involving biomarkers seeing huge growth. Available from: http://www.amplion.com/biomarker-trends/chart-of-the-week-how-many-trials-will-be-using-biomarkers-in-2020. [2016-02-05].

[4] Vasan RS. Biomarkers of cardiovascular disease: molecular basis and practical considerations. Circulation. 2006; 113(19):2335–62. DOI: 10.1161/CIRCULATIONAHA.104.482570.

[5] Adela R, Banerjee SK. GDF-15 as a target and biomarker for diabetes and cardiovascular diseases: a translational prospective. J Diabetes Res. 2015; 2015:490842. DOI: 10.1155/2015/490842. Epub 2015 Jul 27.

[6] Kaur J. A comprehensive review on metabolic syndrome. Cardiol Res Pract. 2014; 2014:943162. DOI: 10.1155/2014/943162.

[7] Sivitz WI. Lipotoxicity and glucotoxicity in type 2 diabetes. Effects on development and progression. Postgrad Med. 2001; 109(4):55–9, 63–4.

[8] Seeree P, Pearngam P, Kumkate S, Janvilisri T.An omics perspective on molecular biomarkers for diagnosis, prognosis, and therapeutics of cholangiocarcinoma. Int J Genomics. 2015; 2015:179528. DOI: 10.1155/2015/179528.

[9] Maynard S, Menown I, Adgey A. Troponin T or troponin I as cardiac markers in ischaemic heart disease. Heart. 2000; 83:371–373. DOI:10.1136/heart.83.4.371

[10] Ucar H, Gur M, Seker T, Kaypakli O, Elbasan Z et al. High-sensitivity cardiac troponin T is associated with SYNTAX score and diabetes mellitus in patients with stable coronary artery disease. J Clin Exp Cardiol. 2013; 4:263. DOI:10.4172/2155-9880.1000263

[11] Everett BM, Brooks MM, Vlachos HE, Chaitman BR, Frye RL, Bhatt DL; BARI 2D Study Group. Troponin and cardiac events in stable ischemic heart disease and diabetes. N Engl J Med. 2015; 373(7):610–20. DOI: 10.1056/NEJMoa1415921.

[12] Bay M, Kirk V, Parner J, Hassager C, Nielsen H, Krogsgaard K, Trawinski J, Boesgaard S, Aldershvile J. NT-proBNP: a new diagnostic screening tool to differentiate between patients with normal and reduced left ventricular systolic function. Heart. 2003; 89(2): 150–4.

[13] Pfutzner A, Forst T. High-sensitivity C-reactive protein as cardiovascular risk marker in patients with diabetes mellitus. Diabetes Technol Ther. 2006; 8(1):28–36.

[14] Yousuf O, Mohanty BD, Martin SS, Joshi PH, Blaha MJ, Nasir K, Blumenthal RS, Budoff MJ. High-sensitivity C-reactive protein and cardiovascular disease: a resolute belief or an elusive link? J Am Coll Cardiol. 2013; 62(5):397–408. DOI: 10.1016/j.jacc.2013.05.016.

[15] Santos AC, Lopes C, Guimaraes JT, Barros H. Central obesity as a major determinant of increased high-sensitivity C-reactive protein in metabolic syndrome. Int J Obes (Lond). 2005; 29(12):1452–6.

[16] Mahajan A, Tabassum R, Chavali S, Dwivedi OP, Bharadwaj M, Tandon N, Bharadwaj D. High-sensitivity C-reactive protein levels and type 2 diabetes in urban North Indians. J Clin Endocrinol Metab. 2009; 94(6):2123–7. DOI: 10.1210/jc.2008-2754.

[17] Hanefeld M, Marx N, Pfützner A, Baurecht W, Lubben G, Karagiannis E, Stier U, Forst T. Anti-inflammatory effects of pioglitazone and/or simvastatin in high cardiovascular risk patients with elevated high sensitivity C-reactive protein: the PIOSTAT Study. J Am Coll Cardiol. 2007; 49(3):290–7.

[18] Pejnovic NN, Pantic JM, Jovanovic IP, Radosavljevic GD, Milovanovic MZ, Nikolic IG, Zdravkovic NS, Djukic AL, Arsenijevic NN, Lukic ML. Galectin-3 deficiency accelerates high-fat diet-induced obesity and amplifies inflammation in adipose tissue and pancreatic islets. Diabetes. 2013; 62(6):1932–44. DOI: 10.2337/db12-0222.

[19] de Boer RA, Yu L, van Veldhuisen DJ.Galectin-3 in cardiac remodeling and heart failure. Curr Heart Fail Rep. 2010; 7(1):1–8. DOI: 10.1007/s11897-010-0004-x.

[20] Karlsen AE, Størling ZM, Sparre T, et al. Immune-mediated beta-cell destruction in vitro and in vivo—a pivotal role for galectin-3. Biochem Biophys Res Commun. 2006; 344:406–415.

[21] Pugliese G, Pricci F, Iacobini C, et al. Accelerated diabetic glomerulopathy in galectin-3/AGE receptor 3 knockout mice. FASEB J. 2001; 15:2471–2479.

[22] Iacobini C, Menini S, Ricci C, et al. Accelerated lipid-induced atherogenesis in galectin-3-deficient mice: role of lipoxidation via receptor-mediated mechanisms. Arterioscler Thromb Vasc Biol. 2009; 29:831–836.

[23] Ohkura T, Fujioka Y, Nakanishi R, Shiochi H, Sumi K, Yamamoto N, Matsuzawa K, Izawa S, Ohkura H, Ueta E, Kato M, Miyoshi E, Taniguchi S ,Yamamoto K. Low serum galectin-3 concentrations are associated with insulin resistance in patients with type 2 diabetes mellitus. Diabetol Metab Syndr. 2014; 6(1):106. DOI: 10.1186/1758-5996-6-106.

[24] Ho JE, Liu C, Lyass A, Courchesne P, Pencina MJ, Vasan RS, Larson MG, Levy D. Galectin-3, a marker of cardiac fibrosis, predicts incident heart failure in the community. J Am Coll Cardiol. 2012; 60(14):1249–56. DOI: 10.1016/j.jacc.2012.04.053.

[25] Ozturk D, Celik O, Satilmis S, Aslan S, Erturk M, Cakmak HA, Kalkan AK, Ozyilmaz S, Diker V, Gul M. Association between serum galectin-3 levels and coronary atherosclerosis and plaque burden/structure in patients with type 2 diabetes mellitus. Coron Artery Dis. 2015; 26(5):396–401. DOI: 10.1097/MCA.0000000000000252.

[26] Chen JQ, Huang YY, Gusdon AM, Qu S.Irisin: a new molecular marker and target in metabolic disorder. Lipids Health Dis. 2015; 14:2. DOI: 10.1186/1476-511X-14-2.

[27] Wang HX, Wu XR, Yang H, Yin CL, Shi LJ. Urotensin II inhibits skeletal muscle glucose transport signalling pathways via the NADPH oxidase pathway. PLoS One. 2013; 8(10):e76796. DOI: 10.1371/journal.pone.0076796.

[28] He WY, Bai Q, A LT, Tang CS, Zhang AH. Irisin levels are associated with urotensin II levels in diabetic patients. J Diabetes Investig. 2015; 6(5):571–6. DOI: 10.1111/jdi.12331.

[29] Crujeiras AB, Zulet MA, Lopez-Legarrea P, de la Iglesia R, Pardo M, Carreira MC, Martínez JA, Casanueva FF. Association between circulating irisin levels and the promotion of insulin resistance during the weight maintenance period after a dietary weight-lowering program in obese patients. Metabolism. 2014; 63(4):520–31. DOI: 10.1016/j.metabol.2013.12.007.

[30] Gouni-Berthold I, Berthold HK, Huh JY, Berman R, Spenrath N, Krone W, Mantzoros CS. Effects of lipid-lowering drugs on irisin in human subjects in vivo and in human skeletal muscle cells ex vivo. PLoS One. 2013; 8(9):e72858. DOI: 10.1371/journal.pone.0072858.

[31] Guilherme A, Virbasius JV, Puri V, Czech MP. Adipocyte dysfunctions linking obesity to insulin resistance and type 2 diabetes. Nat Rev Mol Cell Biol. 2008; 9(5):367–77. DOI: 10.1038/nrm2391.

[32] Handschin C, Spiegelman BM. The role of exercise and PGC1alpha in inflammation and chronic disease. Nature. 2008; 454(7203):463–9. DOI: 10.1038/nature07206.

[33] Yan J, Feng Z, Liu J, Shen W, Wang Y, Wertz K, et al. Enhanced autophagy plays a cardinal role in mitochondrial dysfunction in type 2 diabetic Goto-Kakizaki (GK) rats: ameliorating effects of (−)-epigallocatechin-3-gallate. J Nutr Biochem. 2012; 23(7):716–24. DOI: 10.1016/j.jnutbio.2011.03.014.

[34] Moreno-Navarrete JM, Ortega F, Serrano M, Guerra E, Pardo G, Tinahones F, Ricart W, Fernández-Real JM. Irisin is expressed and produced by human muscle and adipose tissue in association with obesity and insulin resistance. J Clin Endocrinol Metab. 2013; 98(4):E769–78. DOI: 10.1210/jc.2012-2749.

[35] Choi YK, Kim MK, Bae KH, Seo HA, Jeong JY, Lee WK, Kim JG, Lee IK, Park KG. Serum irisin levels in new-onset type 2 diabetes. Diabetes Res Clin Pract. 2013; 100(1):96–101. DOI: 10.1016/j.diabres.2013.01.007.

[36] Sanchis-Gomar F, Alis R, Pareja-Galeano H, Sola E, Victor VM, Rocha M, Hernández-Mijares A, Romagnoli M. Circulating irisin levels are not correlated with BMI, age, and other biological parameters in obese and diabetic patients. Endocrine. 2014; 46(3):674–7. DOI: 10.1007/s12020-014-0170-9.

[37] Liu JJ, Wong MD, Toy WC, Tan CS, Liu S, Ng XW, Tavintharan S, Sum CF, Lim SC. Lower circulating irisin is associated with type 2 diabetes mellitus. J Diabetes Complications. 2013; 27(4):365–9. DOI: 10.1016/j.jdiacomp.2013.03.002.

[38] Aydin S, Aydin S, Kobat MA, Kalayci M, Eren MN, Yilmaz M, Kuloglu T, Gul E, Secen O, Alatas OD, Baydas A. Decreased saliva/serum irisin concentrations in the acute myocardial infarction promising for being a new candidate biomarker for diagnosis of this pathology. Peptides. 2014; 56:141–5. DOI: 10.1016/j.peptides.2014.04.002.

[39] Aronis KN, Moreno M, Polyzos SA, Moreno-Navarrete JM, Ricart W, Delgado E, de la Hera J, Sahin-Efe A, Chamberland JP, Berman R, Spiro A 3rd, Vokonas P, Fernández-Real JM, Mantzoros CS. Circulating irisin levels and coronary heart disease: association with future acute coronary syndrome and major adverse cardiovascular events. Int J Obes (Lond). 2015; 39(1):156–61. DOI: 10.1038/ijo.2014.101.

[40] O'Carroll AM, Lolait SJ, Harris LE, Pope GR. The apelin receptor APJ: journey from an orphan to a multifaceted regulator of homeostasis. J Endocrinol. 2013; 219(1):R13–35. DOI: 10.1530/JOE-13-0227.

[41] Papadopoulos DP, Makris T, Perrea D, Zerva K, Tsioufis C, Faselis C, Papademetriou V. Apelin and relaxin plasma levels in young healthy offspring of patients with essential hypertension. J Clin Hypertens (Greenwich). 2010; 16(3):198–201.DOI: 10.1111/jch.12260.

[42] Than A, Zhang X, Leow MK, Poh CL, Chong SK, Chen P. Apelin attenuates oxidative stress in human adipocytes. J Biol Chem. 2014; 289(6):3763–74. DOI: 10.1074/jbc.M113.526210.

[43] Yue P, Jin H, Aillaud M, Deng AC, Azuma J, Asagami T, Kundu RK, Reaven GM, Quertermous T, Tsao PS. Apelin is necessary for the maintenance of insulin sensitivity. Am J Physiol Endocrinol Metab. 2010; 298(1):E59–67. DOI: 10.1152/ajpendo.00385.2009.

[44] Daviaud D, Boucher J, Gesta S, Dray C, Guigne C, Quilliot D, Ayav A, Ziegler O, Carpene C, Saulnier-Blache JS, Valet P, Castan-Laurell I. TNF alpha up-regulates apelin expression in human and mouse adipose tissue. FASEB J. 2006; 20(9):1528–30.

[45] Attane C, Foussal C, Le Gonidec S, Benani A, Daviaud D, Wanecq E, Guzmán-Ruiz R, Dray C, Bezaire V, Rancoule C, Kuba K, Ruiz-Gayo M, Levade T, Penninger J, Burcelin R, Pénicaud L, Valet P, Castan-Laurell I. Apelin treatment increases complete fatty acid oxidation, mitochondrial oxidative capacity, and biogenesis in muscle of insulin-resistant mice. Diabetes. 2012; 61(2):310–20. DOI: 10.2337/db11-0100.

[46] Ma WY, Yu TY, Wei JN, Hung CS, Lin MS, Liao YJ, Pei D, Su CC, Lu KC, Liu PH, Lin CH, Chuang LM, Kao HL, Lin JW, Chuang YJ, Li HY. Plasma apelin: a novel biomarker for predicting diabetes. Clin Chim Acta. 2014; 435:18–23. DOI: 10.1016/j.cca.2014.03.030.

[47] Akinci B, Celtik A, Tunali S, Genc S, Yuksel F, Secil M, Ozcan MA, Bayraktar F. Circulating apelin levels are associated with cardiometabolic risk factors in women

with previous gestational diabetes. Arch Gynecol Obstet. 2014; 289(4):787–93. DOI: 10.1007/s00404-013-3070-y.

[48] Abd-Elbaky AE, Abo-ElMatty DM, Mesbah NM, Ibrahim SM. Associations of serum omentin and apelin concentrations with obesity, diabetes mellitus type 2 and cardiovascular diseases in Egyptian population. Endocrinol Metab Synd. 2015; 4:171. DOI: 10.4172/2161-1017.1000171.

[49] McPherron AC. Metabolic functions of myostatin and GDF-11. Immunol Endocr Metab Agents Med Chem. 2010; 10(4):217–231.

[50] Fadini GP, Menegazzo L, Bonora BM, Mazzucato M, Persano S, Kreutzenberg SV, Avogaro A. Effects of age, diabetes, and vascular disease on growth differentiation factor 11: first-in-human study. Diabetes Care. 2015:e1–e2.

[51] Sinha M, Jang YC, Oh J, Khong D, Wu EY, Manohar R et al. Restoring systemic GDF11 levels reverses age-related dysfunction in mouse skeletal muscle. Science. 2014; 344 (6184):649–652.

[52] Loffredo FS, Steinhauser ML, Jay SM, Gannon J, Pancoast JR et al. Growth differentiation factor 11 is a circulating factor that reverses age-related cardiac hypertrophy. Cell. 2013; 153(4):828–39.

[53] Harmon EB, Apelqvist AA, Smart NG, Gu X, Osborne DH, Kim SK. GDF-11 modulates NGN3+ islet progenitor cell number and promotes beta-cell differentiation in pancreas development. Development. 2004; 131(24):6163–74.

[54] Egerman MA ,Cadena SM , Gilbert JA, Meyer A, Nelson HN, Swalley SE et al. GDF11 increases with age and inhibits skeletal muscle regeneration. Cell Metab. 2015; 22(1): 164–74.

[55] Poggioli T, Vujic A, Yang P, Macias-Trevino C, Uygur A, Loffredo FS, Pancoast JR, Cho M, Goldstein J, Tandias RM, Gonzalez E, Walker RG, Thompson TB , Wagers AJ, Fong YW, Lee RT. Circulating Growth Differentiation Factor 11/8 Levels Decline With Age. Circ Res. 2016; 118(1):29–37. DOI: 10.1161/CIRCRESAHA.

[56] Heidecker B, Olson K, Beatty A, Dubin R, Kato S, Lawn R, Murthy A, Regan M, Sterling D, Whooley M, Ganz P. Low levels of growth differentiation factor 11 and high levels of its inhibitor follistatin-like 3 are associated with adverse cardiovascular outcomes in humans. JACC. 2015; 65(10S): A999.

[57] Olson K, Beatty A, Heidecker B, Regan M, Whooley M, Ganz P. High levels of growth differentiation factor 11 are associated with lower prevalence of left ventricular hypertrophy: data from the heart and soul study. JACC. 2014; 63(12):A780

[58] Adela R, Reddy PN, Banerjee SK. Alteration of plasma gdf-11 levels in type 2 diabetes patients with cardiovascular complications: A pilot study. J Pract Cardiovasc Sci 2015; 1:262–6. Doi:10.4103/2395-5414.177246

[59] Seizer P, Gawaz M, May AE. Cyclophilin A and EMMPRIN (CD147) in cardiovascular diseases. Cardiovasc Res. 2014; 102(1):17–23. DOI: 10.1093/cvr/cvu035.

[60] Satoh K. Cyclophilin A in cardiovascular homeostasis and diseases. Tohoku J Exp Med. 2015; 235(1):1–15. DOI: 10.1620/tjem.235.1.

[61] Tsai SF, Su CW, Wu MJ, Chen CH, Fu CP, Liu CS, Hsieh M. Urinary cyclophilin A as a new marker for diabetic nephropathy: a cross-sectional analysis of diabetes mellitus. Medicine (Baltimore). 2015; 94(42):e1802. DOI: 10.1097/MD.0000000000001802.

[62] Ramachandran S, Venugopal A, Sathisha K, Reshmi G, Charles S, Divya G, Chandran NS, Mullassari A, Pillai MR, Kartha CC. Proteomic profiling of high glucose primed monocytes identifies cyclophilin A as a potential secretory marker of inflammation in type 2 diabetes. Proteomics. 2012; 12(18):2808–21. DOI: 10.1002/pmic.201100586.

[63] Ramachandran S, Venugopal A, Kutty VR, A V, G D, Chitrasree V, Mullassari A, Pratapchandran NS, Santosh KR, Pillai MR, Kartha CC. Plasma level of cyclophilin A is increased in patients with type 2 diabetes mellitus and suggests presence of vascular disease. Cardiovasc Diabetol. 2014; 13:38. DOI: 10.1186/1475-2840-13-38.

[64] Ramachandran S, Kartha CC. Cyclophilin-A: a potential screening marker for vascular disease in type-2 diabetes. Can J Physiol Pharmacol. 2012; 90(8):1005–15. DOI: 10.1139/y2012-038.

[65] Wang T, Lu J, Xu Y, Li M, Sun J, Zhang J, Xu B, Xu M, Chen Y, Bi Y, Wang W, Ning G. Circulating prolactin associates with diabetes and impaired glucose regulation: a population-based study. Diabetes Care. 2013; 36(7):1974–80. DOI: 10.2337/dc12-1893.

[66] Pereira-Lima JF, Leães CG, Freitas Neto FM, Barbosa MV, da Silva ALM, Oliveira MDC. Hyperprolactinemia and body weight: prevalence of obesity and overweight in patients with hyperprolactinemia. Res J Endocrinol Metab. 2013; 1:2. DOI: 10.7243/2053-3640-1-2

[67] Arnold E, Rivera JC, Thebault S, Moreno-Páramo D, Quiroz-Mercado H, Quintanar-Stéphano A, Binart N, Martínez de la Escalera G, Clapp C. High levels of serum prolactin protect against diabetic retinopathy by increasing ocular vasoinhibins. Diabetes. 2010; 59(12):3192–7. DOI: 10.2337/db10-0873.

[68] Balbach L, Wallaschofski H, Völzke H, Nauck M, Dorr M, Haring R. Serum prolactin concentrations as risk factor of metabolic syndrome or type 2 diabetes? BMC Endocr Disord. 2013; 13:12. DOI: 10.1186/1472-6823-13-12

[69] Carrero JJ, Kyriazis J, Sonmez A, Tzanakis I, Qureshi AR, Stenvinkel P, Saglam M, Stylianou K, Yaman H, Taslipinar A, Vural A, Gok M, Yenicesu M, Daphnis E, Yilmaz MI. Prolactin levels, endothelial dysfunction, and the risk of cardiovascular events and mortality in patients with CKD. Clin J Am Soc Nephrol. 2012; 7(2):207–15. DOI: 10.2215/CJN.06840711.

[70] Reuwer AQ, Twickler MT, Hutten BA, Molema FW, Wareham NJ, Dallinga-Thie GM, Bogorad RL, Goffin V, Smink-Bol M, Kastelein JJ, Boekholdt SM, Khaw KT. Prolactin

levels and the risk of future coronary artery disease in apparently healthy men and women. Circ Cardiovasc Genet. 2009; 2:389–395. DOI: 10.1161/CIRCGENETICS.109.853572.

[71] Hsieh DJ, Huang CY, Pai P, Wang SG, Tsai YL, Li CN, Kuo WW, Huang CY. Prolactin protects cardiomyocytes against intermittent hypoxia-induced cell damage by the modulation of signaling pathways related to cardiac hypertrophy and proliferation. Int J Cardiol. 2015; 181:255–66. DOI: 10.1016/j.ijcard.2014.11.154.

[72] Landberg E, Dahlström U, Alehagen U. Serum prolactin and macroprolactin in heart failure: no relation to established laboratory or clinical parameters. Ann Clin Biochem. 2011; 48(Pt 1):51–6. DOI: 10.1258/acb.2010.010164.

[73] Hilfiker-Kleiner D, Kaminski K, Podewski E, Bonda T, Schaefer A, Sliwa K, Forster O, Quint A, Landmesser U, Doerries C, Luchtefeld M, Poli V, Schneider MD, Balligand JL, Desjardins F, Ansari A, Struman I, Nguyen NQ, Zschemisch NH, Klein G, Heusch G, Schulz R, Hilfiker A, Drexler H. A cathepsin D-cleaved 16 kDa form of prolactin mediates postpartum cardiomyopathy. Cell. 2007; 128(3):589–600.

[74] Bartoszewicz Z, Kondracka A, Jaźwiec R, Popow M, Dadlez M, Bednarczuk T. Can we accurately measure the concentration of clinically relevant vitamin D metabolites in the circulation? The problems and their consequences. Endokrynol Pol. 2013; 64(3):238–45.

[75] Talaei A, Mohamadi M, Adgi Z. The effect of vitamin D on insulin resistance in patients with type 2 diabetes. Diabetol Metab Syndr. 2013; 5(1):8.

[76] Mozos I, Marginean O. Links between vitamin D deficiency and cardiovascular diseases. Biomed Res Int. 2015; 2015:109275.

[77] Vishwanath P, Kulkarni P, Prashant A. Vitamin D deficiency in India: are we overconcerned? Int J Health Allied Sci. 2014; 3:77–8.

[78] Goswami R, Gupta N, Goswami D, Marwaha RK, Tandon N, Kochupillai N. Prevalence and significance of low 25-hydroxyvitamin D concentrations in healthy subjects in Delhi. Am J Clin Nutr. 2000; 72(2):472–5.

[79] Harinarayan CV, Ramalakshmi T, Prasad UV, Sudhakar D. Vitamin D status in Andhra Pradesh: a population based study. Indian J Med Res. 2008; 127(3):211–8.

[80] Goswami R, Kochupillai N, Gupta N, Goswami D, Singh N, Dudha A. Presence of 25(OH) D deficiency in a rural North Indian village despite abundant sunshine. J Assoc Physicians India. 2008; 56:755–7.

[81] Garg MK, Tandon N, Marwaha RK, Menon AS, Mahalle N. The relationship between serum 25-hydroxy vitamin D, parathormone and bone mineral density in Indian population. Clin Endocrinol (Oxf). 2014; 80(1):41–6.

[82] Roy A, Lakshmy R, Tarik M, Tandon N, Reddy KS, Prabhakaran D. Independent association of severe vitamin D deficiency as a risk of acute myocardial infarction in Indians. Indian Heart J. 2015; 67(1):27–32.

[83] Bonakdaran S, Nejad AF, Abdol-Reza V, Hatefi A, Shakeri M. Impact of oral 1,25-dihydroxy vitamin D (calcitriol) replacement therapy on coronary artery risk factors in type 2 diabetic patients. Endocr Metab Immune Disord Drug Targets. 2013; 13(4):295–300.

[84] Tarcin O, Yavuz DG, Ozben B, et al. Effect of vitamin D deficiency and replacement on endothelial function in asymptomatic subjects. J Clin Endocrinol Metab. 2009; 94:4023–30. DOI: 10.1210/jc.2008-1212.

[85] Li YC, Qiao G, Uskokovic M, Xiang W, Zheng W, Kong J. Vitamin D: a negative endocrine regulator of the renin–angiotensin system and blood pressure. J Steroid Biochem Mol Biol. 2004; 89–90(1–5):387–92.

[86] Oh J, Riek AE, Darwech I, Funai K, Shao J, Chin K, Sierra OL, Carmeliet G, Ostlund RE Jr, Bernal-Mizrachi C. Deletion of macrophage vitamin d receptor promotes insulin resistance and monocyte cholesterol transport to accelerate atherosclerosis in mice. Cell reports. 2015; 10(11):1872–1886.

[87] Pellitero S, Reverter JL, Granada ML, Pizarro E, Pastor MC, Tàssies D, Reverter JC, Salinas I, Sanmartí A. Association of the IGF1/pregnancy-associated plasma protein-A system and adipocytokine levels with the presence and the morphology of carotid plaques in type 2 diabetes mellitus patients with stable glycaemic control. Eur J Endocrinol. 2009; 160(6):925–32.

[88] Bayes-Genis A, Conover CA, Schwartz RS: The insulin-like growth factor axis: a review of atherosclerosis and restenosis. Circ Res. 2000; 86:125–130.

[89] Bayes-Genis A, Conover CA, Overgaard MT, Bailey KR, Christiansen M, Holmes DR, Virmani R, Oxvig C, Schwartz RS: Pregnancy-associated plasma protein A as a marker of acute coronary syndromes. N Engl J Med. 2001; 345:1022–1029.

[90] Cosin-Sales J, Kaski JC, Christiansen M, Kaminski P, Oxvig C, Overgaard MT, Cole D, Holt DW: Relationship among pregnancy associated plasma protein-A levels, clinical characteristics, and coronary artery disease extent in patients with chronic stable angina pectoris. Eur Heart J. 2005; 26:2093–2098.

[91] Conti E, Andreotti F, Zuppi C: Pregnancy-associated plasma protein-A as predictor of outcome in patients with suspected acute coronary syndromes. Circulation. 2004; 109:e211–e212.

[92] Crea F, Andreotti F: Pregnancy associated plasma protein-A and coronary atherosclerosis: marker, friend, or foe? Eur Heart J. 2005; 26:2075–2076.

[93] Piñon P, Kaski JC: Inflammation, atherosclerosis and cardiovascular disease risk: PAPP-A, Lp-PLA2 and cystatin C: new insights or redundant information? Rev Esp Cardiol. 2006; 59:247–258.

[94] Harrington SC, Simari RD, Conover CA. Genetic deletion of pregnancy-associated plasma protein-A is associated with resistance to atherosclerotic lesion development in apolipoprotein E-deficient mice challenged with a high-fat diet. Circ Res. 2007; 100(12):1696–702.

[95] Pellitero S, Reverter JL, Pizarro E, Pastor MC, Granada ML, Tàssies D, Reverter JC, Salinas I, Sanmartí A. Pregnancy-associated plasma protein-A levels are related to glycemic control but not to lipid profile or hemostatic parameters in type 2 diabetes. Diabetes Care. 2007; 30(12):3083–5.

[96] Hjortebjerg R, Lindberg S, Hoffmann S , Jensen JS, Oxvig C, Bjerre M, Frystyk J . PAPP-A and IGFBP-4 fragment levels in patients with ST-elevation myocardial infarction treated with heparin and PCI. Clin Biochem. 2015; 48(4–5):322–8. DOI: 10.1016/j.clinbiochem.2014.11.022

[97] Conover CA, Bale LK, Oxvig C.Targeted Inhibition of Pregnancy Associated Plasma Protein A Activity Reduces Atherosclerotic Plaque Burden in Mice. J Cardiovasc Transl Res. 2016; 9(1):77–9. Doi: 10.1007/s12265-015-9666-9.

[98] Wang-Sattler R, Yu Z, Herder C, Messias AC, Floegel A, He Y, Heim K, Campillos M, Holzapfel C, Thorand B, Grallert H, Xu T et al. Novel biomarkers for pre-diabetes identified by metabolomics. Mol Syst Biol. 2012; 8:615. DOI: 10.1038/msb.2012.43.

[99] Rao PV, Reddy AP, Lu X, Dasari S, Krishnaprasad A, Biggs E, Roberts CT, Nagalla SR. Proteomic identification of salivary biomarkers of type-2 diabetes. J Proteome Res. 2009; 8(1):239–45. DOI: 10.1021/pr8003776.

[100] Arora P. Metabolomics yield a novel biomarker for predicting diabetes mellitus risk in humans. Circ Cardiovasc Genet. 2014; 7(1):95–6. DOI: 10.1161/circgenetics.114.000528

[101] Stegemann C, Pechlaner R, Willeit P, Langley SR, Mangino M, Mayr U, Menni C, Moayyeri A, Santer P, Rungger G, Spector TD, Willeit J, Kiechl S, Mayr M.. Lipidomics profiling and risk of cardiovascular disease in the prospective population-based Bruneck study. Circulation. 2014; 129(18):1821–31. DOI: 10.1161/CIRCULATIONAHA.113.002500

[102] Rauschert S, Uhl O, Koletzko B, Kirchberg F, Mori TA, Huang RC, Beilin LJ, Hellmuth C, Oddy WH. Lipidomics reveals associations of phospholipids with obesity and insulin resistance in young adults. J Clin Endocrinol Metab. 2015:jc20153525. [Epub ahead of print].

[103] Wurtz P, Havulinna AS, Soininen P, Tynkkynen T, Prieto-Merino D, Tillin T, Ghorbani A, Artati A, Wang Q, Tiainen M et al. Metabolite profiling and cardiovascular event

risk: a prospective study of 3 population-based cohorts. Circulation. 2015; 131(9):774–85. DOI: 10.1161/CIRCULATIONAHA.114.013116.

[104] Shah SH, Sun JL, Stevens RD, Bain JR, Muehlbauer MJ, Pieper KS, Haynes C, Hauser ER, Kraus WE, Granger CB, Newgard CB, Califf RM, Newby LK. Baseline metabolomic profiles predict cardiovascular events in patients at risk for coronary artery disease. Am Heart J. 2012; 163(5):844–850.

[105] Lappas M, Mundra PA, Wong G, Huynh K, Jinks D, Georgiou HM, Permezel M, Meikle PJ. The prediction of type 2 diabetes in women with previous gestational diabetes mellitus using lipidomics. Diabetologia. 2015; 58(7):1436–42. DOI: 10.1007/s00125-015-3587-7.

Chapter 6

# Biomarkers, Obesity, and Cardiovascular Diseases

Monica Navarro Meza and
Jesus Alcala-Bejarano Carrillo

Additional information is available at the end of the chapter

http://dx.doi.org/10.5772/62555

**Abstract**

Obesity and overweight are among the major health problems in the world today. The excessive accumulation of fat in adipose tissue is accompanied by low-grade inflammation, adipokine secretion dysregulation, oxidative stress, and an alteration of the secretion of gut hormones and food intake related to peptides. This is related to the development of cardiovascular diseases, which have been increased worldwide during the last 15 years approximately. The biomarkers are tremendously important to predict, diagnose, and observe the therapeutic success of common complex multifactorial metabolic diseases, such as obesity and cardiovascular diseases. This chapter presents a review of the most common biomarkers that have been used in the prevention, treatment, prognosis, and diagnosis of obesity and cardiovascular diseases.

**Keywords:** biomarkers, cardiovascular disease, obesity, genetic markers, serum markers

## 1. Introduction

### 1.1. Overweight and obesity

Obesity and overweight have greatly become a stigma in most of the countries around the world since the middle of the past century, depending on the location, but it was not recognized as a disease until 2013 [1]. Its presence and the difficulty to eradicate it, it is mainly due to the multifactorial nature of this trait that depends on genetic and environmental factors as well as stimuli, learning, reward, and representation of food processing at high centers of the nervous system, which results in an increase of energy intake and subsequently body fat [2]. The most recent estimations (2014) by World Health Organization (WHO) have pointed out that more than 1.9 billion adults who were 18 years old or more (39%) suffered overweight and more than 600 million were obese (13%). Predictions about this epidemic growth do not seem to be very promising with a theoretical increase of 33% in obesity prevalence and a 130% increase in severe obesity prevalence by 2030 [3].

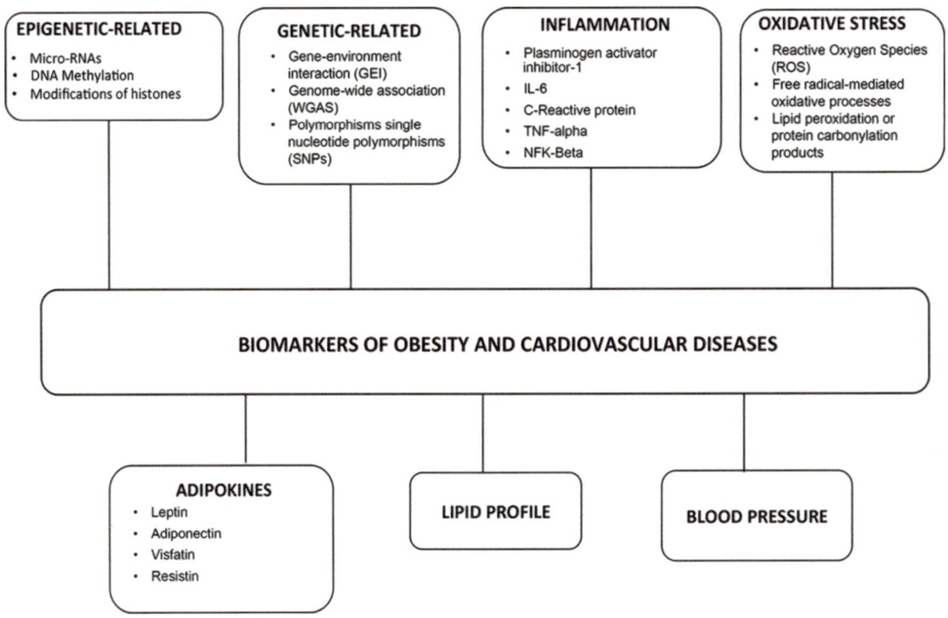


The WHO defines overweight as an abnormal or excessive fat accumulation that represents a health risk [4]. This disproportionate fat in the adipose tissue includes a low grade of inflammation, adipokine secretion dysregulation, hypoxia, oxidative stress, and an alteration of the secretion of gut hormones and food intake-related peptides [5]. All of these disturbances are associated to a wide variety of disorders such as diabetes, cardiovascular diseases (CVDs), cancer, depression, conception and respiratory problems, and musculoskeletal disorders [6].

Body mass index (BMI) is a measure of weight adjusted to height and calculates weight as in kilograms divided by the square of height in meters (kg/m$^2$). Although BMI is often considered an indicator of body fatness, it is a surrogate measure of body fat because it measures excess weight rather than excess fat. Despite this fact, studies have shown that BMI is correlated with more direct measures of body fat, such as underwater weighing and dual-energy X-ray absorptiometry. The clinical limitations of BMI should be considered. Factors such as age, sex, ethnicity, and muscle mass can influence the relationship between BMI and body fat [7]. Considerable literature has grown up around the theme and suggests that other measures of body fat, such as skinfold thicknesses, bioelectrical impedance, and/or dual-energy X-ray absorption may be more accurate than BMI, for example, waist circumference (sometimes divided by height) is a simple measure of fat distribution. The main problem of standardization is that the cost of it tends to be highly overpriced, intrusive, not widely available, or difficult to standardize across observers or devices. Therefore, the procedures previously mentioned are considered not suitable for a regular physician exercise purpose. In addition, most of the literature concerning obesity health risks is based on several BMI studies and their outcomes, yet there are not enough standardized frames to calculate body fatness which may compromising the measurement of the fat amount that an individual may preserve.

Nowadays, just one of the anti-obesity therapies was approved; bariatric surgery can effectively lead to considerable weight loss sustained over the long-term period [8]. However, it has largely been rendered impractical as a useful anti-obesity approach, mostly due to its cost and its mortality rate. In general, obesity alters the perfectly co-ordinated homeostatic system that regulates food intake, leading to an increase, decrease, or absence of change of the signals that are involved in this function such as adipokines, metabolites, gastrointestinal, central peptides, and other factors. There is awareness regarding those effects, but discovering the contribution of each one of those aspects and its relation to food intake is still obscure.

### 1.2. Cardiovascular diseases (CVDs)

Cardiovascular diseases refer to a disorder of the heart or blood vessels; there are three main types of CVDs depending on the grade of affectation and organ that is being disturb: heart could suffer acute coronary syndromes, angina, arrhythmia, cardiomyopathy, coronary heart disease, heart failure, inflammatory heart disease, ischemic heart disease, etc.

The brain could suffer cerebrovascular disease, hemorrhagic stroke, ischemic stroke, and/or the circulatory system, deep vein thrombosis, hypertensive heart disease, peripheral artery disease and pulmonary embolism [9].

The most recent data show that global death rate caused by CVDS increased by 41% from 1990 to 2013 (except 39% out of that 41% decreases at specific age death rates) [10] and it has become the first death cause of all noncommunicable diseases (NCDs) by 17.5 million people annually. Factors such as smoking, physical inactivity, alcohol ingest, and unhealthy diets increase the risk of suffering NCDs [11]. Heart attacks and strokes can be prevented if high-risk individuals are detected and treated early. For eligible subjects aged from 40 to 79 years, a prescription where aspirin and/or statin to lower blood pressure has been estimated to prevent about one-fifth of cardiovascular deaths. This instruction can be assigned to a prospect population with an increase tendency of suffering NCDs (including those with hypertension, diabetes, and other cardiovascular risk factors) where an integrated primary program care is implemented [12]. Several mechanisms have been proposed to be linked to CVDs with obesity, along with the state of inflammation, oxidative stress, and gut microbiome [13]. Thus, there is significant evidence of association with central obesity and coronary artery disease [14] and stroke [15]. Nevertheless, in the last decade, there is no consensus about the relation between obesity and mortality due to CVDs. In this decade, the hypothesis called "obesity paradox" has shown that mild obese people have healthier cardiovascular profile than average weight individuals [16]. This chapter gathers the most significant information concerning validated or well-correlated biomarkers and its relation with obesity and CVDs.

## 2. Indicators and biomarkers

### 2.1. Definition and classification

The term biomarker was presented in 1989 as a Medical Subject Heading (MeSH) and defined in 2001 as *"a characteristic that is objectively measured and evaluated as an indicator of normal biological processes, pathogenic processes, or pharmacologic responses to a therapeutic treatment* [17]." The tern biomarker itself may refer to different concepts; for example, interleukin-6 (IL-6) could classified as a marker of inflammation, obesity, or CVDs.

It should be quite clear the difference between a biomarker and an endpoint. A biomarker, because of the nature of its definition, is objective and may not related to a patient's emotions and sense of well-being. Thus, an endpoint defines how a subject in a study or clinical trial "*feels, functions or survives.*" In some trials, they use biomarkers as surrogate endpoints, but it is mandatory to obtain solid, scientific evidence (eg epidemiological, therapeutic, and/or pathophysiological) [18]. Depending on the function of the biomarker, it can be classified into markers of exposure, effect, and/or susceptibility [19]. Other classifications are based on their biochemical or biological properties (e.g., metabolites, hormones, adipokines) or the disease of interest (e.g., CVDs, obesity) [20].

### 2.2. Relevance and validity

An important aspect of a biomarker is that it refers to its relevance, a term commonly used for Biomarkers, which have significant impact on public health Matters. Due to the use of them in research or risk Assessments, they can contribute to provide useful information that cannot be obtained accurately with the implementation of other approaches such as surveys, environmental measurements, or record revisions.

During the past decade, there has been noticed a rapid development of the study of the validity of biomarkers since then it is still being debated. To validate them, it is required either laboratory and epidemiological support, and even more specifically, a case of control and cohort studies with prospective studies as a key to its investigation to provide estimates of the risk of disease in individuals with and without a particular biomarker which the cost is the main problem [19]. Recently, in order to evaluate the adequacy of a biomarker, it is important to take into consideration three important matters: the analytical validity, clinical validity, and clinical utility [21]. A tool that is highly recommended and needed for evaluating a potential biomarker is the receiver-operating characteristics curve (ROC) analysis, which is well-explained in a study [22] and that can be summarized as a statistical tool that allows the determination of the threshold which can be considered as a "*positive*" or "*non-positive*" in relation to a specific biomarker and a particular disease; ROC is based on the concept of sensitivity that describes the portion of subjects with the trait that have been determined as "*positive*" and specificity that tell us the portion of subjects without the trait that have been identified as "*negative.*" This tool is essential for biomarkers that are detected with metabolomics techniques.

A case of a scale used to classify the validity of biomarkers is the one proposed by the European Society of Cardiology (ESC) which establishes a range from I to III, considering the evidence and/or in agreement to the scientific literature as well as it considers the level of evidence depending on the type of the articles that were conducted [23, 24].

### 2.3. Biomarkers in obesity and CVDs

Biomarkers for obesity and CVDs can be used for three different purposes: study the tendency a prevalence, facilitating the identification of a target population that could require an approach to lower the risk of obesity development or future weight management, and improving the understanding of this complex trait which will help to find the adequate treatment [25].

When speaking about obesity, there are not enough validated biomarkers to be used as a diagnostic tool. That situation probably is mainly due to this trait has different levels of complexity and as we aforementioned, there are numerous traits associated with obesity which each one has its own characteristics that could also vary among the types of populations; such fact probably determines the specific alteration of the physiology and thus the biomarkers. As a matter of fact, there are some biomarkers that have shown strong correlation and signs of reliability related to BMI and/or body fat, which are going to be described hereafter.

In the case of CVDs, there are a wide variety of traits that can be caused and/or either by influenced common factors or specific ones. This chapter focuses on diseases such atherosclerosis, stroke, and heart attack as the most influence mortality traits and well-known biomarkers.

## 3. Genetics-related biomarkers

It has been proposed that genetic modifications could be involved in predisposition to obesity [26]; investigations of gene expression regulatory mechanisms during the evolution of obesity could be applied in prevention and early diagnosis, and treatment. This disease is associated with oxidative stress, insulin resistance, systemic inflammation, endothelial cell dysfunction [25]. The obesity and CVDs are the result from a complex interplay of many genetic and environmental factors [27]. Epidemiological and clinical studies have examined the roles of lifestyle, diet habits, and genetic factors in the development of this disease; studies related to the gene-environment interaction (GEI) have increased rapidly.

However, preliminary results regarding GEI on obesity are mostly inconclusive [28]. Obesity has become one of the most serious health problems, and its occurrence is attributed to the interplay between environmental and genetic factors. Over 40% of the variation in obesity-related phenotypes is estimated to be Heritable. Genetic studies and knockout mouse models have uncovered new obesity-associated genes [29].

Epidemiological and clinical studies trials have examined roles of lifestyle and dietary factors in obesity prevention and weight control; it has been suggested that alterations in adipocyte growth, differentiation, and apoptosis could contribute to changes in fat mass involved in obesity. Recent studies indicate that the turnover rate of pre-adipocytes is low [2].

The increase in fat mass can develop adipocyte hypertrophy or hyperplasia; larger fat cells are closely linked to a greater fat mass rate and production of inflammatory cytokines [29]. This is because it proposed a possible approach, which aims to reduce fat mass and is by performing a therapeutically regulate adipocyte differentiation; however, cellular and molecular mechanisms that are involved are not completely understood in the adipogenesis. In the lasted years, this connection has been connected and concerned in the role of Micro-RNAs (miRNAs) and the fat cell development [30]. There is limited evidence of genetic involvement in the development of obesity.

Advanced studies of genome-wide association (WGAS) and obesity disorders stated that this field has a great potential to identify human genetics-related biomarkers and the contribution to elucidate the genetic mechanisms in the development of obesity. In this matter, it has been reported several genes involved in fat mass and obesity (FTO) such melanocortin-4 receptor (MC4R) which can be identified with GWA scans that have been convincingly associated with obesity risk in a variety of subjects population [31]. However, it has suggested and indicated that replication of genetic-related biomarkers may fail in small samples or in subjects exposed to other environmental factors; obesity is a multifactorial disorder that has a genetic basis but requires environmental influences in order to be able to manifest itself.

An estimation from 40 to 60% of the variation in obesity-related phenotypes BMI and sum of skinfold thickness, fat mass, and leptin levels are thought to be heritable [32]. Studies that show a sequel to discover the specific loci or genes involved in obesity, primarily through the combination of linkage scan and candidate gene-based association, have been performed to identify and examining the co-segregation of genetic markers distributed evenly in genome with the disease within families. It is highly important to mention that there are 253 quantitative-trait loci (QTLs) identified in 61 genome-wide scans, and 52 genomic regions contain QTLs, yet there are limitations in the linkage of the studies. The candidate-gene association analyses focus on identifying loci which are functional or positional; approximately 120 genes are different candidate that have been associated with obesity phenotypes [33]. Such candidate genes are categorized either to be knowledgeable or proposed to be a role that could be influence of adipogenesis, lipid turnover, insulin signaling, mitochondrion and energy expenditure, and adipokine secretion [34]. Some examples of genetic-related biomarkers prohormone convertase are (1/3) PCSK, PPARG (peroxisoma proliferadores-activados receptor gamma), UCP1 (disociación de proteínas 1), UCP2, UCP3, ADRB2 (receptor beta-adrenérgico 2), ADRB3 y PLIN (perilipina) [35–38].

The majority of association studies of candidate genes in obesity focus on only a limited number of single-nucleotide polymorphisms (SNPs) [39]. The narrow topography of genome variation has impeded the candidate gene approach [2, 40].

There were found significant associations with SNP which is mapped in a biological candidate gene for monogenic obesity and fat mass and obesity risk [41]. Studies demonstrated that different shapes of genes variants might cause either monogenic or common form obesity that shares the same pathophysiological changes.

Recent findings have reemphasized the importance of *epistasis*, or gene–gene interactions as a contributing factor to the unexplained heritability of obesity; methods such as statistical epistasis networks (SEN) provide a reference that is likely to be used to address a computing challenge of studying pair-wise interactions among thousands of genetic variants. The outcomes have drawn a heritability rate estimated from 40 to 70% [42]. Still, genetic loci that have been found to be associated with BMI can partially explain its variation. Epistasis or gene–gene interactions are a possible contributing factors to this "*missing heritability*" [43]; meanwhile, some studies suggest to analyze pair-wise interactions that are associated with BMI among SNPs from twelve genes robustly associated with obesity [44]. The most prevalent leptin/leptin receptor genes (LEP/LEPR) and ghrelin/ghrelin receptor genes (GHRL/GHSR) SNP studied were LEP G-2548A, LEPR Q223R, and Leu72-Met [45, 46].

## 4. Epigenetic-related biomarkers

Previous literature has indicated that epigenetics heritable changes in concordance with the individual DNA sequence, while meta-analysis papers related with the genome have proposed a tool to assess the genetic variants of obesity and epigenetic modifications that can be influenced by environmental factors.

Some of the major genetic mechanisms that could be mentioned to help to regulate a gene expression are DNA methylation of guanine-followed cytokines, hypermethylation, modifications of histone, and RNA non-coding.

### 4.1. DNA methylation

The GWAs have identified 55 genetic loci that were associated with either obesity or BMI, but they only explain 1.18–1.45% of the variation observed in BMI. It has been validated the use of blood leukocytes method to categorize the epigenetic modifications that could be used as molecular markers to predict physiological changes linked with obesity and insulin resistance, which are closely associated with methylation and weight status [47].

Newest data have shown that alterations in global DNA methylation may significantly influence the risk incidence of cancer and CVDs [48]. The increased epigenetic variances may be reflected during the adaptation to the environmental risk factors. The obesity is the result of the interplay between external (environmental) and internal (genetic) factors [13]. The methylated CpG sites (DMCs) and differentially variable CpG sites (DVCs) may be related to the development and growth of obesity as well as CVDs [49]. The recent epigenome-wide association studies (EWAS) have identified several DMCs related to obesity [50].

The literature focused on studies in epigenetic sites and proposed intron DNA methylation are able to indirectly prevent a transcription [51]. The DNA methylation is an epigenetic process that influences a wide variety of biological mechanisms including gene expression, chromosomal stability, imprinting, and cellular differentiation [52].

The abnormal DNA methylation patterns, including genome-wide hypomethylation, gene-specific hypo- and hypermethylation, have been shown to be associated with a range of health outcomes. In order to know the global levels of DNA, there are several methods available [total content of 5-methylcytosine (5-mC)] [53].

It has been suggested that obese individuals are likely to possess unique epigenetic patterns that tend to vary with weight. On the other hand, studies that have examined the methylation patterns in leukocytes showed a variation in individuals who lost enough weight from a certain level of obesity to normal weight [54]. The studies related to DNA methylation and obesity that had primarily focused on gene-specific methylation [55, 53] as well as recent global recent methylation levels studies in DNA from blood and BMI [55, 56].

The bioinformatics analysis of the search for the CpG islands promoter obesity-related genes sites has identified a high CpGs density that are implicated with adipogenesis such as human peroxisome proliferator-activated receptor gamma coactivator 1 (PPARGC1), the small heterodimer partner (NROB2), the glucocorticoid receptor (NR3C1), the peroxisome proliferator-activated receptor gamma (PPARG), the basic fibroblast growth factor (FGF2), the phosphatase and tensin homolog (PTEN), the cyclin-dependent kinase inhibitor 1A (CDKN1A), as well as at the estrogen receptor 1 (ESR1) [57–59].

It has been displayed that the same methylation frequency than subjects are likely to show in CpG sites located at 51 and 31 depending on the transcription of the starting site of the LEP gene [60]. Three CpG sites involved in BMI are 1. CpG7 (46801672, cg16672562) 2. CpG1, and 3. CpG5 [61].

The HIF3A regulates the transcriptional activity of some genes related to adipocytes [73]. The increased level of methylation in HIF3A relates to increasing BMI [62–64]; a BMI linked to DNA methylation might play a role in obesity [53].

**4.2. Modifications of histones**

Epidemiological studies that link epigenetic gene regulation and obesity outcomes are needed to understand the effects of the exposure development and identification of epigenetic biomarkers of latent onset of obesity [65].

Such modifications occur through various mechanisms, for instance, the post-translational histone modifications that can cause a transcriptional suppression.

Environmental stimuli where diet and exercise are meant to regulate these mechanisms might have inflammation as a probable contributory factor [66]. Recent literature in the field of epigenomics has led to the first epigenetic potential markers to detect obesity at birth which provides important foundations to determine the effects of exposure developmental to obesogenic [65]. During early stages, the relative expression of genes determines whether mesenchyme stem cells differentiate either osteocytes or adipocytes that potentially predispose the body to fat accumulation [67]. Furthermore, obesity-related chronic low-grade inflammation is implicated with an epigenetic level in the development of some forms of cancer [68].

### 4.3. RNA non-coding and obesity (Micro-RNAs)

Research focused on the gene expression regulatory mechanisms in obesity evolution, and CVDS will have crucial applications in prevention, early diagnosis, and treatment. The miRNAs are small molecular, non-coding, 21–23 nucleotide long RNAs that negatively regulate gene expression by pairing with the 3'-untranslated region (UTR) of their target miRNAs [69]. The miRNAs are involved in highly regulated processes such as proliferation, differentiation, apoptosis, and metabolic processes. The discovery of non-coding miRNAs which can post-transcriptionally regulate thousands of genes has generated enormous research interest [26]. Several studies have highlighted the significance of miRNAs in maintaining metabolic homeostasis [70, 71].

Furthermore, miRNAs have been found in tissues, in serum, in plasma, and other body fluids that have a stable form that is protected from an endogenous RNase activity. Because of these unique characteristics of circulating miRNAs, a possible useful biomarker for supplemental diagnosis can be inferred. The study of serum samples miRNAs can play the role of a potential biomarker as well as provide them since these have shown the ability to induce heritable modifications of several morphological, physiological, and behavioral phenotypes. Data concerning miRNAs imply that five types (miR-142-3p, miR-140-5p, miR-15a, miR-520c-3c, and miR-423-5p) may be primal biomarkers for risk estimation and classification in obese patients [72]. On the other hand, there have been studies in adipocyte-specific mRNAs that also have detected in isolated exosomes and microvesicles from rat serum. In recent researching, miRNA biomarkers have been found in many chronic diseases, for example, cancer, CVDs, and type 2 diabetes [82, 73]; probable future miRNA biomarkers may assist in the early diagnosis of chronic diseases and also provide new therapeutic targets [74]. Furthermore, the impact of extracellular factors such as inflammatory cytokines on adipocyte miRNAs might be considered [75].

The understanding of role miRNAs in proliferation and differentiation of adipocytes during fat cell development could provide new therapeutic targets for anti-obesity drugs [76–77]. The alterations in the number and size of adipocytes are typically accompanied by changes in the expression patterns for miRNAs subsets [78].

The expression of the majority of these miRNAs is known to be controlled by certain cytokines and adipokines that downgrade miR-103 and miRNAs-143 and upgrade miRNAs-221 and miRNAs-222 [79]. The levels of miRNAs-103, miRNAs-107, miRNAs-143, and miRNAs-185 were upgraded in the lean state but downgraded in the obese state [80]. Nevertheless, from the miRNAs analyzed until now, just miRNAs-34a has been found to be positively correlated with the rate of adipocyte differentiation and development of the BMI [81].

Moreover, the miRNAs have also been recognized as regulators of adipocyte metabolic integration, energy homeostasis, and differentiation [83, 84]. Further studies have shown widespread regulation of protein levels caused by miRNAs in cellular and animal models [85].

Several miRNAs, such as miR-126, miR-132, miR-146, miR-155, and miR-221, have emerged as important transcriptional regulators of some inflammation-related mediators [86]. These non-coding RNAs are emerging as biomarkers with diagnosis value in prognosis protocols in personalized treatment of inflammation. The non-coding RNAs and the administration of exogenous miRNAs could be soon a promising therapeutic strategy in the treatment of inflammation-related diseases, for example, obesity [87]. There is also increasing evidence that non-coding miRNAs are critically involved in post-transcriptional regulation of cell functions, including oxidative stress, inflammation, regulation of cell proliferation, adipocyte differentiation, angiogenesis, and apoptosis [88].

## 5. Inflammatory biomarkers in obesity and CVDS

The inflammatory process is a very complex reaction since it is necessary to conduct further research for a better understanding of biological inflammatory biomarkers activity [89]. The obesity-induced chronic inflammation is a component during a pathogenesis of insulin resistance and metabolic syndrome. The pro-inflammatory cytokines can cause insulin resistance in adipose tissue, skeletal muscle, and liver by inhibiting the insulin signal transduction.

The initiating factors of this inflammatory response remain to be fully determined, and chronic inflammation in tissues that liver and fat could cause is localized in insulin resistance through an autocrine/paracrine cytokine signaling, and systemic insulin resistance through an endocrine cytokine signaling, which contribute to an abnormal metabolic phase. The role of inflammation in CVDs is to support the development of pharmacological strategies that aim to reduce inflammation [90]. The studies are mostly focused on the effectors of the inflammatory program, but not on the underlying causes, which initiates the pro-inflammatory stage; some candidates meant to be markers in the inflammatory response are cytokines/chemokines and C-reactive protein (CRP).

In addition, it has been proposed that pro-inflammatory cytokines formed increase the hepatic synthesis of an acute-phase protein. However, it is still unknown how the inflammation of low intensity contributes to increase the risk of suffering CVDs in overweight and obese individuals [91].

The identification of inflammatory markers improves insulin sensitivity and glucose control in insulin-resistant patients, and they are responsible of the reducing risk of CVDs and its complications [92]. It is known that obesity mechanisms, particularly visceral fat that are related to morbi-mortality include increasing in and releasing of expression adipose tissue cytokines that are crucial in the phase proteins.

The resistin, leptin, and adiponectin adipokines, which are secreted by adipocytes, are capable to also affect the inflammation and insulin resistance. When is the case of a chronic and low-intensity inflammatory process, chemokines locally secreted attract pro-inflammatory macrophages to the adipose tissue and they will stimulate the cytokines release, which will activate the inflammatory way in adipocytes and adjacent tissues (autocrine and paracrine effect) that aggravate the inflammation and insulin resistance [87]. The result of an internal environment in adipose tissue is lipotoxic and pro-inflammatory; therefore, it is important to consider that local environmental cues that related the initial inflammatory response in obesity and insulin resistance mechanisms [93].

### 5.1. Plasminogen activator inhibitor-1

The PAI-1 is a protein that inhibits the residual plasminogen activator, which cleaves the plasmin to plasminogen; thus, it is the first physiological inhibitor of fibrinolysis in situ; this occurs while presenting the capacity to inhibit the plasmin forerunner that has as a function the rupture of fibrin network, thus avoiding a thrombus formation [94]. The PAI-1 is produced in several types of tissues, including liver and adipocytes. Many factors contribute to increase the expression and release of PAI-1 in adipose tissue (especially, visceral fat), among them the insulin, TGF-β, and IL-6, [95, 96]. These factors associated with the increase of body fat can explain theirs enhanced concentration in individuals obese and insulin resistant [97].

### 5.2. Interleukin-6 (IL-6)

Recent studies suggest that inflammation markers may reflect different aspects in the risk of developing CVDs and they may correlated with its grade of severity. Furthermore, it has been suggested that interleukin-6 (IL-6) might represent a major mediator of acute-phase protein response while it is a multifunctional cytokine produced by a variety of hematopoietic and non-hematopoietic cells [98, 99]. The IL-6 upgrades and regulates several acute-phase proteins such as CRP, fibrinogen, $\alpha$1-antitrypsin, and serum amyloid [99]. This cytokine regulates lipid metabolism and C-reactive protein (CRP) production and the increase in obesity as well as it is related to insulin resistance [100, 102]. Additionally, it has been shown an association with BMI and fat [103].

### 5.3. C-reactive protein (CRP)

The C-reactive protein (CRP) has been extensively studied in individuals with CVDs, including those that apparently to be healthy. The features related to high CRP levels risk factors and CVDs are dyslipidemia, hypertension, diabetes mellitus, obesity, smoking, and sedentary lifestyle. The CRP used as an inflammatory marker detection of CVDs in plasma, the concentration is easy to determine, and it has the best clinical and epidemiological correlation until now. Another pro-inflammatory cytokines are IL-1-type cytokines that could be stimulated in the liver production of CRP. High levels of certain inflammatory markers such as IL-6, tumor necrosis factor alpha (TNFa) and CRP are also associated with visceral fat [104].

### 5.4. Tumor necrosis factor alpha (TNF-alpha)

The TNF-a is a cytokine that mediates inflammatory responses and is implicated in pathogenesis such as cancer, diabetes, and obesity. The TNF-a is secreted by adipose tissue in obesity [106]; the major pathways activated by TNF-a include caspases, nuclear factor kappa-light-chain-enhancer of activated B cells (NFκB), and mitogen-activated protein kinases (MAP kinases) The TNF-a increases its expression in adipocytes associated with obesity and is related to increased visceral fat deposition and insulin resistance [107]; other studies was associated with glucose uptake and insulin resistance [105], partly through increased expression of cytokines in muscle [108, 109].

### 5.5. NFK-beta (nuclear factor kappa-light-chain-enhancer of activated B cells)

The NF-κB has an important role in regulation of immune response, and its dysregulation has been linked to cancer, inflammatory, and autoimmune diseases. Moreover, it was proposed that is an important cellular regulator in different mechanisms associated with cytokines and nutrients. Regarding nutrients that act via the mechanism, which is independent from NF-κB, demonstrate that obesity promotes the survival of inflammatory, possibly through NF-κB regulated macrophage mechanism [110, 111]. The activation of NF-κB creates a connection with a decrease of expression of proteins specific to β-cells, insulin, glucose transporter 2 (GLUT-2), pancreatic, and the increase in activity of iNOS [112].

The involvement of NF-κB in metabolic pathways comes from a complex network that involves a vast number of factors and post-transcriptional processes [113, 114]. This factor is related to obesity and CVDs mainly because its involvement in the promotion of the inflammatory factors expression (and could be anti-inflammatory as well) [106], insulin resistance, and adipokines such as visfatin takes place [115], and the microflora can have a role in the inflammation process [118].

## 6. Oxidative stress biomarkers in obesity

Oxidative stress is a major player CVDs and obesity [116, 117], the reactive oxygen species (ROS)-dependent signaling pathways, transcriptional and epigenetic deregulation, inducing chronic low-grade inflammation, platelet activation, and endothelial dysfunction. Because of this, several oxidative biomarkers proposed with the potential to improve current under standing of the mechanisms underlying CVDs [119].

Oxidative stress results from an imbalance between the production of ROS and biological systems ability to detoxify the reactive intermediates or to repair the resulting damages, which can impact all the cell components, including proteins, lipids, and DNA. High levels of ROS generated by hypertrophied adipocytes impact many metabolic signaling pathways as well as

http://dx.doi.org/10.5772/62555

neighboring environment for instance perivascular endothelium or immune residing [121]. Such impairment is further amplified by altered systemic metabolic parameters (hyperglycemia, hyperlipemia, hyperleptinemia, etc.) that also enhance ROS generation. Overall, systemic oxidative stress-associated obesity directly impacts insulin sensitivity of metabolic organs, promotes inflammation, and alters lipid metabolism or endothelial dysfunction. The increased levels of systemic oxidative stress that occur in obesity may contribute to the obesity-associated development of others diseases. Clinical evidences for obesity associated with oxidative stress have been provided by using a biomarker of free radical-mediated oxidative processes [122, 123].

Systemic oxidative stress is part of the numerous biological alterations reported during chronic obesity. Evidences regarding obesity-induced oxidative stress are derived from several clinical studies, which have established correlations with biomarkers, or end-products of free radicals-mediated oxidative stress (lipid peroxidation or protein carbonylation products) and BMI [124, 125]. There is also an inverse relationship between body fat, visceral fat, and antioxidant defense markers in obese individuals; the hypothesis is that oxidative stress is producing the development of metabolic disorders, especially insulin-resistant state, and it has been supported by different studies where treatments reducing ROS production improved insulin sensitivity, hyperlipidemia, and hepatic steatosis [59].

Hypertrophied adipocytes have been reported as a significant source of ROS that promote a significant dysfunction by altering the adipokine production. Furthermore, oxidative stress associated with obesity has also shown to alter the function of many cell types or tissues leading to consider oxidative stress as a contributor in obesity-related metabolic diseases [126]. Other examples of enzymes that have been proposed as biomarkers in oxidative stress, which may be an important contributor to ROS generation, are nitric oxide synthase (NOS) can react with vascular NO- and NAD-dependent deacetylases that will drive antioxidant and anti-inflammatory responses [127, 128].

## 7. Lipid profile

A factor that has more influence in these traits is lipoproteins and its related factors which among them is cholesterol, that is, also a sterol (or modified steroid), a molecule lipid that is biosynthesized by all animal cells, and it is required to maintain both membrane structural integrity and fluidity. This molecule is transported by a low-density lipoprotein with different types that depend on the density which are named as LDL, high-density lipoprotein, or HDL [129].

In case of cholesterol, low-density lipoprotein cholesterol, high-density lipoprotein cholesterol, and triglycerides are the types that are the most studied, accepted, and recommended by *American and European Guidelines* as risk status of cardiovascular issues surrogate endpoints.

These biomarkers joint with others agents (age, smoking, etc.) are used in the *Framingham Score*, which is one of the most used, to estimate the risk of cardiovascular diseases (up to 10 or 30 years). However, there is a slight difference where age taken into consideration; levels of total cholesterol and blood pressure give us a risk of CVDs along with the recommendation of the analysis of the lipid profile. The total amount of cholesterol increased is a major cause of burden disease in both the developed countries and non-developing ones as a risk factor for ischemic heart disease and stroke [130]. When high levels of cholesterol are present, atherosclerotic plaque formation may take place, which can result in the narrowing of the coronary arteries and an increase of a heart attack and stroke due to the increased probability of a rupture. These references for total cholesterol are given by the *American Heart Association* (AHA) that recommends a desirable level of <200 mg/ml with a high risk (twice higher risk than lower levels) of heart attack and stroke if the levels are above 240 mg/ml [131]. LDL cholesterol (LDL-C) is the major cholesterol-carrying lipoprotein, and it makes up the majority of total cholesterol in blood. Moreover, LDL-C deposits in the arterial wall can lead to atherosclerotic plaque formation [132], which are recommended to be between 100 and 159 mg/ml, taking into consideration that a level above is a high risk to suffer cardiac disorders.

HDL cholesterol (HDL-C) is a significant predictor of CVDs risk, and its plasma levels have an inverse correlation with the risk of atherosclerosis and CVDs [132, 133]. It is reported that low levels of HDL are associated with cerebrovascular disorders in several populations (*Framingham Study, the Copenhagen Study, and the Israeli Heart Disease Study*) [134]; in any of the cases, it is not unanimously considered as a surrogate endpoint to CVDs risk due to the complexity of its physiology [126]. Organizations as the European Society of Cardiology recommend levels below 1.0 mmol/L (40 mg/dL) in men and 1.2 mmol/L (45 mg/dL) in women [23, 24].

Triglycerides are majority form of fats in vertebrates, and they consist of an ester of glycerol esterified with three fatty acids which have different physical properties depending on the type of the acid; its physiology, as it is pointed out in the extensive review performed by [135].

Triglycerides have an enormous complexity and are involved in many traits such as CVDs, obesity and diabetes. Although, by itself, it is not atherogenic, it is related to atherogenic factors as atherogenic cholesterol-enriched remnant lipoprotein particles (RLPs) and its relationship has been closer to metabolic syndrome and TD2M. Thus, its consideration as a surrogate endpoint for CVDs despite the fact categorized as general, it is becoming clearer as more studies are being conducted. Nevertheless, there is evidence that non-fasting triglycerides may predict CHD risk better in the post-prandial state [136, 137], but due to the lack of standardization, measuring non-fasting triglycerides is not recommended.

On the other hand, there are recommendations given by AHA (and ATP III) that have been changing as time passes by and based on the ethnic differences. There are not standard recommendations, yet this organization (and the ESC) recommends the following thresholds: Desirable <150 mg/dL, Borderline-high 150–199 mg/dL, High 200–499 mg/dL, and Very High ≥500 mg/dL [138].

## 8. Blood pressure

Elevated blood pressure can cause stress in the walls of the blood vessels, which can vanish the development of arteriosclerosis and increase the risk of myocardial infarction (MI) as well as stroke. Also, due to the increase of the pressure, it could led a coronary artery disease (CAD) and widening of the left ventricle [132].

High blood pressure is one of the leading risk factors for global mortality and is estimated to have caused 9.4 million deaths in 2010. A meta-analysis which includes 1 million individuals has indicated that death from both CHD and stroke increase progressively and linearly from BP levels as low as 115 mmHg systolic and 75 mmHg diastolic upwards [138].

The WHO pointed out that a "reduction in systolic blood pressure of 10 mmHg is associated with a 22% reduction in coronary heart disease, 41% reduction in stroke in randomized trials, and a 41–46% reduction in cardiometabolic mortality in epidemiological studies" [139]. Raised blood pressure is defined as systolic blood pressure ≥140 mmHg and/or diastolic blood pressure ≥90 mmHg among adults (<60 years) [140]. Briefly, the reliability of blood pressure as a surrogate endpoint is supported by an extensive number clinical trials and observational studies [141].

## 9. Adipokines

### 9.1. Leptin

This peptide belongs to the adipokine family, it has a molecular weight of 16 KDa, and it consists of 146 amino acids. It was first discover in 1994 after the naming its gene as the *ob* because of the link between a mutation of it and the subsequent development of obesity. Thus, its receptor was subsequently named as the Ob-R and has several variants due to alternatives splicing that combined with the fact that they can act via different signaling pathways, (JAK/STAT, phosphoinositol-3-kinase, etc.), making possible the involvement of this peptide in a wide spectrum of functions in the body. Leptin is mostly secreted in adipose tissue with a correlation with the amount of it in the body. The leptin levels in human and rodent are the measurement of plasma leptin and ob RNA in obese and weight-reduced subjects. Serum immunoreactive-leptin concentrations are found in normal weight and obese humans but recent data show that it is also released by the placenta, skeletal muscle, and stomach [142].

Plasma concentrations vary mainly due to fat amount in the body by an average of 1300–1600 pg/ml in rats [143] and between 6000–10,000 pg/ml in humans [144]. These levels are altered in obesity (until now it is not clear if it is a cause or a consequence), and it seems that there is a state of leptin resistance [145] and the levels decreased with a mild weight lost [146].

It has an anorexigenic effect and the lack of it increase food intake [147]. This peptide is still not validate as a surrogate endpoint for any CVDs, but there are several studies that show an involvement on CVDs with a pro-atherogenic effect due to its involvement in vascular proliferation and smooth muscle migration [148].

Although it is a useful tool, but it is not consider as a surrogate endpoint neither for the risk nor for the severity of obesity, but it is a good candidate for future studies. Thus, we suggest more precise studies to establish the exact role of this hormone in specific traits with detailed metabolic conditions.

### 9.2. Adiponectin

Adiponectin is an adipocyte-specific secretory protein that circulates in the blood in relatively high concentrations (2–30 μg/mL) in at least three forms: low molecular weight, middle molecular weight, and high molecular weight; being the latter considered as the active form of adiponectin [149, 150].

Adiponectin levels are reported to have a positive correlation with insulin sensitivity and lipid metabolism; therefore, they could be involved in metabolic syndrome, type 2 diabetes mellitus, obesity, and atherosclerosis [143].

Despite the beneficial role of adiponectin on vascular homeostasis, studies suggest that increased levels of circulating adiponectin are inversely related to myocardial infarction in men [151]. However, results from subsequent studies lack of unanimity about this correlation in similar conditions, while others show a decrease of this correlation when they were adjusted by other factors, for example, HDL cholesterol [152].

Referred to its role in obesity, it has been shown a decrease of the levels in the obese state and an inverse correlation with the amount of visceral fat [151]. Furthermore, there are several studies that show an increase of adiponectin levels after weight loss [153].

It is too prompt to say that adiponectin can be used as a biomarker or surrogate endpoint in CVDs and obesity. There is needed more research in order to understand the complexity of the metabolic network of this peptide. Lastly, it should be noted from several studies the utility of the leptin/adiponectin ratio and its possible role as a predictor of a cardiovascular events [152].

### 9.3. Resistin

Resistin is an adipokine secreted by white adipose tissue that has been proposed as a biomarker due to the accumulated clinical evidence Showed in very extensive reviews [154], which demonstrates its association with obesity and CVDs complications such as atherosclerotis. However, the validation of this peptide as a cardiovascular marker seems to be complicated due to its dual function as an inflammatory cytokine and a metabolic hormone. Therefore, additional studies are necessary to clearly define resistin as a new biomarker in atherosclerotic diseases.

### 9.4. Visfatin/Nampt

Visfatin/Nampt was discovered in 2005 and later became the newest adipokine unveiled until now [155]. Since then, it has been related to pathogenesis of diabetes, obesity, renal failure, and CVDs, although there are conflicting results about its relationship with atherosclerosis [156].

The complexity of the metabolism of this adipokine, the possible existence of isoforms, and the lack of unanimity about the assays to its measure, which complicates its study consequently research is needed to understand and validate it as a biomarker of obesity and/or CVDs.

## 10. Others

Furthermore, it has to be mentioned that actually B-type natriuretic peptide is used as a diagnostic biomarker for *Acute Decompensate Heart Failure* (ADHF) as well as myeloperoxidase (MPO) for a heart failure, and troponin T for cardiac injuries [157]. Regarding coronary artery disease, there are some emergent indicators such as lectin-like oxidized low-density lipoprotein receptor-1, nuclear factor-kappa B, osteoprotegerin, osteocalcin, osteopontin, CD40, pentraxin-3, amyloid A, fibrinogen, myeloperoxidase, myeloid-related protein 8/14, or PAPP-A that require further investigation [158].

## 11. Conclusion

During the past years, the field of biomarkers and surrogate endpoints has been constantly growing along with greater advances in genetic and physiology knowledge of obesity and associated traits as CVDs. All of these biomarkers are a heterogeneously group that is related mainly with the mechanisms relate to obesity as inflammation, oxidative stress, adipocyte physiology, and regulation of food intake ingest. These biomolecules represent a key role in the identification, treatment, and follow-up of these traits; however, the complexity of the networks that are involved hampers the validation of them as a biomarker of risk, diagnostic and/or prognostic. The genetic modifications could be involved in predisposition to obesity and CVDs; the investigations of genetic and epigenetic in regulatory mechanisms during the evolution of these diseases could have applications in the prevention, early diagnosis, and treatment. Finally, the understanding of development of oxidative stress and inflammation related to obesity and CVDs, their biological role as well as potential therapeutic implications would be transformed into consistent benefits for their effective prevention, intervention, and treatment.

## 12. Future perspectives

The present and future of this area is and will be based on the emergent "*omics*" strategies as metabolomics, transcriptomics, proteomics, etc. These data will enable a complete description of the interactions between metabolites, proteins, transcripts, and genes toward a better understanding of the physiology of disease. The ability of metabolic profiling to provide non- or slight-invasive translational biomarkers provides it an important role in the move toward a better assessment of the risk, prognosis, as well as diagnosis.

## Author details

Monica Navarro Meza[1*] and Jesus Alcala-Bejarano Carrillo[2]

*Address all correspondence to: monica.navarro@cusur.udg.mx

1 Department of Health and Welfare, Laboratory of Molecular Biology and Immunology, Research Center for Eating Behavior, South University Center, University of Guadalajara, Guzman, City, Jalisco, Mexico

2 Faculty of Pharmacy, Department of Animal Physiology, University of Granada, Granada, Spain

## References

[1] Pollack A. A.M.A. Recognizes obesity as a disease. [Internet]. 2013. Available from: http://www.nytimes.com/2013/06/19/business/ama-recognizes-obesity-as-a-disease.html [Accessed 13th February 2016].

[2] Qi L, Cho YA. Gene-environment interaction and obesity. Nutr Rev. 2008;66(12):684–94.

[3] Finkelstein EA, Khavjou OA, Thompson H, Trogdon JG, Pan L, Sherry B, et al. Obesity and severe obesity forecasts through 2030. Am J Prev Med. 2012;42(6):563–70.

[4] World Health Organization. Obesity and Overweight. Available from: http://www.who.int/mediacentre/factsheets/fs311/en/www.who.int/topics/obesity/en. [Accessed 13th February 2016].

[5] Fernández-Fernández L, Comes G, Bolea I, Valente T, Ruiz J, Murtra P, et al. LMN diet, rich in polyphenols and polyunsaturated fatty acids, improves mouse cognitive decline associated with aging and Alzheimer's disease. Behav Brain Res. 2012;228(2):261–71.

[6] Berenson GS, Bogalusa Heart Study group. Health consequences of obesity. Pediatr Blood Cancer. 2012;58(1):117–21.

[7] Centers For Disease Control And Prevention. Body Mass Index: Considerations for Practitioners. Available from: http://www.cdc.gov/obesity/downloads/bmiforpactitioners.pdf#sthash.vvX6k6kc.dpuf [Accessed 13th February 2016]

[8] Murphy SP, Rose D, Hudes M, Viteri FE. Demographic and economic factors associated with dietary quality for adults in the 1987–88 Nationwide Food Consumption Survey. J Am Diet Assoc. 1992;92(11):1352–7.

[9] World Heart Federation. Cardiovascular Disease Terms. Available from: http://www.world-heart-federation.org/heart-facts/fact-sheets/cardiovascular-disease-terms [Accessed 13th February 2016].

[10] Roth GA, Forouzanfar MH, Moran AE, Barber R, Nguyen G, Feigin VL, et al. Demographic and epidemiologic drivers of global cardiovascular mortality. N Engl J Med. 2015;372(14):1333–41.

[11] World Health Organization. Noncommunicable Diseases. Available from: http://www.who.int/mediacentre/factsheets/fs355/en/. [Accessed 13th February 2016].

[12] World Health Organization. Globalization, Diets and Noncommunicable Diseases. Dietary Transition in Developing Countries: Challenges for Chronic Disease Prevention. Geneva: WHO, 2002.

[13] Lovren F, Teoh H, Verma S. Obesity and atherosclerosis: mechanistic insights. Can J Cardiol. 2015;31(2):177–83.

[14] Coutinho T, Goel K, Corrêa de Sá D, Kragelund C, Kanaya AM, Zeller M, et al. Central obesity and survival in subjects with coronary artery disease: a systematic review of the literature and collaborative analysis with individual subject data. J Am Coll Cardiol. 2011;57(19):1877–86.

[15] Strazzullo P, D'Elia L, Cairella G, Garbagnati F, Cappuccio FP, Scalfi L. Excess body weight and incidence of stroke: meta-analysis of prospective studies with 2 million participants. Stroke J Cereb Circ. 2010;41(5):e418–26.

[16] Lavie CJ, McAuley PA, Church TS, Milani RV, Blair SN. Obesity and cardiovascular diseases: implications regarding fitness, fatness, and severity in the obesity paradox. J Am Coll Cardiol. 2014;63(14):1345–54.

[17] Biomarkers Definitions Working Group. Biomarkers and surrogate endpoints: preferred definitions and conceptual framework. Clin Pharmacol Ther. 2001;69(3):89–95.

[18] Strimbu K, Tavel JA. What are biomarkers? Curr Opin HIV AIDS. 2010;5(6):463–6.

[19] World Health Organization. Biomarkers and Risk Assessment: Concepts and Principles. Available from: http://www.inchem.org/documents/ehc/ehc/ehc155.htm [Accessed 13th February 2016].

[20] Schulte PA, Waters M. Using molecular epidemiology in assessing exposure for risk assessment. Ann N Y Acad Sci. 1999;895:101–11.

[21] Bossuyt P. Defining biomarker performance and clinical validity. J Med Biochem. 2011;30(3):193–200.

[22] Xia J, Broadhurst DI, Wilson M, Wishart DS. Translational biomarker discovery in clinical metabolomics: an introductory tutorial. Metabolomics. 2013;9(2):280–99.

[23] Yumuk V, Tsigos C, Fried M, Schindler K, Busetto L, Micic D, et al. European guidelines for obesity management in adults. Obes Facts. 2015;8(6):402–24.

[24] Perk J, De Backer G, Gohlke H, Graham I, Reiner Z, Verschuren WMM, et al. [European guidelines on cardiovascular disease prevention in clinical practice (version 2012). The Fifth Joint Task Force of the European Society of Cardiology and other societies on cardiovascular disease prevention in clinical practice (constituted by representatives of nine societies and by invited experts)]. G Ital Cardiol 2006. 2013;14(5):328–92.

[25] Katsareli EA, Dedoussis GV. Biomarkers in the field of obesity and its related comorbidities. Expert Opin Ther Targets. 2014;18(4):385–401.

[26] Trynka G, Sandor C, Han B, Xu H, Stranger BE, Liu XS, et al. Chromatin marks identify critical cell types for fine mapping complex trait variants. Nat Genet. 2013;45(2):124–30.

[27] Manna P, Jain SK. Obesity, oxidative stress, adipose tissue dysfunction, and the associated health risks: causes and therapeutic strategies. Metab Syndr Relat Disord. 2015;13(10):423–44.

[28] Bondia-Pons I, Ryan L, Martinez JA. Oxidative stress and inflammation interactions in human obesity. J Physiol Biochem. 2012;68(4):701–11.

[29] Pollex RL, Hegele RA. Genetic determinants of the metabolic syndrome. Nat Clin Pract Cardiovasc Med. 2006;3(9):482–9.

[30] McGregor RA, Choi MS. microRNAs in the regulation of adipogenesis and obesity. Curr Mol Med. 2011;11(4):304–16.

[31] Trevaskis JL, Butler AA. Double leptin and melanocortin-4 receptor gene mutations have an additive effect on fat mass and are associated with reduced effects of leptin on weight loss and food intake. Endocrinology. 2005;146(10):4257–65.

[32] Lyon HN, Hirschhorn JN. Genetics of common forms of obesity: a brief overview. Am J Clin Nutr. 2005;82(1 Suppl):215S–217S.

[33] Rankinen T, Zuberi A, Chagnon YC, Weisnagel SJ, Argyropoulos G, Walts B, et al. The human obesity gene map: the 2005 update. Obes Silver Spring Md. 2006;14(4):529–644.

[34] Lohmueller KE, Pearce CL, Pike M, Lander ES, Hirschhorn JN. Meta-analysis of genetic association studies supports a contribution of common variants to susceptibility to common disease. Nat Genet. 2003;33(2):177–82.

[35] Creemers JWM, Choquet H, Stijnen P, Vatin V, Pigeyre M, Beckers S, et al. Heterozygous mutations causing partial prohormone convertase 1 deficiency contribute to human obesity. Diabetes. 2012;61(2):383–90.

[36] Viana Abranches M, Esteves de Oliveira FC, Bressan J. Peroxisome proliferator-activated receptor: effects on nutritional homeostasis, obesity and diabetes mellitus. Nutr Hosp. 2011;26(2):271–9.

[37] Tews D, Fischer-Posovszky P, Fromme T, Klingenspor M, Fischer J, Rüther U, et al. FTO deficiency induces UCP-1 expression and mitochondrial uncoupling in adipocytes. Endocrinology. 2013;154(9):3141–51.

[38] Burguete-Garcia AI, Martinez-Nava GA, Valladares-Salgado A, Bermudez Morales VH, Estrada-Velasco B, Wacher N, et al. Association of β1 and β3 adrenergic receptors gene polymorphisms with insulin resistance and high lipid profiles related to type 2 diabetes and metabolic syndrome. Nutr Hosp. 2014;29(6):1327–34.

[39] Graff M, Gordon-Larsen P, Lim U, Fowke JH, Love S-A, Fesinmeyer M, et al. The influence of obesity-related single nucleotide polymorphisms on BMI across the life course: the PAGE study. Diabetes. 2013;62(5):1763–7.

[40] Wiegand S, Krude H. [Monogenic and syndromic symptoms of morbid obesity. Rare but important]. Internist. 2015;56(2):111–2, 114–20.

[41] Paracchini V, Pedotti P, Taioli E. Genetics of leptin and obesity: a HuGE review. Am J Epidemiol. 2005;162(2):101–14.

[42] Speliotes EK, Willer CJ, Berndt SI, Monda KL, Thorleifsson G, Jackson AU, et al. Association analyses of 249,796 individuals reveal 18 new loci associated with body mass index. Nat Genet. 2010;42(11):937–48.

[43] Manolio TA, Collins FS, Cox NJ, Goldstein DB, Hindorff LA, Hunter DJ, et al. Finding the missing heritability of complex diseases. Nature. 2009;461(7265):747–53.

[44] De R, Hu T, Moore JH, Gilbert-Diamond D. Characterizing gene-gene interactions in a statistical epistasis network of twelve candidate genes for obesity. BioData Min. 2015;8:45.

[45] Hinuy HM, Hirata MH, Sampaio MF, Armaganijan D, Arazi SS, Salazar LA, et al. Relationship between variants of the leptin gene and obesity and metabolic biomarkers in Brazilian individuals. Arq Bras Endocrinol Metabol. 2010;54(3):282–8.

[46] Gueorguiev M, Lecoeur C, Meyre D, Benzinou M, Mein CA, Hinney A, et al. Association studies on ghrelin and ghrelin receptor gene polymorphisms with obesity. Obes Silver Spring Md. 2009;17(4):745–54.

[47] Wen W, Zheng W, Okada Y, Takeuchi F, Tabara Y, Hwang J-Y, et al. Meta-analysis of genome-wide association studies in East Asian-ancestry populations identifies four new loci for body mass index. Hum Mol Genet. 2014;23(20):5492–504.

[48] Baccarelli A, Rienstra M, Benjamin EJ. Cardiovascular epigenetics: basic concepts and results from animal and human studies. Circ Cardiovasc Genet. 2010;3(6):567–73.

[49] Xu X, Su S, Barnes VA, De Miguel C, Pollock J, Ownby D, et al. A genome-wide methylation study on obesity: differential variability and differential methylation. Epigenetics. 2013;8(5):522–33.

[50] Wang X, Zhu H, Snieder H, Su S, Munn D, Harshfield G, et al. Obesity related methylation changes in DNA of peripheral blood leukocytes. BMC Med. 2010;8:87.

[51] Gelfman S, Cohen N, Yearim A, Ast G. DNA-methylation effect on cotranscriptional splicing is dependent on GC architecture of the exon-intron structure. Genome Res. 2013;23(5):789–99.

[52] Keating ST, El-Osta A. Epigenetics and metabolism. Circ Res. 2015;116(4):715–36.

[53] Na YK, Hong HS, Lee DH, Lee WK, Kim DS. Effect of body mass index on global DNA methylation in healthy Korean women. Mol Cells. 2014;37(6):467–72.

[54] Duggan C, Xiao L, Terry MB, McTiernan A. No effect of weight loss on LINE-1 methylation levels in peripheral blood leukocytes from postmenopausal overweight women. Obes Silver Spring Md. 2014;22(9):2091–6.

[55] Carless MA, Kulkarni H, Kos MZ, Charlesworth J, Peralta JM, Göring HHH, et al. Genetic effects on DNA methylation and its potential relevance for obesity in Mexican Americans. Plos One. 2013;8(9):e73950.

[56] van Driel LMJW, Eijkemans MJC, de Jonge R, de Vries JHM, van Meurs JBJ, Steegers EAP, et al. Body mass index is an important determinant of methylation biomarkers in women of reproductive ages. J Nutr. 2009;139(12):2315–21.

[57] Davé V, Yousefi P, Huen K, Volberg V, Holland N. Relationship between expression and methylation of obesity-related genes in children. Mutagenesis. 2015;30(3):411–20.

[58] Martínez JA, Milagro FI, Claycombe KJ, Schalinske KL. Epigenetics in adipose tissue, obesity, weight loss, and diabetes. Adv Nutr Bethesda Md. 2014;5(1):71–81.

[59] Ellis A, Crowe K, Lawrence J. Obesity-related inflammation: implications for older adults. J Nutr Gerontol Geriatr. 2013;32(4):263–90.

[60] Yokomori N, Tawata M, Onaya T. DNA demethylation modulates mouse leptin promoter activity during the differentiation of 3T3-L1 cells. Diabetologia. 2002;45(1):140–8.

[61] Dick KJ, Nelson CP, Tsaprouni L, Sandling JK, Aïssi D, Wahl S, et al. DNA methylation and body-mass index: a genome-wide analysis. Lancet Lond Engl. 2014;383(9933):1990–8.

[62] Hatanaka M, Shimba S, Sakaue M, Kondo Y, Kagechika H, Kokame K, et al. Hypoxia-inducible factor-3alpha functions as an accelerator of 3T3-L1 adipose differentiation. Biol Pharm Bull. 2009;32(7):1166–72.

[63] Huang T, Zheng Y, Qi Q, Xu M, Ley SH, Li Y, et al. DNA Methylation Variants at HIF3A Locus, B-Vitamin Intake, and Long-term Weight Change: Gene-Diet Interactions in Two U.S. Cohorts. Diabetes. 2015;64(9):3146–54.

[64] Heidbreder M, Qadri F, Jöhren O, Dendorfer A, Depping R, Fröhlich F, et al. Non-hypoxic induction of HIF-3alpha by 2-deoxy-D-glucose and insulin. Biochem Biophys Res Commun. 2007;352(2):437–43.

[65] Stel J, Legler J. The role of epigenetics in the latent effects of early life exposure to obesogenic endocrine disrupting chemicals. Endocrinology. 2015;156(10):3466–72.

[66] Horsburgh S, Robson-Ansley P, Adams R, Smith C. Exercise and inflammation-related epigenetic modifications: focus on DNA methylation. Exerc Immunol Rev. 2015;21:26–41.

[67] Bhan A, Hussain I, Ansari KI, Bobzean SAM, Perrotti LI, Mandal SS. Histone methyltransferase EZH2 is transcriptionally induced by estradiol as well as estrogenic endocrine disruptors bisphenol-A and diethylstilbestrol. J Mol Biol. 2014;426(20):3426–41.

[68] Liu L, Zhao X, Kang S, Zhang D. An association between -866G/A polymorphism in the promoter of UCP2 and obesity: a meta-analysis. Gene. 2013;514(1):41–7.

[69] Mansoori B, Mohammadi A, Shirjang S, Baradaran B. Micro-RNAs: The new potential biomarkers in cancer diagnosis, prognosis and cancer therapy. Cell Mol Biol Noisy Gd Fr. 2015;61(5):1–10.

[70] Choi S-W, Claycombe KJ, Martinez JA, Friso S, Schalinske KL. Nutritional epigenomics: a portal to disease prevention. Adv Nutr Bethesda Md. 2013;4(5):530–2.

[71] Duarte FV, Palmeira CM, Rolo AP. The emerging role of MitomiRs in the pathophysiology of human disease. Adv Exp Med Biol. 2015;888:123–54.

[72] Ortega FJ, Mayas D, Moreno-Navarrete JM, Catalán V, Gómez-Ambrosi J, Esteve E, et al. The gene expression of the main lipogenic enzymes is downregulated in visceral adipose tissue of obese subjects. Obes Silver Spring Md. 2010;18(1):13–20.

[73] Campión J, Milagro F, Martínez JA. Epigenetics and obesity. Prog Mol Biol Transl Sci. 2010;94:291–347.

[74] Romaine SPR, Tomaszewski M, Condorelli G, Samani NJ. MicroRNAs in cardiovascular disease: an introduction for clinicians. Heart Br Card Soc. 2015;101(12):921–8.

[75] Campión J, Milagro FI, Martínez JA. Individuality and epigenetics in obesity. Obes Rev. 2009;10(4):383–92.

[76] Tilkorn DJ, Benna S Al-, Hauser J, Ring A, Steinau HU, Tannapfel A, et al. Sarcoma cells induce alteration in adipogenic differentiation. Anticancer Res. 2012;32(4):1167–73.

[77] Kajimoto K, Naraba H, Iwai N. MicroRNA and 3T3-L1 pre-adipocyte differentiation. RNA N Y N. 2006;12(9):1626–32.

[78] Fei J, Tamski H, Cook C, Santanam N. MicroRNA regulation of adipose derived stem cells in aging rats. Plos One. 2013;8(3):e59238.

[79] Xie H, Lim B, Lodish HF. MicroRNAs induced during adipogenesis that accelerate fat cell development are downregulated in obesity. Diabetes. 2009;58(5):1050–7.

[80] Ge Q, Gérard J, Noël L, Scroyen I, Brichard SM. MicroRNAs regulated by adiponectin as novel targets for controlling adipose tissue inflammation. Endocrinology. 2012;153(11):5285–96.

[81] Ameling S, Kacprowski T, Chilukoti RK, Malsch C, Liebscher V, Suhre K, et al. Associations of circulating plasma microRNAs with age, body mass index and sex in a population-based study. BMC Med Genom. 2015;8:61.

[82] Lawson C, Vicencio JM, Yellon DM, Davidson SM. Microvesicles and exosomes: new players in metabolic and cardiovascular disease. J Endocrinol. 2016;228(2):R57–71.

[83] Oger F, Gheeraert C, Mogilenko D, Benomar Y, Molendi-Coste O, Bouchaert E, et al. Cell-specific dysregulation of microRNA expression in obese white adipose tissue. J Clin Endocrinol Metab. 2014;99(8):2821–33.

[84] Lovis P, Roggli E, Laybutt DR, Gattesco S, Yang J-Y, Widmann C, et al. Alterations in microRNA expression contribute to fatty acid-induced pancreatic beta-cell dysfunction. Diabetes. 2008;57(10):2728–36.

[85] Grandjean V, Fourré S, De Abreu DAF, Derieppe M-A, Remy J-J, Rassoulzadegan M. RNA-mediated paternal heredity of diet-induced obesity and metabolic disorders. Sci Rep. 2015;5:18193.

[86] Marques-Rocha JL, Samblas M, Milagro FI, Bressan J, Martínez JA, Marti A. Noncoding RNAs, cytokines, and inflammation-related diseases. FASEB J. 2015;29(9):3595–611.

[87] Lamb RE, Goldstein BJ. Modulating an oxidative-inflammatory cascade: potential new treatment strategy for improving glucose metabolism, insulin resistance, and vascular function. Int J Clin Pract. 2008;62(7):1087–95.

[88] Santilli F, Guagnano MT, Vazzana N, La Barba S, Davi G. Oxidative stress drivers and modulators in obesity and cardiovascular disease: from biomarkers to therapeutic approach. Curr Med Chem. 2015;22(5):582–95.

[89] Pinheiro Volp AC, Santos Silva FC, Bressan J. Hepatic inflammatory biomarkers and its link with obesity and chronic diseases. Nutr Hosp. 2015;31(5):1947–56.

[90] Iantorno M, Campia U, Di Daniele N, Nistico S, Forleo GB, Cardillo C, et al. Obesity, inflammation and endothelial dysfunction. J Biol Regul Homeost Agents. 2014;28(2): 169–76.

[91] Gallagher EJ, Leroith D, Karnieli E. Insulin resistance in obesity as the underlying cause for the metabolic syndrome. Mt Sinai J Med N Y. 2010;77(5):511–23.

[92] Esser N, Paquot N, Scheen AJ. Inflammatory markers and cardiometabolic diseases. Acta Clin Belg. 2015;70(3):193–9.

[93] Ros Pérez M, Medina-Gómez G. [Obesity, adipogenesis and insulin resistance]. Endocrinol Nutr Órgano Soc Esp Endocrinol Nutr. 2011;58(7):360–9.

[94] Yasar Yildiz S, Kuru P, Toksoy Oner E, Agirbasli M. Functional stability of plasminogen activator inhibitor-1. Sci World J. 2014;2014:858293.

[95] Dan T, Ichimura A, Pelisch N, Miyata K, Akahori K, Miyata T. Plasminogen activator inhibitor-1 (PAI-1) molecule: new physiological roles and clinical applications. Rinshō Ketsueki Jpn J Clin Hematol. 2014;55(4):396–404.

[96] Pieterse C, Schutte R, Schutte AE. Leptin links with plasminogen activator inhibitor-1 in human obesity: the SABPA study. Hypertens Res. 2015;38(7):507–12.

[97] de Luca C, Olefsky JM. Inflammation and insulin resistance. FEBS Lett. 2008;582(1):97–105.

[98] Kishimoto T, Akira S, Narazaki M, Taga T. Interleukin-6 family of cytokines and gp130. Blood. 1995;86(4):1243–54.

[99] Naka T, Nishimoto N, Kishimoto T. The paradigm of IL-6: from basic science to medicine. Arthritis Res. 2002;4 Suppl 3:S233–42.

[100] Vozarova B, Weyer C, Hanson K, Tataranni PA, Bogardus C, Pratley RE. Circulating interleukin-6 in relation to adiposity, insulin action, and insulin secretion. Obes Res. 2001;9(7):414–7.

[101] González F, Rote NS, Minium J, O'leary VB, Kirwan JP. Obese reproductive-age women exhibit a proatherogenic inflammatory response during hyperglycemia. Obes Silver Spring Md. 2007;15(10):2436–44.

[102] Berthier M-T, Paradis A-M, Tchernof A, Bergeron J, Prud'homme D, Després J-P, et al. The interleukin 6-174G/C polymorphism is associated with indices of obesity in men. J Hum Genet. 2003;48(1):14–9.

[103] Ouchi N, Kihara S, Funahashi T, Matsuzawa Y, Walsh K. Obesity, adiponectin and vascular inflammatory disease. Curr Opin Lipidol. 2003;14(6):561–6.

[104] Tangvarasittichai S, Pongthaisong S, Tangvarasittichai O. Tumor necrosis factor-A, interleukin-6, C-reactive protein levels and insulin resistance associated with type 2 diabetes in abdominal obesity women. Indian J Clin Biochem IJCB. 2016;31(1):68–74.

[105] Hotamisligil GS, Spiegelman BM. Tumor necrosis factor $\alpha$: a key component of the obesity-diabetes link. Diabetes. 1994;43:1271–1278.

[106] Wybrańska I, Malczewska-Malec M, Niedbał S, Naskalski JW, Dembińska-Kieć A. The TNF-alpha gene NcoI polymorphism at position -308 of the promoter influences insulin

resistance, and increases serum triglycerides after postprandial lipaemia in familiar obesity. Clin Chem Lab Med. 2003;41(4):501–10.

[107] Ishikawa K, Takahashi K, Bujo H, Hashimoto N, Yagui K, Saito Y. Subcutaneous fat modulates insulin sensitivity in mice by regulating TNF-alpha expression in visceral fat. Horm Metab Res Horm Stoffwechs Horm Métab. 2006;38(10):631–8.

[108] Vlahakos DV, Dalamaga M, Marouga A, Bacharaki D, Drakou A, Dimas C. 1C.09: Serum resistin as an independent biomarker associated with all-cause and cardiovascular mortality in elderly hypertensive, non-diabetic patients with chronic kidney disease (CKD). J Hypertens. 2015;33 Suppl 1:e11–2.

[109] Keshk WA, Zineldeen DH, Wasfy REL -saye., El-Khadrawy OH. Fatty acid synthase/oxidized low-density lipoprotein as metabolic oncogenes linking obesity to colon cancer via NF-kappa B in Egyptians. Med Oncol Northwood Lond Engl. 2014;31(10): 192.

[110] Hill AA, Anderson-Baucum EK, Kennedy AJ, Webb CD, Yull FE, Hasty AH. Activation of NF-κB drives the enhanced survival of adipose tissue macrophages in an obesogenic environment. Mol Metab. 2015;4(10):665–77.

[111] Papaccio G, Graziano A, Aquino R D', Valiante S, Naro F. A biphasic role of nuclear transcription factor (NF)-kappaB in the islet beta-cell apoptosis induced by interleukin (IL)-1beta. J Cell Physiol. 2005;204(1):124–30.

[112] Perkins ND. Post-translational modifications regulating the activity and function of the nuclear factor kappa B pathway. Oncogene. 2006;25(51):6717–30.

[113] Yin MJ, Yamamoto Y, Gaynor RB. The anti-inflammatory agents aspirin and salicylate inhibit the activity of I(kappa)B kinase-beta. Nature. 1998;396(6706):77–80.

[114] Paneni F, Costantino S, Cosentino F. Insulin resistance, diabetes, and cardiovascular risk. Curr Atheroscler Rep. 2014;16(7):419.

[115] Gosmanova EO, Le N-A. Cardiovascular complications in CKD patients: role of oxidative stress. Cardiol Res Pract. 2011;2011:156326.

[116] Jeong J-J, Kim K-A, Jang S-E, Woo J-Y, Han MJ, Kim D-H. Orally administrated Lactobacillus pentosus var. plantarum C29 ameliorates age-dependent colitis by inhibiting the nuclear factor-kappa B signaling pathway via the regulation of lipopolysaccharide production by gut microbiota. Plos One. 2015;10(2):e0116533.

[117] Kelly D, Campbell JI, King TP, Grant G, Jansson EA, Coutts AGP, et al. Commensal anaerobic gut bacteria attenuate inflammation by regulating nuclear-cytoplasmic shuttling of PPAR-gamma and RelA. Nat Immunol. 2004;5(1):104–12.

[118] Spychalowicz A, Wilk G, Śliwa T, Ludew D, Guzik TJ. Novel therapeutic approaches in limiting oxidative stress and inflammation. Curr Pharm Biotechnol. 2012;13(13): 2456–66.

[119] Matsuoka T, Narumoto J, Shibata K, Taga C, Fukui K. Jealous delusions and dysfunction of the right parietal lobe in early-onset Alzheimer's disease. J Neuropsychiatry Clin Neurosci. 2011;23(4):E29–30.

[120] Santilli F, Guagnano MT, Vazzana N, La Barba S, Davi G. Oxidative stress drivers and modulators in obesity and cardiovascular disease: from biomarkers to therapeutic approach. Curr Med Chem. 2015;22(5):582–95.

[121] Catalán V, Gómez-Ambrosi J, Rodríguez A, Frühbeck G. Role of extracellular matrix remodelling in adipose tissue pathophysiology: relevance in the development of obesity. Histol Histopathol. 2012;27(12):1515–28.

[122] Jiang CY, Wang W, Tang JX, Yuan ZR. The adipocytokine resistin stimulates the production of proinflammatory cytokines TNF-$\alpha$ and IL-6 in pancreatic acinar cells via NF-κB activation. J Endocrinol Investig. 2013;36(11):986–92.

[123] Rani V, Deep G, Singh RK, Palle K, Yadav UCS. Oxidative stress and metabolic disorders: pathogenesis and therapeutic strategies. Life Sci. 2016;148:183–193.

[124] Lee AL, Ogle WO, Sapolsky RM. Stress and depression: possible links to neuron death in the hippocampus. Bipolar Disord. 2002;4(2):117–28.

[125] Grenier-Larouche T, Galinier A, Casteilla L, Carpentier AC, Tchernof A. Omental adipocyte hypertrophy relates to coenzyme Q10 redox state and lipid peroxidation in obese women. J Lipid Res. 2015;56(10):1985–92.

[126] Harrell JW, Johansson RE, Evans TD, Sebranek JJ, Walker BJ, Eldridge MW, et al. Preserved microvascular endothelial function in young, obese adults with functional loss of nitric oxide signaling. Front Physiol. 2015;6:387.

[127] Vendrov AE, Vendrov KC, Smith A, Yuan J, Sumida A, Robidoux J, et al. NOX4 NADPH oxidase-dependent mitochondrial oxidative stress in aging-associated cardiovascular disease. Antioxid Redox Signal. 2015;23(18):1389–409.

[128] Health & Disability: Reports, News & Medical Conditions. Cholesterol: Management & Information. Available from:http://www.disabled-world.com/health/cardiovascular/cholesterol/.[Accessed 15th February 2016].

[129] Rasnake CM, Trumbo PR, Heinonen TM. Surrogate endpoints and emerging surrogate endpoints for risk reduction of cardiovascular disease. Nutr Rev. 2008;66(2):76–81.

[130] Bangalore S, Fayyad R, Kastelein JJ, Laskey R, Amarenco P, DeMicco DA, et al. 2013 cholesterol guidelines revisited: percent LDL Am J Med. 2016 Apr;129(4):384-91. doi: 10.1016/j.amjmed.2015.10.024. Epub 2015 Nov 6

[131] Gyárfás I, Keltai M, Salim Y. [Effect of potentially modifiable risk factors associated with myocardial infarction in 52 countries in a case-control study based on the INTERHEART study]. Orv Hetil. 2006;147(15):675–86.

[132] Upmeier E, Vire J, Korhonen MJ, Isoaho H, Lehtonen A, Arve S, et al. Cardiovascular risk profile and use of statins at the age of 70 years: a comparison of two Finnish birth cohorts born 20 years apart. Age Ageing. 2016;45(1):84–90.

[133] Wannamethee SG, Shaper AG, Ebrahim S. HDL-Cholesterol, total cholesterol, and the risk of stroke in middle-aged British men. Stroke J Cereb Circ. 2000;31(8):1882–8.

[134] Miller M, Stone NJ, Ballantyne C, Bittner V, Criqui MH, Ginsberg HN, et al. Triglycerides and cardiovascular disease: a scientific statement from the American Heart Association. Circulation. 2011;123(20):2292–333.

[135] Fischer S. [Risk adapted therapy of vascular diseases—basic therapy of dys- and hyperlipoproteinemia]. Z Für Kardiologie. 2005;94 Suppl 4:IV/24–7.

[136] Langsted A, Freiberg JJ, Tybjaerg-Hansen A, Schnohr P, Jensen GB, Nordestgaard BG. Nonfasting cholesterol and triglycerides and association with risk of myocardial infarction and total mortality: the Copenhagen City Heart Study with 31 years of follow-up. J Intern Med. 2011;270(1):65–75.

[137] National Cholesterol Education Program (NCEP) Expert Panel on Detection, Evaluation, and Treatment of High Blood Cholesterol in Adults (Adult Treatment Panel III). Third Report of the National Cholesterol Education Program (NCEP) Expert Panel on Detection, Evaluation, and Treatment of High Blood Cholesterol in Adults (Adult Treatment Panel III) final report. Circulation. 2002;106(25):3143–421.

[138] World Health Organization. Global Status Report on Noncommunicable Diseases 2014. Available from: http://www.who.int/nmh/publications/ncd-status-report-2014/en/ [Accessed 13th February 2016].

[139] Van den Hoogen PC, Seidell JC, Menotti A, Kromhout D. Blood pressure and long-term coronary heart disease mortality in the Seven Countries study: implications for clinical practice and public health. Eur Heart J. 2000;21(20):1639–42.

[140] Albert MA. Biomarkers and heart disease. J Clin Sleep Med JCSM. 2011;7(5 Suppl):S9–11.

[141] Richy S, Burlet A, Max J, Burlet C, Beck B. Effect of chronic intraperitoneal injections of leptin on hypothalamic neurotensin content and food intake. Brain Res. 2000;862(1–2): 276–9.

[142] Canpolat S, Sandal S, Yilmaz B, Yasar A, Kutlu S, Baydas G, et al. Effects of pinealectomy and exogenous melatonin on serum leptin levels in male rat. Eur J Pharmacol. 2001;428(1):145–8.

[143] Huang F, Xiong X, Wang H, You S, Zeng H. Leptin-induced vascular smooth muscle cell proliferation via regulating cell cycle, activating ERK1/2 and NF-kappaB. Acta Biochim Biophys Sin. 2010;42(5):325–31.

[144] Knight ZA, Hannan KS, Greenberg ML, Friedman JM. Hyperleptinemia is required for the development of leptin resistance. Plos One. 2010;5(6):e11376.

[145] Rodrigues AM, Radominski RB, Suplicy H de L, De Almeida SM, Niclewicz PA, Boguszewski CL. The cerebrospinal fluid/serum leptin ratio during pharmacological therapy for obesity. J Clin Endocrinol Metab. 2002;87(4):1621–6.

[146] Richy S, Burlet A, Max J, Burlet C, Beck B. Effect of chronic intraperitoneal injections of leptin on hypothalamic neurotensin content and food intake. Brain Res. 2000;862(1–2): 276–9.

[147] Correia MLG, Rahmouni K. Role of leptin in the cardiovascular and endocrine complications of metabolic syndrome. Diabetes Obes Metab. 2006;8(6):603–10.

[148] Chakraborti CK. Role of adiponectin and some other factors linking type 2 diabetes mellitus and obesity. World J Diabetes. 2015;6(15):1296–308.

[149] Sattar N, Wannamethee G, Sarwar N, Tchernova J, Cherry L, Wallace AM, et al. Adiponectin and coronary heart disease: a prospective study and meta-analysis. Circulation. 2006;114(7):623–9.

[150] Yoo HJ, Choi KM. Adipokines as a novel link between obesity and atherosclerosis. World J Diabetes. 2014;5(3):357–63.

[151] Kappelle PJWH, Dullaart RPF, van Beek AP, Hillege HL, Wolffenbuttel BHR. The plasma leptin/adiponectin ratio predicts first cardiovascular event in men: a prospective nested case-control study. Eur J Intern Med. 2012;23(8):755–9.

[152] Abranches MV, Oliveira FCE de, da Conceição LL, Peluzio M do CG. Obesity and diabetes: the link between adipose tissue dysfunction and glucose homeostasis. Nutr Res Rev. 2015;28(2):121–32.

[153] Lazar MA. Resistin- and Obesity-associated metabolic diseases. Horm Metab Res Horm Stoffwechs Horm Métab. 2007;39(10):710–6.

[154] Romacho T, Sánchez-Ferrer CF, Peiró C. Visfatin/Nampt: an adipokine with cardiovascular impact. Mediators Inflamm. 2013;2013:946427.

[155] Chang Y-H, Chang D-M, Lin K-C, Shin S-J, Lee Y-J. Visfatin in overweight/obesity, type 2 diabetes mellitus, insulin resistance, metabolic syndrome and cardiovascular diseases: a meta-analysis and systemic review. Diabetes Metab Res Rev. 2011;27(6):515–27.

[156] Lubrano V, Balzan S. Consolidated and emerging inflammatory markers in coronary artery disease. World J Exp Med. 2015;5(1):21–32.

[157] Dalzell JR, Jackson CE, McDonagh TA, Gardner RS. Novel biomarkers in heart failure: an overview. Biomark Med. 2009;3(5):453–63.

Chapter 7

# High-Mobility Group Box-1 Protein a Potential Inflammatory Biomarker in Diabetic Retinopathy

Ghulam Mohammad

Additional information is available at the end of the chapter

http://dx.doi.org/10.5772/62524

**Abstract**

Diabetic retinopathy (DR) is the leading cause of acquired blindness, which is one of the most feared complications of diabetes among young adults. The cause of vision loss in DR is complex and remains incompletely understood. One of the earliest changes in the development of retinopathy is breakdown of blood-retinal barrier (BRB) and the formation of acellular capillaries by unknown mechanism. There is an accumulating body of evidence that demonstrated, chronic low-grade subclinical inflammation and retinal leukocyte stasis are responsible for many of the vascular lesions in DR. In the retina, diabetes induced sustained proinflammatory responses by increasing the production of proinflammatory cytokines, chemokines, and other inflammatory mediators leading to damaged vasculature and neovascularization. An emerging issue in DR research is the focus on the mechanistic link between chronic low-grade inflammation and angiogenesis. Recent evidence has revealed that extracellular high-mobility group box-1 (HMGB1) protein acts as a potent proinflammatory cytokine that triggers inflammation and recruits leukocytes to the site of tissue damage, and exhibits angiogenic effects. The expression of HMGB1 is upregulated in epiretinal membranes and vitreous fluid from patients with proliferative DR and in the diabetic retina. HMGB1 mediates inflammation, breakdown of the BRB, and apoptosis in the diabetic retina. The overall objective of this chapter is to provide the up-to-date literature about the crosstalk between extracellular HMGB1 and DR.

**Keywords:** Diabetic retinopathy, HMGB-1, Inflammation, Neurodegeneration, Cytokines

## 1. Introduction

Diabetes is a chronic disease, and it affects more than 230 million people worldwide, and this number is expected to reach 350 million by 2025. Diabetes, a result of body's inability to produce adequate amounts of insulin or to effectively use the insulin which is required to regulate the amount of sugar in the blood resulting in high levels of circulating blood sugar over a prolonged period. Diabetes is a quickly growing metabolic disorder and fourth of the 10 leading causes of death worldwide, which attributed to one death in every 10 seconds [1]. Several epidemiological studies have recognized that hyperglycemia is a main source of this disease in diabetes. High blood sugar over a prolonged period creates complicated consequences related to the glucose acting as a metabolic substrate and as an intracellular mediator which induces biochemical alteration and finally leads to cells dysfunction. High glucose induces cellular injuries that are known to initiate repair or cell death pathways. During hyperglycemia or altered glucose handling, it promotes nonenzymatic glycation reactions between reducing sugars and the free amino groups on proteins generating advanced glycation end products (AGEs). AGEs formation from protein glycation reactions is thought to be the major pathway involved in the development and progression of different types of complications associated with diabetes, including retinopathy [2]. Glycation-derived free radicals can cause protein fragmentation and oxidation of nucleic acids and lipids. Continuous high level of blood glucose in diabetes damages micro and macro blood vessels throughout the body by altering the endothelial cell lining of the blood vessels which causes more intake of glucose than normal and enhances the level of surface glycoproteins than normal, and results in thicker and weaker basement membrane.

### 1.1. Diabetic retinopathy

Diabetes threatens vision, and patients with diabetes develop cataracts at an earlier age and are nearly twice as likely to get glaucoma compared to nondiabetic [3]. More than 75% of patients who have had diabetes mellitus for more than 20 years will develop diabetic retinopathy (DR) [4]. According to Wisconsin epidemiologic study of diabetic retinopathy (WESDR), 3.6% of younger-onset patients (type 1diabetes) and 1.6% of older-onset patients (type 2 diabetes) were legally blind [5].The retina, a light-sensitive nerve layer that lines the back of the eye, is damaged by hyperglycemia, which is manifested as DR, and is the leading cause of acquired blindness, which is one of the most feared complications of diabetes among young adults. DR is a slow progressive retinal disease and occurs as a consequence of long-standing accumulated functional and structural impairment of the retina by diabetes. It is a multifactorial condition arising from the complex interplay between biochemical and metabolic abnormalities occurring in all cells of the retina. DR has been classically regarded as a microangiopathy of the retina, involving changes in the vascular wall leading to capillary occlusion and thereby retinal ischemia and leakage. And more recently, the neural defects in the retina are also being appreciated [6]. DR is classified into three major categories based on its severity: (i) mild to moderate non-proliferative retinopathy (NPDR), (ii) severe NPDR, and (iii) proliferative retinopathy (PDR). PDR is an advanced form of diabetic eye damage that is caused by chronic hyperglycemia in the blood, which is characterized by the epiretinal outgrowth of fibrovascular membranes at the vitreoretinal interface. The formation of fibrovascular tissue or angiogenesis (i.e., the formation of new blood vessels from existing retinal blood vessels in the vitreous humor) often leads to visual loss due to vitreous hemorrhage and/or tractional retinal detachment. Development of DR is a multifarious process where proteases, growth factors, cytokines, and chemokines such as monocyte chemoattractant protein-1 (MCP-1), interleukin-8 (IL-8), intercellular adhesion molecule-1 (ICAM-1), vascular cell adhesion molecule-1 (VCAM-1), stromal cell-derived factor-1$\alpha$ (SDF-1$\alpha$), cyclooxygenase-2 (COX-2) and prostaglandin E2 production, vascular endothelial growth factor (VEGF), matrix metalloproteinases (MMPs), connective tissue growth factor (CTGF), and high-mobility group box-1 (HMGB1) protein are released from retinal cells under hyperglycemia and interact with each other as well as activate several signaling pathway to promote neovascularization and fibrosis in retina [7–11]. In this chapter, a major emphasis is given on diabetes-induced HMGB1 protein in the retina, mediates a range of molecules and pathways involved early in the pathophysiology of DR which is briefly discussed and those major cascades of events are shown in the schematic diagram as depicted in **Figure 1**.

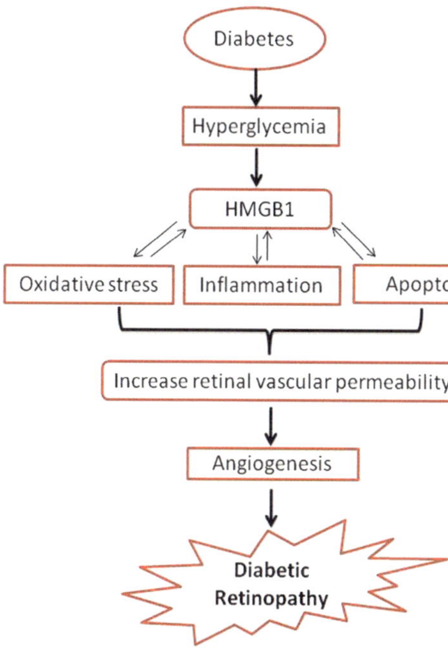


**Figure 1.** Possible signaling cascade of high mobility group box protein-1 (HMGB1) in diabetic retina. Diabetes causes a rise in HMGB1, which results in increased retinal vascular permeability and angiogenesis through enhancing oxidative stress, apoptosis, and inflammation.

### 1.2. Inflammation and diabetic retinopathy

Inflammation is a second-line defense process by which the innate immune system of the body guards from infection with foreign pathogen or antigen. The immune system identifies this foreign pathogen or antigen by specific binding receptors, such as receptor for advanced glycation end products (RAGE) and toll-like receptors (TLRs), and activation of these receptors after binding with an antigen induces the production of cytokines (e.g., IL-1$\beta$, IL8, and TNF-$\alpha$) that further help in the induction or expression of pro-inflammatory mediators [12–14]. As demonstrated by various studies, during the development of DR proinflammatory cytokines, chemokines and other inflammatory mediators play a central role leading to persistent low-grade inflammation, which influx the leukocytes to the damaged retinal vasculature and induce neovascularization [15, 16]. In the retina or vitreous of diabetic animals and patients, many of the molecular and physiological alterations are found consistent with inflammation, and the gene profile patterns from the diabetic retinas of rodents share resemblance with an inflammatory response [17]. The level of proinflammatory cytokines such as TNF-$\alpha$, IL-1$\beta$, and IL-6 and chemokines such as MCP-1, interferon-$\gamma$-inducible protein of 10 kDa (IP-10), SDF-1, and IL-8 in addition to other key inflammatory proteins including iNOS, COX-2, and MMP-9/gelatinase B, are increased in the vitreous fluid of patients with PDR [18] and in the retina of diabetic animal models [19–21]. Much of the attention on production of proinflammatory cytokines has focused on the IKK-beta/nuclear factor (NF)-kappa ($\kappa$)-B pathway, a protein network that enhances transcription of cytokine genes. As inflammation is suggested to be an initiating event of proliferative vitreoretinal disorders, the identification of biomarkers related to leukocyte activities and reflecting the amount of inflammation may provide insight into cellular processes linked to proliferative vitreoretinal disorder progression and would aid in identification of novel targets for therapeutic intervention. Among various cytokines, several recently published studies suggested that HMGB1 protein, a pro-inflammatory cytokine, plays an important role in the development of DR

## 2. HMGB1

HMGB1 (also known as HMG-1 or amphoterin) is a highly conserved non-histone chromosomal protein which functions as a transcriptional activator in the nucleus [22]. However, HMGB1 is also secreted into the extracellular spaces by a variety of cells involved in immune biology and by necrotic cells. Numerous studies have evaluated proinflammatory cytokine-like activities of extracellular HMGB1 during the event of inflammation [22–25]. The HMGB1 structural functional analyses suggested that the specific post-translational modifications regulate the bioactivity of the molecule.

### 2.1. HMGB1 structure and functions

The HMGB1 protein is composed of three domains, two positively charged domains at N-terminal (A and B boxes) and one negatively charged (C-terminal). The structure-specific DNA binding is attributed to the A box while the DNA-bending ability is attributed to the B domain. Whereas the C-terminal (acidic tail) of this protein helps in maintaining the stability and DNA bend and not DNA binding. The A box and B domain are responsible for the specific DNA-binding and DNA-bending ability, respectively, whereas the C-terminal maintains the protein stability [26]. In addition, the primary structure consists of three oxidation-sensitive unpaired cysteine residues, C23, C45, and C106, which facilitates the activities of extracellular HMGB1. During the event of inflammation, HMGB1 exerts its cytokine-like activities, the unpaired C106-residue-containing thiol group is essential for the interaction with TLR4 to generate cytokine-inducing capacity. The inactive form of HMGB1 contains terminally oxidized cysteine residues C23, C45, and C106, causing resolution of inflammation. The chemoattractic activities of HMGB1 are correspond to a fully reduced form all three cysteine residues C23, C45 and C106. Recently, a great deal of research evidence indicated the major role of HMGB1 in the regulation of oxidative stress, apoptosis, inflammation, and angiogenesis in various diseases. HMGB1 binds with multiple receptors including RAGE and TLR2, TLR4, and TLR9. Signaling through these receptors leads to activate various cellular signaling pathways which induce proinflammatory cytokines and chemokines and escalate leukocyte adhesion in various diseases. HMGB1 is not just released in reply to inflammatory stimuli, but itself facilitates the production of inflammatory mediators [27, 28]. In **Figure 2**, the molecular docking shows the interaction between HMGB1 and RAGE. All of this explains the implication of HMGB1 in mediating fundamental cellular events such as transcription, recombination, replication, and tissue damage repair and plays a role in inflammatory reaction through its cytokine-like activities.

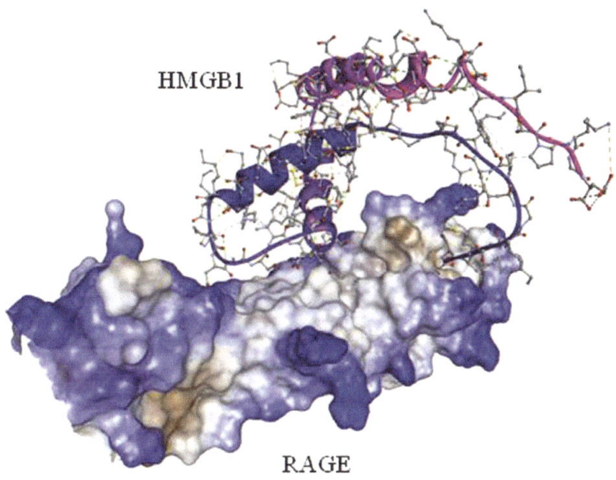


**Figure 2.** The binded form of HMGB1 and receptor for advanced glycation endproducts (RAGE). The most stable bound conformation obtained after the protein-protein docking by using the ZDOCK.

## 2.2. HMGB1 and inflammation

Inflammation is a cascade of biochemical immune responses involving soluble factors, vascular permeability, and leukocyte migration in response to pathophysiology associated to acute or chronic inflammatory conditions. Various leukocytes, which normally reside in blood, must move into the inflamed tissue via extravasation to aid in initiation and maintenance of inflammation. In an event of immune response, HMGB1 is actively secreted from the nucleus to the extracellular space by different leukocytes and endothelial cells and functions as a proinflammatory cytokine. In the culture media of lipopolysaccharide (LPS) -treated cell, HMGB1 could be detected after 8 hours and highest at 18 hours. Similarly, HMGB1 could be released from serum samples after 8–32 hours mice challenged with LPS or TNF-$\alpha$. In addition, recombinant HMGB1 injected intraperitoneally was lethal to LPS-sensitive or LPS-resistant mice. Thus, extracellular HMGB1 seems to have a remarkable proinflammatory effect. Leukocyte transmigration or extravasation is the movement of leukocytes out of the circulatory system, toward the site of tissue damage, or infection is mediated by cascade sequence of adhesion and activation events that ends with extravasation of the leukocyte, whereby the cell exerts its effects on the inflamed site. Extracellular HMGB1 proteins promote the recruitment of leukocytes across endothelial barriers through their effects on integrin signaling mainly involving RAGE, a primary receptors for HMGB1 to mediate chemotaxis, proliferation, and differentiation activities [23, 29]. The receptor-ligand interactions involved in this complex process is mediated through adhesive interactions between leukocytes and endothelial cells. In the time of inflammation, the adhesive glycoproteins expressed on the surface of both leukocytes (CD11/CD18) and endothelial cells ICAM, endothelial-leukocyte adhesion molecule (ELAM) interact and facilitate the leukocyte adherence [30]. In recent years, several published reports have indicated that HMGB1, which is released in an immune response by a variety of cells, involved in immune biology and by necrotic cells, also mediates the leukocyte adherence by inducing inflammatory cytokines [23, 25, 31, 32]. Various studies have suggested that binding of secreted HMGB1 to its receptors activates various signaling pathways leading to activation of transcription factor that induces production of adhesion molecules, cytokines, and chemokines [33–39]. However, the exact mechanism by which HMGB1 mediates leukocyte adhesion has not been defined, but the one possible mechanism can be thought is that extracellularly secreted HMGB1 neutralizes or inactivates the endothelial cell-derived antiadhesive substance. In addition to leukocyte adhesion, recent studies also documented that involvement of extracellular HMGB1 in the disruption of vascular barriers such as breakdown of the blood-brain barrier (BBB) and blood-retinal barrier (BRB). Major cascades of events are shown in the schematic diagram as depicted in **Figure 3**.

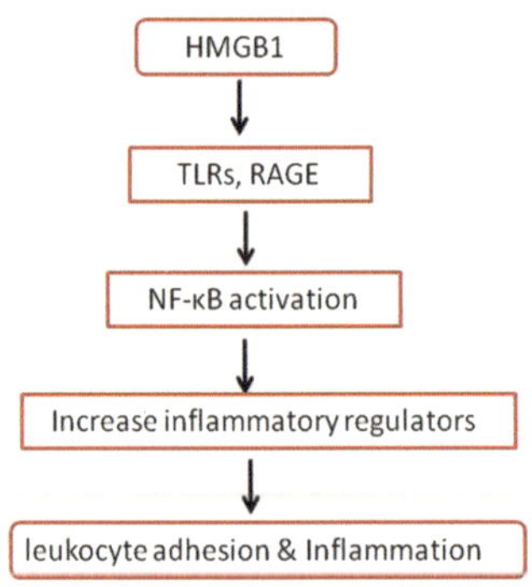


**Figure 3.** Hypothetic diagram of HMGB1 mediated leukocyte adhesion and inflammation in diabetic retina via RAGE or TLR.

### 2.3. HMGB1 as a biomarker in the diseases

The biomarkers are of growing importance in the difficult fields of predict, diagnose, and therapy monitoring in various disease. HMGB1 is one potential biomarker for inflammatory and autoimmune-related diseases, as established by both animal models and clinical studies. In animal models, HMGB1 expression significantly increases and is associated with immune modulation, inflammation, angiogenesis, trauma, cardiac dysfunction, diabetic complications, and metastasis. Clinical studies have also established a relationship between HMGB1 and in immune modulation in many acute and chronic diseases such as trauma, acute inflammation, and autoimmune diseases, making HMGB1 a viable candidate to add to the multiple biomarker lists. Extracellular release of HMGB1 from immunological active cells or necrotic cell plays an essential role in autoimmune diseases like rheumatoid arthritis (RA) and systemic lupus erythematosus (SLE), as well as in acute inflammatory events like sepsis and trauma. It was demonstrated that increased levels of HMGB1 in the serum samples from patients with SLE correlated positively with disease activity measured by SLE disease activity index scores and proteinuria, as well as with levels of anti-HMGB1 antibodies. In addition, the presence of HMGB1-specific antibodies suggests a pathogenetic role of HMGB1/anti-HMGB1 immune complexes in SLE [40]. RA is characterized by enhanced angiogenesis, and HMGB1 was shown to promote angiogenesis in RA by enhanced expression of VEGF and HIF-1$\alpha$ activation [41]. Furthermore, HMGB1-induced angiogenesis was inhibited by cilostazol via SIRT1 activation in synovial fibroblasts from RA [42]. Several studies have shown that HMGB1 levels were elevated in all kinds of trauma such as severe trauma, burn trauma, or iatrogenic trauma [43–46] and suggested that this elevated level of HMGB1 derived from trauma-induced cell death. Anti-neutrophil cytoplasmic antibody (ANCA)-associated vasculitides (AAV) are systemic inflammatory disorders in which the serum level of HMGB1 did not change significantly and remains same level as control suggesting HMGB1 is not a useful biomarker in AAV [47]. Viral hepatitis E clinically ranges between acute self-limiting hepatitis (AVH) and acute liver failure (ALF) in which the mean circulating HMGB1 levels were significantly higher in ALF than AVH [48]. In cancer, HMGB1 regulates the transcription of many cancer genes, such as *E-selectin, TNF-α, insulin receptor*, and *BRCA1* [49–51]. In the serum samples of colorectal carcinoma patients, the HMGB1 level was increased compared to those in healthy controls [52]. In malignant cancer, HMGB1 play an important role in creating a pro-inflammatory microenvironment which resulted in promoting tumor growth, angiogenesis, and metastasis

## 3. HMGB1 and diabetic retinopathy

Extensive experimental data generated in both tissue culture and animal models as well as clinical indicated that the progression of DR development involved alteration in the vascular wall leading to capillary occlusion and promoting ischemia and leakage in the retina. And newly, retinal neurodegeneration is also being greatly appreciated [6]. Many recent research are focused on retinal vascular dysfunction, such as breakdown of the BRB, altered tight junctions, death of capillary cells, and thickening of basement membrane. One of the early pathological sign of retinopathy in experimental diabetes models include increased retinal permeability. The possible mechanism by which diabetes-induced retinal permeability is considering the inflammatory reaction between reactive oxygen species (ROS) and cell-adhesion molecules resulted in breakdown of the BRB and loss of endothelial cells by leukocyte adhesion [53, 54]. The earlier events in diabetic retinal inflammation are the adhesion of leukocytes to the microvasculature which encourages the induction of adhesion molecules such as ICAM-1 and P-selectin, on the endothelium and its leukocyte counter-receptor CD18 [54]. Occludin is a transmembrane protein located at the tight junction which confers the cell-to-cell adhesion and interaction [55]. A high level of occludin was shown to maintain endothelial cells BRB, occludin expression is specific to vascular endothelial cells with strong barrier properties and its down-regulation increases vascular permeability [55–57]. Diabetes increases retinal vascular permeability and reduces the level of occludin in retina; similarly, administration of HMGB1 to normal eye enhances the vascular permeability and lowers the expression of occludin. In addition, retinal endothelial cell exposed to HMGB1 reduces the trans-endothelial electrical resistance [58]. Furthermore, one essential consequence of the inflammatory process by which vascular permeability enhances is the induction of adhesion molecules such as ICAM-1 by leukocyte endothelial cell interaction. The expression of ICAM-1 increases in the diabetic retina and its expression significantly correlated with retinal vascular permeability. Intravitreal injection HMGB1 induces up-regulation of ICAM and blocker of HMGB1 attenuates diabetes-induced ICAM-1 expression in the retina [58]. However, the detailed molecular mechanisms by which HMGB1, leukocyte adhesion, and vascular permeability cross-talk in the development of DR is not discussed much and it needs to be investigated further.

AGEs are key mediators of almost all complications associated with diabetes [59, 60]; hyperglycemic environment facilitates ROS generation which promotes AGEs formation. AGEs damages microvascular and macrovascular by promoting crosslink formation between proteins, which alters their structure and function, as in cellular matrix, basement membranes, and vessel-wall components. In addition, AGEs interact with a variety of cell-surface AGE-binding receptors, leading either to their endocytosis and degradation or to cellular activation and pro-oxidant, pro-inflammatory events. AGEs binding to RAGE induces ROS generation, which in turn activates the pleiotropic transcription signaling factor such as NF-κB, inducing multiple pathological responses [61]. In the diabetic retina, AGEs formation contributes to enhance angiogenesis in retinal microvessels, and endothelial cell incubated with AGE-BSA enhances the production of proangiogenic factor such as VEGF and increases cell proliferation and tube formation through NF-κB activation pathways [62, 63]. Therefore, the contribution of AGEs in regulation a pro-angiogenic factor to enhance angiogenesis in the development of DR cannot be ignored. In fact, epiretinal membranes obtained from PDR patient were shown the expression of AGE, RAGE, and HMGB1 by vascular endothelial cells and stromal cells and its presence correlated with level of vascularization [64]. In the retina of experimental diabetic animals, increased expressions of AGEs, RAGE, and HMGB1 have been documented [11, 65]. In addition, the level of HMGB1, AGE, and RAGE is upregulated and significantly correlated with biomarkers of inflamation in the vitreous of patients with PDR [11, 57, 66]. RAGE is a cell surface receptor that binds AGEs, which are expressed by the endothelial cells that form the inner lining of blood vessels [67]. In the diabetic retina, HMGB1 and RAGE upregulate and interact with each other and activate the extracellular signal-regulated kinase 1 and 2 (ERK1/2) phosphorylation [58], leading to induction of pro-angiogenic molecules such as VEGF, TNF, and IL-8 [11, 68, 69]. In diabetes, HMGB1 up-regulation is associated with microvessel and

http://dx.doi.org/10.5772/62524

macrovessel abnormalities, in the eye it damages retinal function, and its inhibition may be able to improve this retinal defect caused by hyperglycemia [11, 25, 69].

Inflammation all known to cause retinal cells death largely occurs via apoptosis in diabetes and the possible signaling mechanism involved in this is believed to be mediated by activation of NF-κB pathways. In the retina of diabetic animal and retinal capillary cells incubated with high glucose, NF-κB is activated and this causes production of inflammatory cytokines and apoptosis [70]. Thus, activation of NF-κB in the retina is considered as pro-apoptotic factor and its activation is considered as a negative regulator of cell survival [71, 72]. However, in various cancers, activation of NF-κB is considered as an anti-apoptotic factor and positive regulator of cell survival, thus suggesting a differential role of activation of NF-κB in diseases. HMGB1 has been shown that in diabetic retina induces NF-κB activation [58], and recently, it was shown that HMGB1 directly mediates retinal endothelial apoptosis [32]. The possible mechanism by which HMGB1 induces retinal cell death in diabetes may be mediated by ROS via NF-κB activation because it is known that ROS activated NF-κB and induced apoptosis retina. Various studies have drawn a connection between oxidative stress and apoptosis, and in retina, diabetes-induced ROS modulates or activates pro-apoptotic mediators has been shown [1, 68, 72, 73]. Supplementation of antioxidants to diabetic rats prevents the retina from oxidative stress and apoptosis, and also the development of retinopathy [1, 74]. In addition, it was shown that local oxidative stress that has a neurodegenerative influence in the diabetic retina is prevented by constant intake of an antioxidant-supplemented diet such as lutein [75]. Recently, various clinical investigators detect neuronal dysfunction at very early stages of diabetes and numerous abnormalities in the retina can be identified even before the vascular pathology appears [76, 77], thus suggesting a direct effect of diabetes on the neural retina. In streptozotocin (STZ)-induced diabetic mice, capillary lesion occurs at very early stages of DR, which resulted in loss of inner retinal neurons by increasing apoptosis [78]. At the early stage of diabetes, retinal ganalion cell dies by apoptosis, which is necessary to maintain the normal function of retina [79]. The mechanisms by which diabetes induce retinal neurodegeneration involve metabolic stress, altering the regulation of many growth factors which are involved in the process of neuronal death. Recently, it was demonstrated that HMGB1 is the main mediator bridging persistent neuroinflammation and chronic progressive dopaminergic neurodegeneration in neurodegenerative diseases, such as Parkinson's disease [80]. It was also reported that release of HMGB1 to extracellular space arbitrates to postischemic brain and retina damage and that blocking of HMGB1 prevents postischemic neurodegeneration [81]. Neurotrophin are a family of protein which regulates many aspects of neural function, its survival and developments, and it is sensitive toward oxidative stress. Brain-derived neurotrophic factor (BDNF), a protein belonging to the neurotrophin family, is expressed in retinal cells such as ganglion cells and Müller cells [82, 83] and is essential for its development, survival, and its synaptic activity [84]. In retina, diabetes induces retinal neuropathy by reducing the expression of BDNF and can be ameliorated by an exogenous administration [75]. Various study suggested that in the diabetic retina the BDNF levels, and synaptophysin, a synaptic vesicle protein for neurotransmitter is reduced by ROS [73, 85, 86]. Glutamate, the excitatory neurotransmitter in the retina, mediates the transfer of visual signals from the retina to the brain by photoreceptors, bipolar cells, and ganglion cells. Excitotoxicity is a state of high glutamate level, damage to the retinal gangalion cell by activation of ionotropic and metabotropic glutamate receptors [87, 88]. Glutamine synthetase, an enzyme which converts glutamate to glutamine, significantly decreased in the diabetic rat retinas, which resulted in elevated glutamate levels in the diabetic retinas, which might induce retinal neurodegeneration via glutamate excitotoxicity [87, 89]. Synaptophysin protein is decreased in the retina of the STZ-induced diabetes model through the ROS-ERK$_{1/2}$ and suggested the cross-talk between mitogen-activated protein kinases (MAPK) pathway signals and neurodegeneration [75, 90]. Recently, Abu El-Asrar et al. studied the involvement of HMGB1 in retinal neurodegeneration and showed that diabetes and intravitreal administration of HMGB1 induces up-regulation of lipid peroxidation and cleaved caspase-3 and glutamate, whereas BDNF, synaptophysin, tyrosine hydroxylase, glutamine synthetase, and glyoxalase 1 were downregulated in the retinas and inhibitor of HMGB1 attenuates diabetes which induced these changes [85, 91], and they suggested that the early retinal neuropathy induced by diabetes involves HMGB1 and can be ameliorated by inhibition of HMGB1. Thus, targeting the HMGB1-mediated signaling cascade may constitute a new beneficial approach to inhibiting the progress of DR.

## 4. Future perspective of HMGB1 as a biomarker for diabetic retinopathy

Ischemia-induced angiogenesis is the pathological hallmark in PDR and remains a significant cause of vision loss due to vitreous hemorrhage and/or traction retinal detachment. Therapeutic regulation of angiogenesis has emerged as an attractive approach for the treatment of PDR. Recently, extracellular HMGB-1 has been recognized as a potent proinflammatory cytokine that triggers inflammation and recruits leukocytes to the site of tissue damage [11, 23, 25, 92], and exhibits angiogenic effects. The angiogenic potency of HMGB1 has been confirmed in several *in vitro* and *in vivo* model systems providing a strong clinical evidence for the proangiogenic function of HMGB1 [11, 41, 42, 69, 92]. It was demonstrated that HMGB1 localized in vascular endothelial cells and stromal cells in epiretinal fibrovascular membranes from patients with PDR. In addition, increased levels of HMGB1 positively correlated with the levels of the inflammatory biomarkers such as ICAM-1 in the vitreous fluid of PDR patients [11, 64]. Furthermore, intravitreal injection of HMGB1 induces the expression of RAGE, activated ERK1/2 and activated NF-κB in the retinas of rats [58]. VEGF and HIF-1$\alpha$ is the major angiogenic factor in PDR that promotes neovascularization and vascular leakage. HMGB1 was shown to enhance the expression of VEGF and HIF-1$\alpha$ in retinal endothelial cell and in the retina [69]. Retinal leukostasis and leukocyte adhesion to the retinal microvasculature is associated with endothelial cell death, capillary occlusion, and increased vascular permeability, which all contribute to the progression of DR [15, 16, 18, 93]. Administration of HMGB-1 in the vitreous of normal rats has been shown to enhance the retinal vascular permeability, and retinal endothelial cell treated with HMGB1 causes reduction in transendothelial electric resistance [58]. Recently, a great deal of evidence has indicated that diabetes induced ROS generation implicated in the developmental DR and it is considered as important mediator of apoptosis in retina. In diabetic microenvironment, retina and capillary cells experience increased oxidative damage and the therapy which blocks oxidative stress also blocks the progression of retinopathy [1, 72, 74, 75]. A strong relation between oxidative stress and accelerated retinal capillary cells death was observed in the pathogenesis of DR [72, 74]. HMGB1 levels and oxidative stress marker protein carbonyl content levels were significantly correlated in the vitreous fluid of PDR patients [68]. In addition, HMGB1 treatment enhanced ROS generation and up-regulation of retinal apoptotic markers such as poly (ADP-ribose) polymerase (PARP)-1 and cleaved caspase-3 production by human retinal endothelial cells [68]. Similarly, administration of HMGB1 in the vitreous of normal rats increases ROS production and markers of apoptosis [68]. Furthermore, it was demonstrated that the HMGB1 mediates pericyte death via cytotoxic activity of glial cells, whereas it directly induces endothelial cells death and regulates endothelial cell activity [32]. Therefore, HMGB1 may be a potential biomarker because it exerts a multitude of functions in the development of DR.

## 5. Conclusions

As described in this chapter, extensive research progress has been made in investigating the pathophysiology of the disease; however, because early stages of DR is scarcely explored and much of the ophthalmic therapy for DR is focused on severe stages (pre-proliferative stage) of the disease, the exact molecular mechanism has not been elucidated. Here, we describe the potential role of HMGB1 in DR as a result of its pro-inflammatory properties and multiple activities. Because HMGB1 destabilizes the markers of oxidative stress, apoptosis and inflammation in the retina from hyperglycemia, it suggests that early blockade of HMGB1 may be an effective strategy to prevent the progression of DR.

## Acknowledgment and declaration of interest

The authors acknowledge funding from National Plan for Science and Technology (NPST strategic technologies programs, number 12-MED2604-02) in the Kingdom of Saudi Arabia.

## Author details

Ghulam Mohammad

Address all correspondence to: mghulam@ksu.edu.sa, gmkbiochembhu@gmail.com

Dr. Nasser Al-Rasheed Research Chair in Ophthalmology, Department of Ophthalmology, College of Medicine, King Saud University, Riyadh, Saudi Arabia

## References

[1] Kowluru RA, Chan PS. Oxidative stress and diabetic retinopathy. Exp Diabetes Res. 2007;2007:43603.

[2] Negre-Salvayre A, Salvayre R, AugéN, Pamplona R, Portero-Otín M. Hyperglycemia and glycation in diabetic complications. Antioxid Redox Signal. 2009;11(12):3071–109.

[3] Sharma S, Oliver-Fernandez A, Liu W, Buchholz P, Walt J. The impact of diabetic retinopathy on health-related quality of life. Curr Opin Ophthalmol. 2005;16(3):155–9.

[4] BarcelóA, Aedo C, Rajpathak S, Robles S. The cost of diabetes in Latin America and the Caribbean. Bull World Health Organ. 2003;81(1):19–27.

[5] Fong DS, Aiello L, Gardner TW, King GL, Blankenship G, Cavallerano JD, Ferris FL3rd, Klein R, American Diabetes Association. Diabetic retinopathy. Diabetes Care. 2003;26(1):226–9.

[6] Antonetti DA, Barber AJ, Bronson SK, Freeman WM, Gardner TW, Jefferson LS, Kester M, Kimball SR, Krady JK, La Noue KF, Norbury CC, Quinn PG, Sandirasegarane L, Simpson IA, JDRF Diabetic Retinopathy Center Group. Diabetic retinopathy: seeing beyond glucose-induced microvascular disease. Diabetes. 2006;55(9):2401–11.

[7] Aiello LP, Avery RL, Arrigg PG, Keyt BA, Jampel HD, Shah ST, Pasquale LR, Thieme H, Iwamoto MA, Park JE, et al. Vascular endothelial growth factor in ocular fluid of patients with diabetic retinopathy and other retinal disorders. N Engl J Med. 1994;331(22):1480–7.

[8] Canataroglu H, Varinli I, Ozcan AA, Canataroglu A, Doran F, Varinli S. Interleukin (IL)-6, interleukin (IL)-8 levels and cellular composition of the vitreous humor in proliferative diabetic retinopathy, proliferative vitreoretinopathy, and traumatic proliferative vitreoretinopathy. Ocul Immunol Inflamm. 2005;13(5):375–81.

[9] Yuuki T, Kanda T, Kimura Y, Kotajima N, Tamura J, Kobayashi I, Kishi S. Inflammatory cytokines in vitreous fluid and serum of patients with diabetic vitreoretinopathy. J Diabetes Complications. 2001;15(5):257–9.

[10] Vincent AM, Perrone L, Sullivan KA, Backus C, Sastry AM, Lastoskie C, Feldman EL. Receptor for advanced glycation end products activation injures primary sensory neurons via oxidative stress. Endocrinology. 2007;148(2):548–58.

[11] Abu El-Asrar AM, Nawaz MI, Kangave D, Abouammoh M, Mohammad G. High-mobility group box-1 and endothelial cell angiogenic markers in the vitreous from patients with proliferative diabetic retinopathy. Mediators Inflamm. 2012;2012:697489.

[12] Hayashi F, Smith KD, Ozinsky A, Hawn TR, Yi EC, Goodlett DR, Eng JK, Akira S, Underhill DM, Aderem A. The innate immune response to bacterial flagellin is mediated by Toll-like receptor 5. Nature. 2001;410(6832):1099–103.

[13] Hemmi H, Kaisho T, Takeuchi O, Sato S, Sanjo H, Hoshino K, Horiuchi T, Tomizawa H, Takeda K, Akira S. Small anti-viral compounds activate immune cells via the TLR7 My D88-dependent signaling pathway. Nat Immunol. 2002;3(2):196–200.

[14] Huttunen HJ, Fages C, Rauvala H. Receptor for advanced glycation end products (RAGE)-mediated neurite outgrowth and activation of NF-kappa B require the cytoplasmic domain of the receptor but different downstream signaling pathways. J Biol Chem. 1999;274(28):19919–24.

[15] Semeraro F, Cancarini A, dell'Omo R, Rezzola S, Romano MR, Costagliola C. Diabetic retinopathy: vascular and inflammatory disease. J Diabetes Res. 2015;2015:582060.

[16] Rangasamy S, Mc Guire PG, Das A. Diabetic retinopathy and inflammation: novel therapeutic targets. Middle East Afr J Ophthalmol. 2012;19(1):52–9.

[17] Brucklacher RM, Patel KM, Van Guilder HD, Bixler GV, Barber AJ, Antonetti DA, Lin CM, La Noue KF, Gardner TW, Bronson SK, Freeman WM. Whole genome assessment of the retinal response to diabetes reveals a progressive neurovascular inflammatory response. BMC Med Genomics. 2008;1:26.

[18] El-Asrar AM. Role of inflammation in the pathogenesis of diabetic retinopathy. Middle East Afr J Ophthalmol. 2012;19(1):70–4.

[19] Chan PS, Kanwar M, Kowluru RA. Resistance of retinal inflammatory mediators to suppress after reinstitution of good glycemic control: novel mechanism for metabolic memory. J Diabetes Complications. 2010;24(1):55–63.

[20] Du Y, Sarthy VP, Kern TS. Interaction between NO and COX pathways in retinal cells exposed to elevated glucose and retina of diabetic rats. Am J Physiol Regul Integr Comp Physiol. 2004;287(4):R735–41.

[21] Mohammad G, Siddiquei MM. Role of matrix metalloproteinase-2 and -9 in the development of diabetic retinopathy. J Ocul Biol Dis Infor. 2012;5(1):1–8.

[22] Yang H, Wang H, Czura CJ, Tracey KJ. The cytokine activity of HMGB1. J Leukoc Biol. 2005;78:1–8.

[23] van Beijnum JR, Buurman WA, Griffioen AW. Convergence and amplification of toll-like receptor (TLR) and receptor for advanced glycation end products (RAGE) signaling pathways via high mobility group B1 (HMGB1). Angiogenesis. 2008;11:91–9.

[24] Treutiger CJ, Mullins GE, Johansson AS, Rouhiainen A, Rauvala HM, Erlandsson-Harris H, et al. High mobility group 1 B-box mediates activation of human endothelium. J Intern Med 2003;254:375–85.

[25] Fiuza C, Bustin M, Talwar S, Tropea M, Gerstenberger E, Shelhamer JH, et al. Inflammation-promoting activity of HMGB1 on human microvascular endothelial cells. Blood. 2003;101:2652–60.

[26] Belgrano FS, de Abreu da Silva IC, Bastos de Oliveira FM, Fantappié MR, Mohana-Borges R. Role of the acidic tail of high mobility group protein B1 (HMGB1) in protein stability and DNA bending. PLo S One 2013;8:e79572.

[27] Andersson U, Wang H, Palmblad K, Aveberger AC, Bloom O, Erlandsson-Harris H, Janson A, Kokkola R, Zhang M, Yang H, Tracey KJ. High mobility group 1 protein (HMG-1) stimulates proinflammatory cytokine synthesis in human monocytes. J Exp Med. 2000;192(4):565–70.

[28] Park JS, Arcaroli J, Yum HK, Yang H, Wang H, Yang KY, Choe KH, Strassheim D, Pitts TM, Tracey KJ, Abraham E. Activation of gene expression in human neutrophils by high mobility group box 1 protein. Am J Physiol Cell Physiol. 2003;284(4):C870–9.

[29] Rouhiainen A, Kuja-Panula J, Wilkman E, Pakkanen J, Stenfors J, Tuominen RK, Lepäntalo M, Carpén O, Parkkinen J, Rauvala H. Regulation of monocyte migration by amphoterin (HMGB1). Blood. 2004;104(4):1174–82.

[30] Tonnesen MG. Neutrophil-endothelial cell interactions: mechanisms of neutrophil adherence to vascular endothelium. J Invest Dermatol. 1989;93:53S–8S.

[31] Urbonaviciute V, Fürnrohr BG, Meister S, Munoz L, Heyder P, De Marchis F, et al. Induction of inflammatory and immune responses by HMGB1-nucleosome complexes: implications for the pathogenesis of SLE. J Exp Med. 2008;205:3007–18.

[32] Santos AR, Dvoriantchikova G, Li Y, Mohammad G, Abu El-Asrar AM, Wen R, et al. Cellular mechanisms of high mobility group 1 (HMGB-1) protein action in the diabetic retinopathy. PLo S One. 2014;9:e87574.

[33] Lotze MT, De Marco RA. Dealing with death: HMGB1 as a novel target for cancer therapy. Curr Opin Investig Drugs. 2003;4:1405–9.

[34] Yang J, Huang C, Yang J, Jiang H, Ding J. Statins attenuate high mobility group box-1 protein induced vascular endothelial activation: a key role for TLR4/NF-κB signaling pathway. Mol Cell Biochem. 2010;345:189–95.

[35] Kanellakis P, Agrotis A, Kyaw TS, Koulis C, Ahrens I, Mori S, et al. High-mobility group box protein 1 neutralization reduces development of diet-induced atherosclerosis in apolipoprotein e-deficient mice. Arterioscler Thromb Vasc Biol. 2011;31:313–9.

[36] Mollica L, De Marchis F, Spitaleri A, Dallacosta C, Pennacchini D, Zamai M, et al. Glycyrrhizin binds to high-mobility group box 1 protein and inhibits its cytokine activities. Chem Biol. 2007;14:431–41.

[37] Véliz LP, González FG, Duling BR, Sáez JC, Boric MP. Functional role of gap junctions in cytokine-induced leukocyte adhesion to endothelium in vivo. Am J Physiol Heart Circ Physiol. 2008;295:H1056–66.

http://dx.doi.org/10.5772/62524

[38] Zheng QZ, Lou YJ. Pathologic characteristics of immunologic injury in primary cultured rat hepatocytes and protective effect of glycyrrhizin in vitro. Acta Pharmacol Sin. 2003;24:771–7.

[39] Yuan H, Ji WS, Wu KX, Jiao JX, Sun LH, Feng YT. Anti-inflammatory effect of diammonium glycyrrhizinate in a rat model of ulcerative colitis. World J Gastroenterol. 2006;12:4578–81.

[40] Abdulahad DA, Westra J, Bijzet J, Limburg PC, Kallenberg CG, Bijl M. High mobility group box 1 (HMGB1) and anti-HMGB1 antibodies and their relation to disease characteristics in systemic lupus erythematosus. Arthritis Res Ther. 2011;13(3):R71.

[41] Park SY, Lee SW, Kim HY, Lee WS, Hong KW, Kim CD. HMGB1 induces angiogenesis in rheumatoid arthritis via HIF-1$\alpha$ activation. Eur J Immunol. 2015;45(4):1216–27.

[42] Kim HY, Park SY, Lee SW, Lee HR, Lee WS, Rhim BY, Hong KW, Kim CD. Inhibition of HMGB1-induced angiogenesis by cilostazol via SIRT1 activation in synovial fibroblasts from rheumatoid arthritis. PLo S One. 2014;9(8):e104743.

[43] Cohen MJ, Brohi K, Calfee CS, Rahn P, Chesebro BB, Christiaans SC, Carles M, Howard M, Pittet JF. Early release of high mobility group box nuclear protein 1 after severe trauma in humans: role of injury severity and tissue hypoperfusion. Crit Care. 2009;13(6):R174.

[44] Wang XW, Karki A, Du DY, Zhao XJ, Xiang XY, Lu ZQ. Plasma levels of high mobility group box 1 increase in patients with posttraumatic stress disorder after severe blunt chest trauma: a prospective cohort study. J Surg Res. 2015;193(1):308–15.

[45] Lantos J, Földi V, Roth E, Wéber G, Bogár L, Csontos C. Burn trauma induces early HMGB1 release in patients: its correlation with cytokines. Shock. 2010;33(6):562–7.

[46] Manganelli V, Signore M, Pacini I, Misasi R, Tellan G, Garofalo T, Lococo E, Chirletti P, Sorice M, Delogu G. Increased HMGB1 expression and release by mononuclear cells following surgical/anesthesia trauma. Crit Care. 2010;14(6):R197.

[47] de Souza A, Westra J, Bijzet J, Limburg PC, Stegeman CA, Bijl M, Kallenberg CG. Is serum HMGB1 a biomarker in ANCA-associated vasculitis? Arthritis Res Ther. 2013;15(5):R104.

[48] Majumdar M, Ratho R, Chawla Y, Singh MP. High levels of circulating HMGB1 as a biomarker of acute liver failure in patients with viral hepatitis E. Liver Int. 2013;33(9):1341–8.

[49] Thanos D, Maniatis T. The high mobility group protein HMG I(Y) is required for NF-kappa B-dependent virus induction of the human IFN-beta gene. Cell. 1992;71(5):777–89.

[50] Baldassarre G, Battista S, Belletti B, Thakur S, Pentimalli F, Trapasso F, Fedele M, Pierantoni G, Croce CM, Fusco A. Negative regulation of BRCA1 gene expression by

HMGA1 proteins accounts for the reduced BRCA1 protein levels in sporadic breast carcinoma. Mol Cell Biol. 2003;23(7):2225–38.

[51] Fashena SJ, Reeves R, Ruddle NH. A poly(d A-d T) upstream activating sequence binds high-mobility group I protein and contributes to lymphotoxin (tumor necrosis factor-beta) gene regulation. Mol Cell Biol. 1992;12(2):894–903.

[52] Lee H, Song M, Shin N, Shin CH, Min BS, Kim HS, Yoo JS, Kim H. Diagnostic significance of serum HMGB1 in colorectal carcinomas. PLo S One. 2012;7(4):e34318.

[53] Joussen AM, Poulaki V, Le ML, Koizumi K, Esser C, Janicki H, Schraermeyer U, Kociok N, Fauser S, Kirchhof B, Kern TS, Adamis AP. A central role for inflammation in the pathogenesis of diabetic retinopathy. FASEB J. 2004;18(12):1450–2.

[54] Adamis AP, Berman AJ. Immunological mechanisms in the pathogenesis of diabetic retinopathy. Semin Immunopathol. 2008;30(2):65–84.

[55] Matter K, Balda MS. Occludin and the functions of tight junctions. Int Rev Cytol. 1999;186:117–46.

[56] Fanning AS, Mitic LL, Anderson JM. Transmembrane proteins in the tight junction barrier. J Am Soc Nephrol. 1999;10(6):1337–45.

[57] Nawaz MI, Mohammad G. Role of high-mobility group box-1 protein in disruption of vascular barriers and regulation of leukocyte-endothelial interactions. J Recept Signal Transduct Res. 2015;35(4):340–5.

[58] Mohammad G, Siddiquei MM, Othman A, Al-Shabrawey M, Abu El-Asrar AM. High-mobility group box-1 protein activates inflammatory signaling pathway components and disrupts retinal vascular-barrier in the diabetic retina. Exp Eye Res. 2013;107:101–9.

[59] Kim W, Hudson BI, Moser B, Guo J, Rong LL, Lu Y, Qu W, Lalla E, Lerner S, Chen Y, Yan SS, D'Agati V, Naka Y, Ramasamy R, Herold K, Yan SF, Schmidt AM. Receptor for advanced glycation end products and its ligands: a journey from the complications of diabetes to its pathogenesis. Ann N Y Acad Sci. 2005;1043:553–61.

[60] Singh VP, Bali A, Singh N, Jaggi AS. Advanced glycation end products and diabetic complications. Korean J Physiol Pharmacol. 2014;18(1):1–14.

[61] Goldin A, Beckman JA, Schmidt AM, Creager MA. Advanced glycation end products: sparking the development of diabetic vascular injury. Circulation. 2006;114(6):597–605.

[62] Yamagishi S, Yonekura H, Yamamoto Y, Katsuno K, Sato F, Mita I, Ooka H, Satozawa N, Kawakami T, Nomura M, Yamamoto H. Advanced glycation end products-driven angiogenesis in vitro. Induction of the growth and tube formation of human microvascular endothelial cells through autocrine vascular endothelial growth factor. J Biol Chem. 1997;272(13):8723–30.

[63] Okamoto T, Yamagishi S, Inagaki Y, Amano S, Koga K, Abe R, Takeuchi M, Ohno S, Yoshimura A, Makita Z. Angiogenesis induced by advanced glycation end products and its prevention by cerivastatin. FASEB J. 2002;16(14):1928–30.

[64] El-Asrar AM, Missotten L, Geboes K. Expression of high-mobility groups box-1/receptor for advanced glycation end products/osteopontin/early growth response-1 pathway in proliferative vitreoretinal epiretinal membranes. Mol Vis. 2011;17:508–18.

[65] Zong H, Ward M, Stitt AW. AGEs, RAGE, and diabetic retinopathy. Curr Diab Rep. 2011;11(4):244–52.

[66] Zhou J, Wang S, Xia X. Role of intravitreal inflammatory cytokines and angiogenic factors in proliferative diabetic retinopathy. Curr Eye Res. 2012;37(5):416–20.

[67] Ramasamy R, Yan SF, Schmidt AM. The RAGE axis and endothelial dysfunction: maladaptive roles in the diabetic vasculature and beyond. Trends Cardiovasc Med. 2005;15(7):237–43.

[68] Mohammad G, Alam K, Nawaz MI, Siddiquei MM, Mousa A, Abu El-Asrar AM. Mutual enhancement between high-mobility group box-1 and NADPH oxidase-derived reactive oxygen species mediates diabetes-induced upregulation of retinal apoptotic markers. J Physiol Biochem. 2015;71(3):359–72.

[69] Abu El-Asrar AM, Mohammad G, Nawaz MI, Siddiquei MM. High-mobility group box-1 modulates the expression of inflammatory and angiogenic signaling pathways in diabetic retina. Curr Eye Res. 2015;40(11):1141–52.

[70] Du X, Stocklauser-Färber K, Rösen P. Generation of reactive oxygen intermediates, activation of NF-kappa B, and induction of apoptosis in human endothelial cells by glucose: role of nitric oxide synthase? Free Radic Biol Med. 1999;27(7–8):752–63.

[71] Romeo G, Liu WH, Asnaghi V, Kern TS, Lorenzi M. Activation of nuclear factor-kappa B induced by diabetes and high glucose regulates a proapoptotic program in retinal pericytes. Diabetes. 2002;51(7):2241–8.

[72] Kowluru RA, Koppolu P, Chakrabarti S, Chen S. Diabetes-induced activation of nuclear transcriptional factor in the retina, and its inhibition by antioxidants. Free Radic Res. 2003;37(11):1169–80.

[73] Mohammad G, Siddiquei MM, Abu El-Asrar AM. Poly (ADP-ribose) polymerase mediates diabetes-induced retinal neuropathy. Mediators Inflamm. 2013;2013:510451.

[74] Kowluru RA, Menon B, Gierhart DL. Beneficial effect of zeaxanthin on retinal metabolic abnormalities in diabetic rats. Invest Ophthalmol Vis Sci. 2008;49(4):1645–51.

[75] Sasaki M, Ozawa Y, Kurihara T, Kubota S, Yuki K, Noda K, Kobayashi S, Ishida S, Tsubota K. Neurodegenerative influence of oxidative stress in the retina of a murine model of diabetes. Diabetologia. 2010;53(5):971–9.

[76] Han Y, Adams AJ, Bearse MAJr, Schneck ME. Multifocal electroretinogram and short-wavelength automated perimetry measures in diabetic eyes with little or no retinopathy. Arch Ophthalmol. 2004;122(12):1809–15.

[77] Bearse MAJr, Han Y, Schneck ME, Barez S, Jacobsen C, Adams AJ. Local multifocal oscillatory potential abnormalities in diabetes and early diabetic retinopathy. Invest Ophthalmol Vis Sci. 2004;45(9):3259–65.

[78] Feit-Leichman RA, Kinouchi R, Takeda M, Fan Z, Mohr S, Kern TS, Chen DF. Vascular damage in a mouse model of diabetic retinopathy: relation to neuronal and glial changes. Invest Ophthalmol Vis Sci. 2005;46(11):4281–7.

[79] van Dijk HW, Kok PH, Garvin M, Sonka M, Devries JH, Michels RP, van Velthoven ME, Schlingemann RO, Verbraak FD, Abràmoff MD. Selective loss of inner retinal layer thickness in type 1 diabetic patients with minimal diabetic retinopathy. Invest Ophthalmol Vis Sci. 2009;50(7):3404–9.

[80] Gao HM, Zhou H, Zhang F, Wilson BC, Kam W, Hong JS. HMGB1 acts on microglia Mac1 to mediate chronic neuroinflammation that drives progressive neurodegeneration. J Neurosci. 2011;31(3):1081–92.

[81] Kim ID, Shin JH, Kim SW, Choi S, Ahn J, Han PL, Park JS, Lee JK. Intranasal delivery of HMGB1 si RNA confers target gene knockdown and robust neuroprotection in the postischemic brain. Mol Ther. 2012;20(4):829–39.

[82] Seki M, Nawa H, Fukuchi T, Abe H, Takei N. BDNF is upregulated by postnatal development and visual experience: quantitative and immunohistochemical analyses of BDNF in the rat retina. Invest Ophthalmol Vis Sci. 2003;44(7):3211–8.

[83] Martin KR, Quigley HA, Zack DJ, Levkovitch-Verbin H, Kielczewski J, Valenta D, Baumrind L, Pease ME, Klein RL, Hauswirth WW. Gene therapy with brain-derived neurotrophic factor as a protection: retinal ganglion cells in a rat glaucoma model. Invest Ophthalmol Vis Sci. 2003;44(10):4357–65.

[84] Binder DK, Scharfman HE. Brain-derived neurotrophic factor. Growth Factors. 2004;22(3):123–31.

[85] Abu El-Asrar AM, Nawaz MI, Siddiquei MM, Al-Kharashi AS, Kangave D, Mohammad G. High-mobility group box-1 induces decreased brain-derived neurotrophic factor-mediatedneuroprotection in the diabetic retina. Mediators Inflamm. 2013;2013:863036.

[86] KiveläT, Tarkkanen A, Virtanen I. Synaptophysin in the human retina and retinoblastoma. An immunohistochemical and Western blotting study. Invest Ophthalmol Vis Sci. 1989;30(2):212–9.

[87] Lieth E, La Noue KF, Antonetti DA, Ratz M. Diabetes reduces glutamate oxidation and glutamine synthesis in the retina. The Penn State Retina Research Group. Exp Eye Res. 2000;70(6):723–30.

[88] Li Q, Puro DG. Diabetes-induced dysfunction of the glutamate transporter in retinal Müller cells. Invest Ophthalmol Vis Sci. 2002;43(9):3109–16.

[89] Yu XH, Zhang H, Wang YH, Liu LJ, Teng Y, Liu P. Time-dependent reduction of glutamine synthetase in retina of diabetic rats. Exp Eye Res. 2009;89(6):967–71.

[90] Ozawa Y, Kurihara T, Sasaki M, Ban N, Yuki K, Kubota S, Tsubota K. Neural degeneration in the retina of the streptozotocin-induced type 1 diabetes model. Exp Diabetes Res. 2011;2011:108328.

[91] Abu El-Asrar AM, Siddiquei MM, Nawaz MI, Geboes K, Mohammad G. The proinflammatory cytokine high-mobility group box-1 mediates retinal neuropathy induced by diabetes. Mediators Inflamm. 2014;2014:746415.

[92] Mitola S, Belleri M, Urbinati C, Coltrini D, Sparatore B, Pedrazzi M, Melloni E, Presta M. Cutting edge: extracellular high mobility group box-1 protein is a proangiogenic cytokine. J Immunol. 2006;176(1):12–15.

[93] Zhang W, Liu H, Al-Shabrawey M, Caldwell RW, Caldwell RB. Inflammation and diabetic retinal microvascular complications. J Cardiovasc Dis Res. 2011;2(2):96–103.

Chapter 8

# Potential Biomarkers for Physical Exercise-Induced Brain Health

Suk Yu Yau, Ang Li, Xin Sun, Christine J. Fontaine,
Brian R. Christie and Kwok-Fai So

Additional information is available at the end of the chapter

http://dx.doi.org/10.5772/62458

**Abstract**

Physical exercise has long been recognized as an effective and economic strategy to promote brain health in humans. The cellular and structural changes in the brains of exercised animals, including enhancements of neurogenesis and synaptogenesis, dendritic remodeling, and synaptic plasticity, have been considered as the key biological alterations accounting for exercise-elicited benefits to brain health. However, what transduces body movements into the above-mentioned changes remains largely unknown. Emerging theories indicate that physical activity triggers the release of various factors into the circulation from skeletal muscle (neurotrophins, myokines, and cytokines) and/or adipose tissue (adipokines). In this chapter, we review several of these molecules that are potentially implicated in this process, including neurotrophic factors (BDNF, IGF-1, and VEGF), adipokines (adiponectin and irisin), and myokines/cytokines (IL-15). The relationship, either causal or concomitant, between levels of these molecules (particularly in the blood) and brain function after exercise may help to identify biomarkers that can serve as objective indicators to evaluate exercise therapy on diseased or ageing brain. In addition, unmasking biomarkers may be instrumental in elucidating the mechanisms mediating exercise-induced brain health, thereby contributing to novel drug discovery for treatments to maintain brain health.

**Keywords:** biomarkers, brain health, cognition, hippocampal plasticity, physical exercise

## 1. Introduction

With an ageing population worldwide, there is an increasing interest in interventions that allow for healthy ageing. Currently, physical exercise is the best known intervention that can effectively maintain or even enhance brain health. Physical exercise is beneficial to brain health and cognitive function, especially in elderly people [1]. Clinical studies have demonstrated that more physical activity is associated with a lower risk of ageing-related neurodegenerative disorders, such as Alzheimer's disease (AD) [2] and Parkinson's disease (PD) [3]. Owing to the heterogeneity of exercise *per se* (in terms of the duration, frequency, intensity, type, physical fitness, and diseased state of human subjects), it is difficult to prescribe physical exercise with optimal effects on brain health in a customized way. Therefore, more research is needed to maximize exercise-elicited benefits to counteract brain ageing. In line with this goal, identification of biological markers (biomarkers) would substantially facilitate the evaluation and monitoring of the clinical effectiveness of physical exercise therapy on brain health. This information will also help with the discovery of exercise-mimetic treatments for dealing with neurodegenerative diseases, considering that there is no commercial pharmaceutical drug that can exert preventative effects on neurodegenerative diseases in ageing brains at this moment.

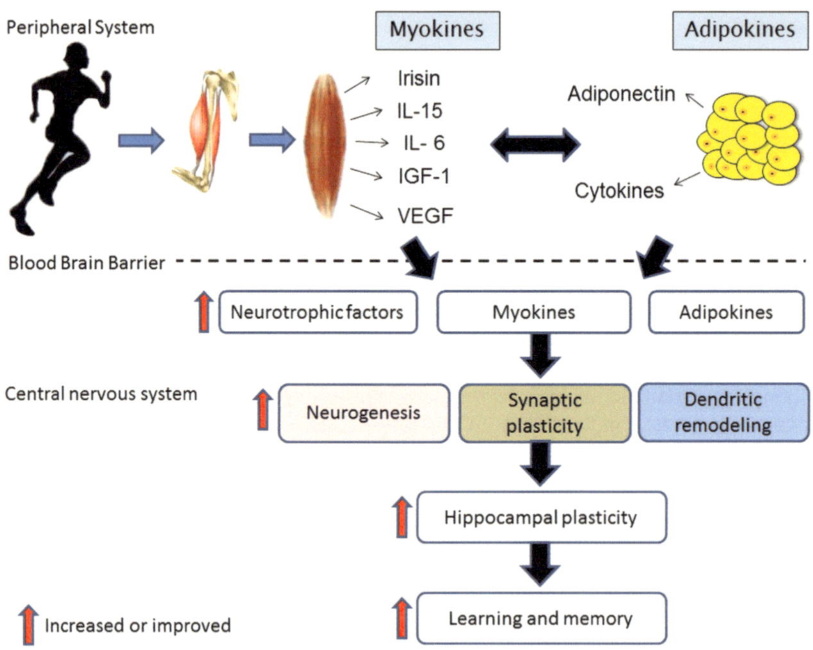


**Figure 1.** Exercise enhances hippocampal plasticity and hence improves cognitive performance.Physical activities promote the production and release of a variety of mediators in both central and periphery nervous systems, such as neurotrophic factors, myokines, adipokines, and cytokines. These molecules enter the brain and regulate hippocampal plasticity by affecting neurogenesis, synaptic plasticity, and dendritic remodeling, eventually improving learning and memory performance.

Effects of physical exercise on the brain are most apparent in the hippocampus, a brain region involved in learning and memory. Animal studies have indicated that physical exercise robustly improves hippocampal structural and functional plasticity by enhancing the generation of adult-born neurons (adult neurogenesis) in the hippocampal dentate gyrus (DG) [4, 5], increasing dendritic complexity and spine density [6-8], as well as promoting synaptic plasticity [5]. It is thought that important mediators for these exercise-triggered beneficial effects include neurotrophic factor produced in the brain such as brain-derived neurotrophic factor (BDNF) [9], as well as factors secreted by peripheral organs, such as insulin-like growth factor 1 (IGF-1) [10] and vascular endothelial growth factor (VEGF) [11]. In addition to these well-known factors, emerging evidence has suggested that many other peripheral molecules known to be induced by physical exercise may also affect brain health, particularly those secreted by skeletal muscle and/or adipose tissues, termed myokines (e.g., irisin), cytokines (e.g., interleukin-5 (IL-15)), and adipokines (e.g., adiponectin)(**Figure 1**).

Biomarkers are measurable indicators of normal biological and pathogenic states, as well as pharmacological responses to treatment intervention [12]. They can be used for clinical assessment of treatment effect or disease state. The biomarker should be present at baseline and its levels should be changed in response to treatment or disease state such that its levels can be used to predict the ultimate response. The ideal biomarkers should be easy to measure and quantify, and most importantly, they should closely correlate with the parameters being measured. Unfortunately, there are no conclusions on any one of the biomarkers that can fulfill the characteristics so far. Multiple biomarkers are likely needed for measurements in clinical studies, since using multiple biomarkers may be able to increase sensitivity, specificity, and predictive abilities for clinical diagnosis [13]. With the necessity to develop a biomarker panel to better evaluate exercise-induced cognitive enhancement, in this chapter, we first summarize the influences of physical exercise training on brain health, involving both animals and humans, and discuss the possible underlying mechanisms. Next, we summarize the effect of physical exercise on regulating potential peripheral biomarker candidates. Finally, we address the relationship between exercise-biomarkers and hippocampal plasticity with available literatures.

## 2. Beneficial effect of physical exercise on learning and memory in animals and humans

Extensive evidence from animal studies has reliably shown that the enhancement of adult-born neurons in the hippocampus, termed as hippocampal neurogenesis, may underlie the exercise-induced improvements on cognitive function. Seminal studies by van Praag and collaborators (1999) have shown that exercise in the form of wheel running not only increased hippocampal neurogenesis [4, 5], but also improved performance in the Morris water maze, and selectively increased the long-term potentiation (LTP) in the mouse DG [5]. These initial studies showed that not only does physical activity upregulate hippocampal neurogenesis, but it can also improve the capacity for hippocampal neurons to undergo synaptic plasticity and facilitate hippocampal-dependent learning and memory behavior in the same animals. Three months of physical exercise in humans was correlated with the increased blood volume in the DG, as measured by functional magnetic resonance imaging (fMRI) and improved cognitive function [14]. Exercise is indeed known to increase the cerebral blood flow [15], blood-brain-barrier permeability [16], and angiogenesis [17-20]. Given the relationship between angiogenesis and neurogenesis [21, 22], cognition improvement [14] following exercise can be interpreted as a result of increased hippocampal angiogenesis and therefore neurogenesis.

The beneficial effects of physical exercise on cognitive function imply that it may be used as a treatment to prevent of cognitive decline in age-related neurodegenerative diseases. Exercise has been shown to prevent a number of factors that decline with age, such as the decreases in hippocampal cell proliferation, neurogenesis [23], LTP, and neurotrophin levels [24]. Moreover, in aged mice, physical exercise can enhance hippocampal-dependent learning [25]. The benefits of exercise are not limited to midlife or aged adulthood, as rats submitted to a physical exercise regime during early postnatal development retained increases in hippocampal neurogenesis and improvement in spatial memory into their adult loves [26], highlighting the long-lasting benefits of physical exercise on brain plasticity throughout the lifespan [27].

Physical exercise has emerged in recent years as one of the most effective, affordable, and simple strategies for healthy aging, and therefore has the potential as a preventative treatment for cognitive decline associated with neurodegenerative diseases [28]. A meta-analysis has shown that 1–12 months of exercise in healthy adults is associated with significant behavioral benefits including ameliorated memory, processing speed, and attention [29]. Moreover, a regular exercise regime during not only adulthood [30], but also midlife [31] reduce the risk of developing dementia and preserve cognition later in life, which suggests that physical exercise may play a role in preventing age-related cognitive decline. In fact, a recent observational study has found a reduction in the risk of developing AD and other forms of dementia in individuals that exercise regularly, as opposed to those that did not engage in physical activity [32]. Physical exercise is beneficial to cognition across the life span, with its most significant effect on cognitive tasks involving the prefrontal cortex and the hippocampus [33].

## 3. Mechanism of physical exercise-induced hippocampal plasticity

Animal studies have suggested that physical exercise increases structural (e.g., neurogenesis and dendritic remodeling) and functional plasticity (e.g., synaptic plasticity) in the hippocampus (**Figure 2**).

### 3.1. Neurogenesis

Running distance is used as the physical assessment of voluntary running in animal studies, where a positive correlation between running distance and levels of neurogenesis in the hippocampus have been reliably shown in the literature using mice [34-36]. However, running distance is not the only variable that can affect the exercise-induced increases in hippocampal neurogenesis. Additional factors such as the genetic background [34, 37], age of the animals [38, 39], whether the running is forced or voluntary [4, 40-42], whether the animals are housed alone or in a group [43], and the duration of the running regime [44] can all affect neurogenesis following exercise. While there is some variability among studies of exercise, increases in neurogenesis are consistently reported in the literature [4, 25, 45, 46]. Long-term wheel running (2–4 months) with female C57 mice significantly increases the process of neuronal survival and neurogenesis concomitant with enhanced synaptic plasticity and improved performance

http://dx.doi.org/10.5772/62458

in the Morris water maze [4]. Others have found that there appear to be discrete stages at which voluntary running affects cell proliferation and differentiation. Namely, voluntary running in adult male C56B/L mice results in an increase in proliferating cells that peaks at 3 days following short-term running, which returns to basal levels following running for 32 [47] or 35 days [48]. Meanwhile, significant increases in neuronal differentiation are only observed following 10 days of voluntary running [23]. These data indicate that voluntary-running-induced increases in cell proliferation occurs during the earliest stages of running while a longer period of running promotes neuronal differentiation of adult-born cells.

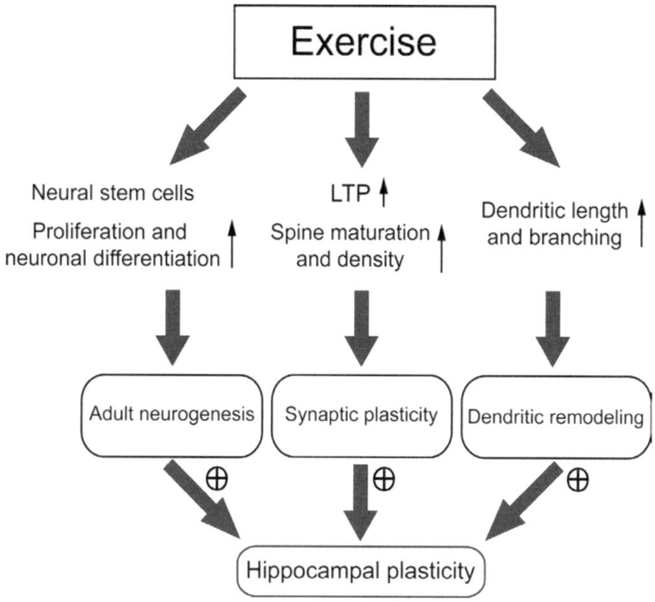


**Figure 2.** Potential mechanisms mediating exercise-induced hippocampal plasticity.Adult neurogenesis in the dentate gyrus of hippocampus is enhanced by exercise through increasing proliferation and neuronal differentiation of neural stem cells. Physical activities also alter synaptic plasticity by facilitating the induction of long-term potentiation and promoting the spine density and maturation in the hippocampus. Additionally, exercise modulates dendritic complexity by increasing the length and branching of dendrites. The above-mentioned changes may contribute to exercise-exerted effects on hippocampal plasticity.

### 3.2. Synaptic plasticity

Synaptic plasticity refers to changes in the way in which neurons communicate as a result of prior experience. Two forms of synaptic plasticity have been shown in the hippocampus, the LTP, where synaptic responses to a particular input are increased following a conditioning episode for memory formation, and the long-term depression (LTD), where synaptic responses to an input are decreased following a conditioning episode, which is recently implicated in memory clearance. The effects of exercise on *in vitro* hippocampal DG recordings were first shown in female mice by van Praag and colleagues in 1999, where 1 week of voluntary wheel running resulted in a greater LTP in the DG. Enhancement of LTP in the DG by exercise may occur by lowering the induction threshold for LTP [49]. However, a longer period of running is required to observe the exercise effect on synaptic plasticity in the DG [50] and CA3 [51] of rats.

### 3.3. Dendritic remodeling and synaptogenesis

In addition to increasing neurogenesis in the DG, voluntary wheel running can promote increased dendritic complexity or spine density in hippocampal subregions including the DG, CA1, CA3, and entorhinal cortex (EC) subregions [8]. Retroviral labeling of newborn neurons in the DG showed that voluntary running accelerates spine maturation with increased proportions of mushroom spines [52], which suggests that running may enhance the functional integration of newborn neurons into existing neuronal circuits. Moreover, voluntary wheel running increases both spine density and dendritic length of dentate granule cells [7]. Particularly, running increases the proportion of cells with higher dendritic complexity [53]. Two months of voluntary running also increase spine density in the CA1 subregion and layer III of the EC [8]. However, a longer period of running may be needed to trigger structural changes in the CA3 region because running for 2 weeks increases spine density in the DG and CA1 regions, but not in the CA3 region [54]. Increases of dendritic branching and spine density of CA3 pyramidal neurons are only observed after running for 4 weeks [55].

## 4. Potential biomarkers of physical exercise-promoted brain health

### 4.1. Neurotrophic factors

#### *4.1.1. BDNF*

##### *4.1.1.1. Animal studies*

BDNF levels can be increased by exercise [56, 57], with the increase occurring as early as 2–7 days of running [56], and it remains elevated for the whole duration of running [9], even extending to an additional 2 weeks following the end of the running period [58]. Increases in BDNF are important not only for the promotion of neurogenesis but also the enhancement of functional plasticity in the forms of LTP and behavioral learning and memory performance [5, 59, 60]. A direct link between BDNF and neurogenesis has been revealed by acutely knocking down BDNF in the DG by the lentivirus-mediated RNA interference, which resulted in a remarkable reduction in adult neurogenesis [61]. Additionally, 1 month following 2 weeks of BDNF overexpression significantly increases neuronal differentiation [62].

##### *4.1.1.2. Human studies*

Erickson and colleagues reported that physical exercise as an intervention for the aging population not only attenuated the age-related loss of hippocampal volume but also increased the serum levels of BDNF in these individuals [63]. Increases in hippocampal BDNF levels are thought to contribute to the upregulation of hippocampal neurogenesis seen with antidepressant treatment [64]. In fact, clinical studies have reported decreased serum BDNF levels in depressive patients, which were improved following treatment with antidepressants [65]. Given the well-established link between neurotrophins and adult hippocampal neurogenesis, it is reasonable to speculate that peripheral levels of these factors may be used as biomarkers of hippocampal neurogenesis. While the exact relationship between peripheral levels of neurotrophic factors and hippocampal neurogenesis has not reliably been established, progress has been made in this respect. Rasmussen and colleagues provided the first evidence that BDNF in the brain is a major contributor to the increase in plasma BDNF in response to exercise [66]. More recently, Yau and colleagues (2012) investigated the interaction of hippocampal neurogenesis, plasma neurotrophin levels, and cognitive performance in a rat stress model. They found that acute stress enhanced spatial learning as well as both hippocampal and plasma BDNF levels, but these findings were independent of hippocampal neurogenesis [67]. When chronic stress was administered, it significantly decreased hippocampal BDNF levels, hippocampal neurogenesis, and impaired spatial learning without affecting plasma BDNF levels [67]. While 28 days of voluntary running increased hippocampal neurogenesis and spatial learning, plasma BDNF levels were not significantly altered by exercise in rats [67]. While there is still possibility to use peripheral levels of neurotrophins as biomarkers correlating to changes in hippocampal neurogenesis, the interaction between these two factors remains to be understood and is far from a simple, linear relationship. It is possible that in order to fully depict changes in hippocampal neurogenesis at the periphery, we must examine multiple neurotrophins simultaneously, as peripheral BDNF changes may only be evident once substantial changes in BDNF levels have first occurred in the brain. This dissociation between central and peripheral BDNF levels shown in animals has also been reported in human subjects. Following 3 months of endurance training in healthy individuals, blood samples from the internal jugular vein but not the peripheral vessels showed increased BDNF levels [68]. Understandably, the responses of plasma or serum levels of BDNF varied considerably between studies; however, many reported a transient increase in plasma/serum levels of BDNF following exercise [69]. Lee and colleagues (2014) recently showed that adolescent athletes have lower resting serum levels of both BDNF and VEGF, and also showed improved brain function in the medial-temporal and frontal areas specifically compared to age-matched controls [70].

#### *4.1.2. IGF-1*

##### *4.1.2.1. Animal studies*

IGF-1 is another important growth factor that is shown to increase as a result of exercise [10]. This growth factor is taken up by the hippocampus from the bloodstream; however, if this process is blocked by subcutaneous infusions of IGF-1 antiserum, the exercise-mediated increase in neurogenesis is inhibited [10]. When IGF-1 is injected systemically in sedentary rats, it can mimic the effects of exercise and lead to enhancements in neurogenesis [71]. When IGF-1 is taken up by neurons, it can lead to increased firing and sensitivity of the neuron, which may stimulate BDNF and c-fos expression [71], which can, in turn, increase neurogenesis in the surrounding area.

*4.1.2.2. Human studies*

IGF-1 is a neurotrophic factor that is primarily secreted from the liver [72] that can readily be transported across the blood-brain and blood-cerebrospinal fluid barriers [73]. In the brain, IGF-1 plays a critical role in the creation of new neurons and synapses where transgenic overexpression of IGF-1 promotes neurogenesis and synaptogenesis in the hippocampus during postnatal development [74]. Both 6 and 20 days after exogenous IGF-1 is administered, there is an increase in the number of hippocampal cell proliferation [75]. Clinical studies have established a positive correlation between serum IGF-1 levels and cognitive function [76-78]. Additionally, following two 60-minute cycling sessions, middle-aged men show increased peripheral IGF-1 levels [79], which has also been replicated in road cyclists [80]. While there is evidence to suggest that there is a link among peripheral IGF-1, exercise and cognitive function, a direct relationship among peripheral IGF-1, brain IGF-1, hippocampal neurogenesis, and hippocampus-specific function has yet to be established. In contrast to studies of acute exercise, sustained physical exercise has been shown to either have no effect [81] or reduce peripheral IGF-1 levels in healthy subjects [82], regardless of previous experience as athletes [70] or exercise intensity [83]. As with BDNF, the relationship between IGF-1 in the body and brain in response to exercise is ambiguous.

*4.1.3. VEGF*

*4.1.3.1. Animal studies*

Angiogenesis and vascular function are enhanced in response to exercise in many brain areas, which may improve normal neural function, and also potentially offer protection during insult [84]. Magnetic resonance imaging of both mice and humans has suggested a correlation between exercise, DG blood flow, and neurogenesis; however, histological examination of the vasculature did not show exercise-induced changes in mice [14]. Increased blood flow can also increase the exposure to growth factors [56, 85] that can influence neurogenesis, such as VEGF. This neurotrophin, which is known for its role in stimulating angiogenesis, is increased following exercise [11] and may play a role in enhancing neurogenesis [21, 86]. Interestingly, new neurons in the DG tend to cluster around the local microvasculature [11, 87], and if VEGF is blocked, the exercise-induced increase in neurogenesis is abolished [11].

*4.1.3.2. Human studies*

VEGF is a 45-kDa heparin-binding homodimeric glycoprotein that is secreted by skeletal muscles and can be released into the vascular system [88]. Levels of VEGF have been shown to increase in skeletal muscle following acute physical exercise [89, 90]. VEGF mRNA expression in human muscle is elevated after 30 minutes of exercise [89]. Plasma VEGF levels are decreased in the femoral vein following 3 hours of two-legged kicking exercise meanwhile skeletal muscle VEGF mRNA expression was increased [91]. Similarly, arterial VEGF plasma levels are decreased following 10 days of exercise [89]. Kraus and colleagues have reported increased plasma VEGF levels following 2 hours of exercise in well-trained endurance athletes, but not sedentary controls at any time points [92]. The first link between exercise-induced functional improvements in the temporal cortex and changes of BDNF, IGF-1, and VEGF has recently been reported in healthy elderly subjects [93]. Following a 7-week regime of aerobic exercise, there was increased connectivity between the bilateral parahippocampi and the bilateral temporal gyri, which was associated with increased peripheral levels of BDNF, IGF-1, and VEGF. In teens that exercise regularly, Lee and colleagues showed improved frontal and temporal lobe cognitive function when compared to age-matched teens that did not exercise [70]. In contrast to what was seen in the study of elderly subjects, in the teen study there was a negative correlation between peripheral levels of BDNF and VEGF with temporal and frontal lobe functions. These studies raise critical questions regarding the type and duration of exercise as well as the age and previous exercise experience of the subjects.

## 5. Changes of other potential peripheral factors in response to physical exercise

Skeletal muscle and adipose tissues have recently been identified as major secretory organs in the maintenance of metabolic functions of the body. Myokines are identified as peptides and cytokines that are released by muscle fibers and can act in a paracrine or endocrine manner [94]. Adipokines are identified as hormones that are involved in metabolic functions and mediate the crosstalk between adipose tissues and the brain [95]. In response to physical exercise, these factors may have a crosstalk to regulate the secretion of myokines and adipokines, and work in concert to regulate many biological activities such as immune responses, neuroplasticity, and neurogenesis. Although linkage between hippocampal neurogenesis and levels of myokines or adipokines are still unclear, emerging animal studies have given us hints regarding their potential role in mediating the effect of exercise on regulating hippocampal plasticity.

### 5.1. Adipokine-adiponectin

#### *5.1.1. Animal studies*

Adiponectin, which is a protein secreted by adipose tissue, is well-known for its effects on metabolism and the cardiovascular system including antidiabetic, antiinflammatory, and antiatherosclerosis functions [96, 97]. Recent work has uncovered a role for adiponectin, as a peripheral factor mediating exercise-induced hippocampal cell proliferation [46]. Adiponectin has previously been shown to stimulate proliferation but not differentiation of adult hippocampal progenitor cells *in vitro* [98]. Acute administration via intracerebroventricular injections of either recombinant adiponectin [99] or an adenovirus expressing recombinant adiponectin [46] mimics the antidepressant effects of physical exercise. In the adenovirus experiment, administration also increased hippocampal neurogenesis, while knocking out adiponectin attenuated the antidepressant and neurogenic effects of physical exercise [46]. Following 14 days of running in mice, hippocampal adiponectin levels are elevated paired with increases in hippocampal cell proliferation [46]. Lower levels of adiponectin are associated with cognitive dysfunction [100]. Knockdown of adiponectin in aged animals results in cognitive deficits and AD pathogenesis such as Aβ-aggregate deposition, Tau hyperphosphorylation, excess neuroinflammation, and synaptic loss in frontal cortex [101], suggesting adiponectin may have an important influence on ageing-associated neurodegeneration.

#### *5.1.2. Human studies*

Levels of plasma adiponectin are positively correlated with physical activity [102]. However, effects of acute or chronic exercise training on modulating adiponectin levels are inconsistent and require further study. Circulating concentrations of adiponectin in normal individuals range from 5 to 20 μg/ml [103]. In clinical studies of acute exercise training, the reported levels of adiponectin have been varied, where some groups report increases [104, 105], decreases [106], or no changes [107-109]. The effect of exercise on adiponectin seems to be intensity dependent, because the acute effect of exercise in the form of volume-extended rowing training significantly increases adiponectin levels in elite athletes immediately and 30 minutes postexercise, but leads to decreased adiponectin levels in less elite athletes [106]. Both aerobic and resistance training with moderate to high intensity have been reported to significantly increase adiponectin levels [110], suggesting that the intensity of physical exercise is important to modulate adiponectin levels. Since adequate duration and intensity of physical training may be needed to augment circulating adiponectin levels, more detailed examinations of how adiponectin levels are manipulated by different forms and durations of exercise are necessary to provide insight regarding the role of adiponectin as a useful biomarker for evaluating the beneficial effects of physical exercise on the brains.

### 5.2. Adipokine-FNDC5/Irisin

#### *5.2.1. Animal studies*

In 2012, irisin was discovered as a novel exercise hormone for mediating the beneficial effects of exercise on metabolism [111]. Irisin is encoded by the *Fndc5* gene and is produced with the cleavage of its precursor FNDC5, and is then secreted from muscle during exercise [111]. Bostrom and colleagues identified irisin as a peroxisome proliferator-activated receptor $\gamma$ coactivator-1$\alpha$ (PGC-1$\alpha$)-dependent myokine secreted by skeletal muscle. In response to exercise, it circulates in the blood stream to reach fat tissue, where it triggers the browning of white adipose tissue [111]. Emerging animal studies have implicated irisin as a potential mediator for exercise-induced brain health. Irisin facilitates glucose and lipid metabolism in human muscle through AMP kinase phosphorylation [112]. It is known that administration of an AMPK agonist in wild-type mice, but not skeletal muscle-specific AMPK mutant mice, improves brain plasticity and memory function [113], suggesting that skeletal muscle-secreted factors that activate AMPK may influence brain and behavior. Irisin promotes cell proliferation in a mouse H19–7 hippocampal cell line in a dose-dependent manner [114]. Irisin was elevated in serum and skeletal muscle immediately after acute exercise [115]; however, whether its levels were increased in the hippocampus has not yet been explored. Notably, its precursor, FNDC5, is elevated by endurance exercise in the mouse hippocampus [116]. Increased FNDC5 in the hippocampus can in turn upregulate PGC-1$\alpha$ and BDNF expressions in the brain [116]. Knockdown of FNDC5 significantly decreases neural differentiation in mouse embryonic stem cells [117] and reduces Bdnf gene expression in hippocampal neurons [116], whereas peripheral delivery of FNDC5 by adenoviral vectors increases BDNF expression in the hippocampus [116]. These findings have suggested that FNDC5 may have a direct or indirect role in regulating hippocampal neurogenesis in response to physical training.

#### *5.2.2. Human studies*

Circulating irisin and its levels in adipose tissue are significantly associated with Fndc5 gene expression in adipose tissue. The Fndc5 gene is more strongly expressed in muscle than in adipose tissue by a 200-fold increase. Of note, obese patients and those with type 2 diabetes have lower circulating levels of irisin and *Fndc5* gene expression in adipose tissue [118, 119]. Circulating levels of irisin in sedentary individuals is ~3.6 ng/ml [120]. Its levels can be reduced in response to a 12-week training, and increased (~1.2-fold) just after acute exercise; however, FNDC5 and serum irisin levels did not change after acute aerobic and long-term endurance training. Interestingly, salivary and serum irisin increased significantly after moderate exercise [121]. Circulating irisin increased immediately after high-intensity interval exercise and declined 1 hour postexercise, suggesting that the increase in irisin levels may be transient and dose-/duration-dependent in humans.

### 5.3. Myokines/cytokine-interleukin 15 (IL-15)

#### *5.3.1. Animal studies*

IL-15 is a proinflammatory cytokine which can be secreted by muscle cells. IL-15 is stable in the circulation and can reach the parenchyma through the blood-brain barrier [122]. Beck and colleagues observed increases in hippocampal IL-15 expression and concurrent neurogenesis in IL-2-null mice [123]. Direct administration of IL-15 modulated neuronal differentiation of rat neural stem cells *in vitro* [124]. The suppression on olfactory neurogenesis was also found in a mouse model lacking the IL-15 receptor (IL-15R) [125]. Furthermore, IL-15 was shown to regulate neural stem cell proliferation through the MEK and JAK pathways [126]. In terms of depression-like behaviors, IL-15 treatment in wild-type mice shortened immobility time in the forced swim test. Conversely, IL-15R-deficient mice displayed increased immobility in the tail suspension and the forced swim tests, indicating that IL-15 signaling is essential to prevent neuropsychiatric symptoms [127]. Additionally, the IL-15/IL-15R pathway is also important for maintaining normal hippocampal activity and reducing anxiety-like behaviors in mice [128, 129].

*5.3.2. Human studies*

How IL-15 level is modulated by physical exercise is still unclear. An acute endurance exercise failed to elevate muscle IL-15 levels [130], whereas acute resistance exercise was reported to increase IL-15 mRNA expression without affecting its protein content in muscle [131]. Interestingly, a prolonged 12-week endurance exercise only raised the muscle IL-15 protein content without any changes at its mRNA levels [130]. This suggests divergent regulatory mechanisms mediating IL-15 production during muscle contraction. Plasma IL-15 concentrations were elevated by acute resistance exercise [132]. However, chronic resistance exercise seemed to have no such effect [133]. Therefore, more studies with the unified training paradigm are needed to identify the dynamic changes of IL-15.

## 6. Conclusion

In summary, the changes of central and/or peripheral neurotrophins, adipokines, myokines, or cytokines in response to physical training are still inconclusive so far. In human subjects, it is important to consider that age, health status, and previous exercise experience as well as general fitness can all play a role. Exercise with insufficient duration or intensity or form may not necessarily affect the expression of the above-mentioned factors. Therefore, answering the questions that by which type of and to what extent the exercise should be performed in the specific population are of particular significance. Further research is required to validate the use of exercise-modulated peripheral factors as the potential biomarkers for monitoring brain health following exercise intervention. Future direction should be focused on characterizing changes of aforementioned potential biomarkers and cognitive performance in different targeted groups. Identifying different biomarker panels may be necessary to examine the beneficial effect of exercise on targeted populations, since this will provide a more complete assessment with a better characterization on the effect of exercise on brain health.

## Acknowledgements

The work is supported by Hong Kong Health and Medical Research Fund and by funds of Leading Talents of Guangdong (2013), and National Natural Science Foundation of China (#81501171).

## Author details

Suk Yu Yau[1], Ang Li[2,3], Xin Sun[2], Christine J. Fontaine[4], Brian R. Christie[4] and Kwok-Fai So[2,3,5*]

*Address all correspondence to: hrmaskf@hku.hk

http://dx.doi.org/10.5772/62458

1 Department of Rehabilitation Sciences, Faculty of Health and Social Sciences, Hong Kong Polytechnic University, Hong Kong SAR, China

2 Guangdong Key Laboratory of Brain Function and Diseases, Guangdong-Hong Kong-Macau Institute of CNS Regeneration, Guangzhou, China

3 State Key Laboratory of Brain and Cognitive Sciences, The University of Hong Kong, Hong Kong SAR, China

4 Division of Medical Sciences, University of Victoria, Victoria, British Columbia, Canada

5 Department of Ophthalmology, LKS Faculty of Medicine, The University of Hong Kong, Hong Kong SAR, China

#These authors contributed equally to this work

## References

[1] Bherer L. Cognitive plasticity in older adults: effects of cognitive training and physical exercise. Ann N Y Acad Sci. 2015;1337:1–6.

[2] Buchman AS, Boyle PA, Yu L, Shah RC, Wilson RS, Bennett DA. Total daily physical activity and the risk of AD and cognitive decline in older adults. Neurology. 2012;78(17):1323–1329.

[3] Chen H, Zhang SM, Schwarzschild MA, Hernan MA, Ascherio A. Physical activity and the risk of Parkinson disease. Neurology. 2005;64(4):664–669.

[4] van Praag H, Kempermann G, Gage FH. Running increases cell proliferation and neurogenesis in the adult mouse dentate gyrus. Nat Neurosci. 1999;2(3):266–270.

[5] van Praag H, Christie BR, Sejnowski TJ, Gage FH. Running enhances neurogenesis, learning, and long-term potentiation in mice. Proc Natl Acad Sci U S A. 1999;96(23): 13427–13431.

[6] Yau SY, Lau BW, Tong JB, Wong R, Ching YP, Qiu G, et al. Hippocampal neurogenesis and dendritic plasticity support running-improved spatial learning and depression-like behaviour in stressed rats. PLoS One. 2011;6(9):e24263.

[7] Eadie BD, Redila VA, Christie BR. Voluntary exercise alters the cytoarchitecture of the adult dentate gyrus by increasing cellular proliferation, dendritic complexity, and spine density. J Comp Neurol. 2005;486(1):39–47.

[8] Stranahan AM, Khalil D, Gould E. Running induces widespread structural alterations in the hippocampus and entorhinal cortex. Hippocampus. 2007;17(11):1017–1022.

[9] Berchtold NC, Chinn G, Chou M, Kesslak JP, Cotman CW. Exercise primes a molecular memory for brain-derived neurotrophic factor protein induction in the rat hippocampus. Neuroscience. 2005;133(3):853–861.

[10] Trejo JL, Carro E, Torres-Aleman I. Circulating insulin-like growth factor I mediates exercise-induced increases in the number of new neurons in the adult hippocampus. J Neurosci. 2001;21(5):1628–1634.

[11] Fabel K, Fabel K, Tam B, Kaufer D, Baiker A, Simmons N, et al. VEGF is necessary for exercise-induced adult hippocampal neurogenesis. Eur J Neurosci. 2003;18(10):2803–2812.

[12] Naylor S. Biomarkers: current perspectives and future prospects. Expert Rev Mol Diagn. 2003;3(5):525–529.

[13] Schmidt HD, Shelton RC, Duman RS. Functional biomarkers of depression: diagnosis, treatment, and pathophysiology. Neuropsychopharmacology. 2011;36(12):2375–2394.

[14] Pereira AC, Huddleston DE, Brickman AM, Sosunov AA, Hen R, McKhann GM, et al. An in vivo correlate of exercise-induced neurogenesis in the adult dentate gyrus. Proc Natl Acad Sci U S A. 2007;104(13):5638–5643.

[15] Yancey SL, Overton JM. Cardiovascular responses to voluntary and treadmill exercise in rats. J App Physiol. 1993;75(3):1334–1340.

[16] Sharma HS, Cervos-Navarro J, Dey PK. Increased blood-brain barrier permeability following acute short-term swimming exercise in conscious normotensive young rats. Neurosci Res. 1991;10(3):211–221.

[17] Black JE, Isaacs KR, Anderson BJ, Alcantara AA, Greenough WT. Learning causes synaptogenesis, whereas motor activity causes angiogenesis, in cerebellar cortex of adult rats. Proc Natl Acad Sci U S A. 1990;87(14):5568–5572.

[18] Isaacs KR, Anderson BJ, Alcantara AA, Black JE, Greenough WT. Exercise and the brain: angiogenesis in the adult rat cerebellum after vigorous physical activity and motor skill learning. J Cerebral Blood Flow Metabol. 1992;12(1):110–119.

[19] Kleim JA, Cooper NR, VandenBerg PM. Exercise induces angiogenesis but does not alter movement representations within rat motor cortex. Brain Research. 2002;934(1): 1–6.

[20] Swain RA, Harris AB, Wiener EC, Dutka MV, Morris HD, Theien BE, et al. Prolonged exercise induces angiogenesis and increases cerebral blood volume in primary motor cortex of the rat. Neuroscience. 2003;117(4):1037–1046.

[21] Jin K, Zhu Y, Sun Y, Mao XO, Xie L, Greenberg DA. Vascular endothelial growth factor (VEGF) stimulates neurogenesis in vitro and in vivo. Proc Natl Acad Sci U S A. 2002;99(18):11946–11950.

[22] Louissaint A, Jr., Rao S, Leventhal C, Goldman SA. Coordinated interaction of neurogenesis and angiogenesis in the adult songbird brain. Neuron. 2002;34(6):945–960.

[23] Kronenberg G, Bick-Sander A, Bunk E, Wolf C, Ehninger D, Kempermann G. Physical exercise prevents age-related decline in precursor cell activity in the mouse dentate gyrus. Neurobiol Aging. 2006;27(10):1505–1513.

[24] O'Callaghan RM, Griffin EW, Kelly AM. Long-term treadmill exposure protects against age-related neurodegenerative change in the rat hippocampus. Hippocampus. 2009;19(10):1019–1029.

[25] van Praag H, Shubert T, Zhao C, Gage FH. Exercise enhances learning and hippocampal neurogenesis in aged mice. J Neurosci. 2005;25(38):8680–8685.

[26] Gomes da Silva S, Unsain N, Masco DH, Toscano-Silva M, de Amorim HA, Silva Araujo BH, et al. Early exercise promotes positive hippocampal plasticity and improves spatial memory in the adult life of rats. Hippocampus. 2012;22(2):347–358.

[27] Leuner B, Gould E, Shors TJ. Is there a link between adult neurogenesis and learning? Hippocampus. 2006;16(3):216–224.

[28] Ahlskog JE, Geda YE, Graff-Radford NR, Petersen RC. Physical exercise as a preventive or disease-modifying treatment of dementia and brain aging. Mayo Clinic Proc. 2011;86(9):876–884.

[29] Smith PJ, Blumenthal JA, Hoffman BM, Cooper H, Strauman TA, Welsh-Bohmer K, et al. Aerobic exercise and neurocognitive performance: a meta-analytic review of randomized controlled trials. Psychosom Med. 2010;72(3):239–252.

[30] Ratey JJ, Loehr JE. The positive impact of physical activity on cognition during adulthood: a review of underlying mechanisms, evidence and recommendations. Rev Neurosci. 2011;22(2):171–185.

[31] Hamer M, Chida Y. Physical activity and risk of neurodegenerative disease: a systematic review of prospective evidence. Psychol Med. 2009;39(1):3–11.

[32] Lautenschlager NT, Cox K, Cyarto EV. The influence of exercise on brain aging and dementia. Biochim Biophys Acta. 2012;1822(3):474–481.

[33] Prakash RS, Voss MW, Erickson KI, Kramer AF. Physical activity and cognitive vitality. Annu Rev Psychol. 2015;66:769–797.

[34] Clark PJ, Kohman RA, Miller DS, Bhattacharya TK, Brzezinska WJ, Rhodes JS. Genetic influences on exercise-induced adult hippocampal neurogenesis across 12 divergent mouse strains. Genes Brain Behav. 2011;10(3):345–353.

[35] Holmes MM, Galea LA, Mistlberger RE, Kempermann G. Adult hippocampal neurogenesis and voluntary running activity: circadian and dose-dependent effects. J Neurosci Res. 2004;76(2):216–222.

[36] Rhodes JS, van Praag H, Jeffrey S, Girard I, Mitchell GS, Garland T, Jr., et al. Exercise increases hippocampal neurogenesis to high levels but does not improve spatial learning in mice bred for increased voluntary wheel running. Behav Neurosci. 2003;117(5):1006–1016.

[37] Merritt JR, Rhodes JS. Mouse genetic differences in voluntary wheel running, adult hippocampal neurogenesis and learning on the multi-strain-adapted plus water maze. Behav Brain Res. 2015;280:62–71.

[38] Kim YP, Kim H, Shin MS, Chang HK, Jang MH, Shin MC, et al. Age-dependence of the effect of treadmill exercise on cell proliferation in the dentate gyrus of rats. Neurosci Lett. 2004;355(1–2):152–154.

[39] Marlatt MW, Potter MC, Lucassen PJ, van Praag H. Running throughout middle-age improves memory function, hippocampal neurogenesis and BDNF levels in female C57Bl/6J mice. Dev Neurobiol. 2012.

[40] Leasure JL, Jones M. Forced and voluntary exercise differentially affect brain and behavior. Neuroscience. 2008;156(3):456–465.

[41] Li H, Liang A, Guan F, Fan R, Chi L, Yang B. Regular treadmill running improves spatial learning and memory performance in young mice through increased hippocampal neurogenesis and decreased stress. Brain Res. 2013;1531:1–8.

[42] Uda M, Ishido M, Kami K, Masuhara M. Effects of chronic treadmill running on neurogenesis in the dentate gyrus of the hippocampus of adult rat. Brain Res. 2006;1104(1):64–72.

[43] Stranahan AM, Khalil D, Gould E. Social isolation delays the positive effects of running on adult neurogenesis. Nat Neurosci. 2006;9(4):526–533.

[44] Snyder JS, Glover LR, Sanzone KM, Kamhi JF, Cameron HA. The effects of exercise and stress on the survival and maturation of adult-generated granule cells. Hippocampus. 2009;19(10):898–906.

[45] van Praag H, Schinder AF, Christie BR, Toni N, Palmer TD, Gage FH. Functional neurogenesis in the adult hippocampus. Nature. 2002;415(6875):1030–1034.

[46] Yau SY, Li A, Hoo RL, Ching YP, Christie BR, Lee TM, et al. Physical exercise-induced hippocampal neurogenesis and antidepressant effects are mediated by the adipocyte hormone adiponectin. Proc Natl Acad Sci U S A. 2014;111(44):15810–15815.

[47] Kronenberg G, Reuter K, Steiner B, Brandt MD, Jessberger S, Yamaguchi M, et al. Subpopulations of proliferating cells of the adult hippocampus respond differently to physiologic neurogenic stimuli. J Comparat Neurol. 2003;467(4):455–463.

[48] Brandt MD, Maass A, Kempermann G, Storch A. Physical exercise increases Notch activity, proliferation and cell cycle exit of type-3 progenitor cells in adult hippocampal neurogenesis. Eur J Neurosci. 2010;32(8):1256–1264.

[49] Schmidt-Hieber C, Jonas P, Bischofberger J. Enhanced synaptic plasticity in newly generated granule cells of the adult hippocampus. Nature. 2004;429(6988):184–187.

[50] Patten AR, Sickmann H, Hryciw BN, Kucharsky T, Parton R, Kernick A, et al. Long-term exercise is needed to enhance synaptic plasticity in the hippocampus. Learning Memory (Cold Spring Harbor, NY). 2013;20(11):642–647.

[51] O'Callaghan RM, Ohle R, Kelly AM. The effects of forced exercise on hippocampal plasticity in the rat: a comparison of LTP, spatial- and non-spatial learning. Behav Brain Res. 2007;176(2):362–366.

[52] Zhao C, Teng EM, Summers RG, Jr., Ming GL, Gage FH. Distinct morphological stages of dentate granule neuron maturation in the adult mouse hippocampus. J Neurosci. 2006;26(1):3–11.

[53] Redila VA, Christie BR. Exercise-induced changes in dendritic structure and complexity in the adult hippocampal dentate gyrus. Neuroscience. 2006;137(4):1299–1307.

[54] Glasper ER, Llorens-Martin MV, Leuner B, Gould E, Trejo JL. Blockade of insulin-like growth factor-I has complex effects on structural plasticity in the hippocampus. Hippocampus. 2010;20(6):706–712.

[55] Lin TW, Chen SJ, Huang TY, Chang CY, Chuang JI, Wu FS, et al. Different types of exercise induce differential effects on neuronal adaptations and memory performance. Neurobiol Learning Memory. 2012;97(1):140–147.

[56] Neeper SA, Gomez-Pinilla F, Choi J, Cotman C. Exercise and brain neurotrophins. Nature. 1995;373(6510):109.

[57] Vaynman S, Gomez-Pinilla F. License to run: exercise impacts functional plasticity in the intact and injured central nervous system by using neurotrophins. Neurorehabilitation Neural Repair. 2005;19(4):283–295.

[58] Berchtold NC, Castello N, Cotman CW. Exercise and time-dependent benefits to learning and memory. Neuroscience. 2010;167(3):588–597.

[59] Bekinschtein P, Oomen CA, Saksida LM, Bussey TJ. Effects of environmental enrichment and voluntary exercise on neurogenesis, learning and memory, and pattern separation: BDNF as a critical variable? Semin Cell Dev Biol. 2011.

[60] Farmer J, Zhao X, van Praag H, Wodtke K, Gage FH, Christie BR. Effects of voluntary exercise on synaptic plasticity and gene expression in the dentate gyrus of adult male Sprague-Dawley rats in vivo. Neuroscience. 2004;124(1):71–79.

[61] Taliaz D, Stall N, Dar DE, Zangen A. Knockdown of brain-derived neurotrophic factor in specific brain sites precipitates behaviors associated with depression and reduces neurogenesis. Mol Psychiat. 2010;15(1):80–92.

[62] Scharfman H, Goodman J, Macleod A, Phani S, Antonelli C, Croll S. Increased neurogenesis and the ectopic granule cells after intrahippocampal BDNF infusion in adult rats. Exp Neurol. 2005;192(2):348–356.

[63] Erickson KI, Voss MW, Prakash RS, Basak C, Szabo A, Chaddock L, et al. Exercise training increases size of hippocampus and improves memory. Proc Natl Acad Sci U S A. 2011;108(7):3017–3022.

[64] Duman RS, Nakagawa S, Malberg J. Regulation of adult neurogenesis by antidepressant treatment. Neuropsychopharmacology. 2001;25(6):836–844.

[65] Shimizu E, Hashimoto K, Okamura N, Koike K, Komatsu N, Kumakiri C, et al. Alterations of serum levels of brain-derived neurotrophic factor (BDNF) in depressed patients with or without antidepressants. Biol Psychiat. 2003;54(1):70–75.

[66] Rachman IM, Unnerstall JR, Pfaff DW, Cohen RS. Estrogen alters behavior and forebrain c-fos expression in ovariectomized rats subjected to the forced swim test. Proc Natl Acad Sci U S A. 1998;95(23):13941–13946.

[67] Yau SY, Lau BW, Zhang ED, Lee JC, Li A, Lee TM, et al. Effects of voluntary running on plasma levels of neurotrophins, hippocampal cell proliferation and learning and memory in stressed rats. Neuroscience. 2012;222:289–301.

[68] Seifert T, Brassard P, Wissenberg M, Rasmussen P, Nordby P, Stallknecht B, et al. Endurance training enhances BDNF release from the human brain. Am J Physiol. 2010;298(2):R372-R377.

[69] Knaepen K, Goekint M, Heyman EM, Meeusen R. Neuroplasticity - exercise-induced response of peripheral brain-derived neurotrophic factor: a systematic review of experimental studies in human subjects. Sports Med. 2010;40(9):765–801.

[70] Lee TM, Wong ML, Lau BW, Lee JC, Yau SY, So KF. Aerobic exercise interacts with neurotrophic factors to predict cognitive functioning in adolescents. Psychoneuroendocrinology. 2014;39:214–224.

[71] Carro E, Nunez A, Busiguina S, Torres-Aleman I. Circulating insulin-like growth factor I mediates effects of exercise on the brain. J Neurosci. 2000;20(8):2926–2933.

[72] Butler AA, LeRoith D. Minireview: tissue-specific versus generalized gene targeting of the igf1 and igf1r genes and their roles in insulin-like growth factor physiology. Endocrinology. 2001;142(5):1685–1688.

[73] Pulford BE, Ishii DN. Uptake of circulating insulin-like growth factors (IGFs) into cerebrospinal fluid appears to be independent of the IGF receptors as well as IGF-binding proteins. Endocrinology. 2001;142(1):213–220.

[74] O'Kusky JR, Ye P, D'Ercole AJ. Insulin-like growth factor-I promotes neurogenesis and synaptogenesis in the hippocampal dentate gyrus during postnatal development. J Neurosci. 2000;20(22):8435–8442.

[75] Aberg MA, Aberg ND, Hedbacker H, Oscarsson J, Eriksson PS. Peripheral infusion of IGF-I selectively induces neurogenesis in the adult rat hippocampus. J Neurosci. 2000;20(8):2896–2903.

[76] Arwert LI, Deijen JB, Drent ML. The relation between insulin-like growth factor I levels and cognition in healthy elderly: a meta-analysis. Growth Hormone IGF Res. 2005;15(6): 416–422.

[77] Aleman A, de Vries WR, de Haan EH, Verhaar HJ, Samson MM, Koppeschaar HP. Age-sensitive cognitive function, growth hormone and insulin-like growth factor 1 plasma levels in healthy older men. Neuropsychobiology. 2000;41(2):73–78.

[78] Aleman A, Verhaar HJ, De Haan EH, De Vries WR, Samson MM, Drent ML, et al. Insulin-like growth factor-I and cognitive function in healthy older men. J Clin Endocrinol Metabol. 1999;84(2):471–475.

[79] Manetta J, Brun JF, Maimoun L, Fedou C, Prefaut C, Mercier J. The effects of intensive training on insulin-like growth factor I (IGF-I) and IGF binding proteins 1 and 3 in competitive cyclists: relationships with glucose disposal. J Sports Sci. 2003;21(3):147–154.

[80] Zebrowska A, Gasior Z, Langfort J. Serum IGF-I and hormonal responses to incremental exercise in athletes with and without left ventricular hypertrophy. J Sports Sci Med. 2009;8(1):67–76.

[81] Cearlock DM, Nuzzo NA. Effects of sustained moderate exercise on cholesterol, growth hormone and cortisol blood levels in three age groups of women. Clin Lab Sci. 2001;14(2):108–111.

[82] Karatay S, Yildirim K, Melikoglu MA, Akcay F, Senel K. Effects of dynamic exercise on circulating IGF-1 and IGFBP-3 levels in patients with rheumatoid arthritis or ankylosing spondylitis. Clin Rheumatol. 2007;26(10):1635–1639.

[83] Nishida Y, Matsubara T, Tobina T, Shindo M, Tokuyama K, Tanaka K, et al. Effect of low-intensity aerobic exercise on insulin-like growth factor-I and insulin-like growth factor-binding proteins in healthy men. Intl J Endocrinol. 2010.

[84] Christie BR, Eadie BD, Kannangara TS, Robillard JM, Shin J, Titterness AK. Exercising our brains: how physical activity impacts synaptic plasticity in the dentate gyrus. Neuromolecular Med. 2008;10(2):47–58.

[85] Spier SA, Delp MD, Meininger CJ, Donato AJ, Ramsey MW, Muller-Delp JM. Effects of ageing and exercise training on endothelium-dependent vasodilatation and structure of rat skeletal muscle arterioles. J Physiol. 2004;556(Pt 3):947–958.

[86] Cao L, Jiao X, Zuzga DS, Liu Y, Fong DM, Young D, et al. VEGF links hippocampal activity with neurogenesis, learning and memory. Nat Genet. 2004;36(8):827–835.

[87] Palmer TD, Willhoite AR, Gage FH. Vascular niche for adult hippocampal neurogenesis. J Comparat Neurol. 2000;425(4):479–494.

[88] Gavin TP, Drew JL, Kubik CJ, Pofahl WE, Hickner RC. Acute resistance exercise increases skeletal muscle angiogenic growth factor expression. Acta Physiologica. 2007;191(2):139–146.

[89] Gustafsson T, Knutsson A, Puntschart A, Kaijser L, Nordqvist AC, Sundberg CJ, et al. Increased expression of vascular endothelial growth factor in human skeletal muscle in response to short-term one-legged exercise training. Pflugers Archiv Eur J Physiol. 2002;444(6):752–759.

[90] Hoffner L, Nielsen JJ, Langberg H, Hellsten Y. Exercise but not prostanoids enhance levels of vascular endothelial growth factor and other proliferative agents in human skeletal muscle interstitium. J Physiol. 2003;550(Pt 1):217–225.

[91] Hiscock N, Fischer CP, Pilegaard H, Pedersen BK. Vascular endothelial growth factor mRNA expression and arteriovenous balance in response to prolonged, submaximal exercise in humans. Am J Physiol Heart Circulat Physiol. 2003;285(4):H1759-H1763.

[92] Kraus RM, Stallings HW, 3rd, Yeager RC, Gavin TP. Circulating plasma VEGF response to exercise in sedentary and endurance-trained men. J Appl Physiol. 2004;96(4):1445–1450.

[93] Voss MW, Erickson KI, Prakash RS, Chaddock L, Kim JS, Alves H, et al. Neurobiological markers of exercise-related brain plasticity in older adults. Brain Behav Immunity. 2013;28:90–99.

[94] Pedersen BK, Akerstrom TC, Nielsen AR, Fischer CP. Role of myokines in exercise and metabolism. J Appl Physiol. 2007;103(3):1093–1098.

[95] Scherer PE. Adipose tissue: from lipid storage compartment to endocrine organ. Diabetes. 2006;55(6):1537–1545.

[96] Chandran M, Phillips SA, Ciaraldi T, Henry RR. Adiponectin: more than just another fat cell hormone? Diabetes Care. 2003;26(8):2442–2450.

[97] Kawano J, Arora R. The role of adiponectin in obesity, diabetes, and cardiovascular disease. J Cardiometab Syndr. 2009;4(1):44–49.

[98] Zhang D, Guo M, Zhang W, Lu XY. Adiponectin stimulates proliferation of adult hippocampal neural stem/progenitor cells through activation of p38 mitogen-activated protein kinase (p38MAPK)/glycogen synthase kinase 3beta (GSK-3beta)/beta-catenin signaling cascade. J Biol Chem. 2011;286(52):44913–44920.

[99] Liu J, Guo M, Zhang D, Cheng SY, Liu M, Ding J, et al. Adiponectin is critical in determining susceptibility to depressive behaviors and has antidepressant-like activity. Proc Natl Acad Sci U S A. 2012;109(30):12248–12253.

[100] Teixeira AL, Diniz BS, Campos AC, Miranda AS, Rocha NP, Talib LL, et al. Decreased levels of circulating adiponectin in mild cognitive impairment and Alzheimer's disease. Neuromol Med. 2013;15(1):115–121.

[101] Ng R. Adiponectin deficiency induced cognitive impairment in aging mice through reductions in insulin sensitivity and AMPK activation (I12–4A). Neurology. 2015;84(14):I12–4A.

[102] St-Pierre DH, Faraj M, Karelis AD, Conus F, Henry JF, St-Onge M, et al. Lifestyle behaviours and components of energy balance as independent predictors of ghrelin and adiponectin in young non-obese women. Diabetes Metab. 2006;32(2):131–139.

[103] Matsuzawa Y. Adiponectin: identification, physiology and clinical relevance in metabolic and vascular disease. Atheroscler Suppl. 2005;6(2):7–14.

[104] Jurimae J, Purge P, Jurimae T. Adiponectin and stress hormone responses to maximal sculling after volume-extended training season in elite rowers. Metabolism. 2006;55(1): 13–19.

[105] Kraemer RR, Aboudehen KS, Carruth AK, Durand RT, Acevedo EO, Hebert EP, et al. Adiponectin responses to continuous and progressively intense intermittent exercise. Med Sci Sports Exercise. 2003;35(8):1320–1325.

[106] Jurimae J, Purge P, Jurimae T. Adiponectin is altered after maximal exercise in highly trained male rowers. Eur J Appl Physiol. 2005;93(4):502–505.

[107] Ferguson MA, White LJ, McCoy S, Kim HW, Petty T, Wilsey J. Plasma adiponectin response to acute exercise in healthy subjects. Eur J Appl Physiol. 2004;91(2–3):324–329.

[108] Jamurtas AZ, Theocharis V, Koukoulis G, Stakias N, Fatouros IG, Kouretas D, et al. The effects of acute exercise on serum adiponectin and resistin levels and their relation to insulin sensitivity in overweight males. Eur J Appl Physiol. 2006;97(1):122–126.

[109] Punyadeera C, Zorenc AH, Koopman R, McAinch AJ, Smit E, Manders R, et al. The effects of exercise and adipose tissue lipolysis on plasma adiponectin concentration and adiponectin receptor expression in human skeletal muscle. Eur J Endocrinol. 2005;152(3):427–436.

[110] Fatouros IG, Tournis S, Leontsini D, Jamurtas AZ, Sxina M, Thomakos P, et al. Leptin and adiponectin responses in overweight inactive elderly following resistance training and detraining are intensity related. J Clin Endocrinol Metab. 2005;90(11):5970–5977.

[111] Bostrom P, Wu J, Jedrychowski MP, Korde A, Ye L, Lo JC, et al. A PGC1-alpha-dependent myokine that drives brown-fat-like development of white fat and thermogenesis. Nature. 2012;481(7382):463–468.

[112] Huh JY, Mougios V, Kabasakalis A, Fatouros I, Siopi A, Douroudos, II, et al. Exercise-induced irisin secretion is independent of age or fitness level and increased irisin may

directly modulate muscle metabolism through AMPK activation. J Clin Endocrinol Metab. 2014;99(11):E2154-E2161.

[113] Kobilo T, Liu QR, Gandhi K, Mughal M, Shaham Y, van Praag H. Running is the neurogenic and neurotrophic stimulus in environmental enrichment. Learning Memory (Cold Spring Harbor, NY). 2011;18(9):605–609.

[114] Moon HS, Dincer F, Mantzoros CS. Pharmacological concentrations of irisin increase cell proliferation without influencing markers of neurite outgrowth and synaptogenesis in mouse H19–7 hippocampal cell lines. Metabolism. 2013;62(8):1131–1136.

[115] Brenmoehl J, Albrecht E, Komolka K, Schering L, Langhammer M, Hoeflich A, et al. Irisin is elevated in skeletal muscle and serum of mice immediately after acute exercise. Int J Biol Sci. 2014;10(3):338–349.

[116] Wrann CD, White JP, Salogiannnis J, Laznik-Bogoslavski D, Wu J, Ma D, et al. Exercise induces hippocampal BDNF through a PGC-1alpha/FNDC5 pathway. Cell Metab. 2013;18(5):649–659.

[117] Hashemi MS, Ghaedi K, Salamian A, Karbalaie K, Emadi-Baygi M, Tanhaei S, et al. Fndc5 knockdown significantly decreased neural differentiation rate of mouse embryonic stem cells. Neuroscience. 2013;231:296–304.

[118] Moreno-Navarrete JM, Ortega F, Serrano M, Guerra E, Pardo G, Tinahones F, et al. Irisin is expressed and produced by human muscle and adipose tissue in association with obesity and insulin resistance. J Clin Endocrinol Metab. 2013;98(4):E769-E778.

[119] Liu JJ, Wong MD, Toy WC, Tan CS, Liu S, Ng XW, et al. Lower circulating irisin is associated with type 2 diabetes mellitus. J Diabetes Complications. 2013;27(4):365–369.

[120] Jedrychowski MP, Wrann CD, Paulo JA, Gerber KK, Szpyt J, Robinson MM, et al. Detection and quantitation of circulating human irisin by tandem mass spectrometry. Cell Metab. 2015;22(4):734–740.

[121] Aydin S, Aydin S, Kuloglu T, Yilmaz M, Kalayci M, Sahin I, et al. Alterations of irisin concentrations in saliva and serum of obese and normal-weight subjects, before and after 45 min of a Turkish bath or running. Peptides. 2013;50:13–18.

[122] Pan W, Hsuchou H, Yu C, Kastin AJ. Permeation of blood-borne IL15 across the blood-brain barrier and the effect of LPS. J Neurochem. 2008;106(1):313–319.

[123] Beck RD, Jr., Wasserfall C, Ha GK, Cushman JD, Huang Z, Atkinson MA, et al. Changes in hippocampal IL-15, related cytokines, and neurogenesis in IL-2 deficient mice. Brain Res. 2005;1041(2):223–230.

[124] Huang YS, Cheng SN, Chueh SH, Tsai YL, Liou NH, Guo YW, et al. Effects of interleukin-15 on neuronal differentiation of neural stem cells. Brain Res. 2009;1304:38–48.

[125] Umehara T, Udagawa J, Takamura K, Kimura M, Ishimitsu R, Kiyono H, et al. Role of interleukin-15 in the development of mouse olfactory nerve. Congenital Anomalies. 2009;49(4):253–257.

[126] Gomez-Nicola D, Valle-Argos B, Pallas-Bazarra N, Nieto-Sampedro M. Interleukin-15 regulates proliferation and self-renewal of adult neural stem cells. Mol Biol Cell. 2011;22(12):1960–1970.

[127] Wu X, Hsuchou H, Kastin AJ, He Y, Khan RS, Stone KP, et al. Interleukin-15 affects serotonin system and exerts antidepressive effects through IL15Ralpha receptor. Psychoneuroendocrinology. 2011;36(2):266–278.

[128] He Y, Hsuchou H, Wu X, Kastin AJ, Khan RS, Pistell PJ, et al. Interleukin-15 receptor is essential to facilitate GABA transmission and hippocampal-dependent memory. J Neurosci. 2010;30(13):4725–4734.

[129] Wu X, He Y, Hsuchou H, Kastin AJ, Rood JC, Pan W. Essential role of interleukin-15 receptor in normal anxiety behavior. Brain Behav Immunity. 2010;24(8):1340–1346.

[130] Rinnov A, Yfanti C, Nielsen S, Akerstrom TC, Peijs L, Zankari A, et al. Endurance training enhances skeletal muscle interleukin-15 in human male subjects. Endocrine. 2014;45(2):271–278.

[131] Nielsen AR, Mounier R, Plomgaard P, Mortensen OH, Penkowa M, Speerschneider T, et al. Expression of interleukin-15 in human skeletal muscle effect of exercise and muscle fibre type composition. J Physiol. 2007;584(Pt 1):305–312.

[132] Riechman SE, Balasekaran G, Roth SM, Ferrell RE. Association of interleukin-15 protein and interleukin-15 receptor genetic variation with resistance exercise training responses. J Appl Physiol (1985). 2004;97(6):2214–2219.

[133] Prestes J, Shiguemoto G, Botero JP, Frollini A, Dias R, Leite R, et al. Effects of resistance training on resistin, leptin, cytokines, and muscle force in elderly post-menopausal women. J Sports Sci. 2009;27(14):1607–1615.

Chapter 9

# Biomarkers in Traumatic Spinal Cord Injury

Stefan Mircea Iencean and Andrei Stefan Iencean

Additional information is available at the end of the chapter

http://dx.doi.org/10.5772/63035

**Abstract**

Spinal cord injury (SCI) is one of the most devastating traumas for an individual because the complete traumatic spinal cord injury leads to paraplegia or tetraplegia. The mechanical injuries directly cause axonal destruction in fiber tracts, destruction of the neurons, and of the glial cells, and their destruction releases substances whose presence, quantity, and dynamics can be lesional biomarkers. The reactions of partially injured cells simultaneously start and the occurring substances and their quantity may be reaction biomarkers. The lesional biomarkers appear immediately post injury and after several hours there are both lesional biomarkers and reaction biomarkers.

In recent years, a number of protein biomarkers have been evaluated to detect neuronal injury and recently there have been studies about their potential diagnostic and predictive value for spinal cord injuries. The most important lesional biomarkers are the phosphorylated neurofilament subunits resulting from the axonal neurofilament destruction. The heavy phosphorylated neurofilament subunit (pNF-H) is a predictive lesional biomarker because its values pattern can show the reducing or stopping of the secondary lesions and the favorable outcome. The complete SCI patients with a favorable development had a specific pattern of daily values of pNF-H: a sudden increase up to a maximum value then a progressive decrease to normal. The patients with unfavorable outcome or neurological stabilization had two patterns: an increase to a plateau of pNF-H values or a progressive increase up to a peak followed by a progressive decrease to quasi-normal values.

**Keywords:** lesional biomarker, microneurosurgery, phosphorylated neurofilament subunit, reactional biomarker, spinal cord injury

INTECH
open science | open minds

# 1. Introduction

Spinal cord injury (SCI) is one of the most devastating traumas for an individual and their family because, depending on the level of injury, the complete traumatic SCI leads to paraplegia or tetraplegia [1].

Immediate traumatic SCI is the primary mechanical injury caused through the direct injury of the neurons, axons, and blood vessels (compression, laceration, shearing, and even transection of the spinal cord). After the injury event, the secondary injury mechanisms begin immediately and the secondary spinal cord lesions consist of hemorrhages, spinal cord edema, vasospasm, and hypoperfusion of the spinal cord and the damage of the spinal cord continues to progress for several days to weeks, and leads to the death of neurons and the interruption of the axonal tracts [2].

Many traumatic spinal cord injuries can be initially incomplete and the secondary damage completes the lesion of the spinal cord. Spinal cord injuries are difficult to treat because of these secondary injuries. Current therapy is unable to act on the primary mechanically lesion, but the secondary injury extension of the spinal cord could be stopped or reduced by an early efficient therapy.

It is necessary to know the type and the evolution of the secondary spinal cord lesions: complete destruction of spinal cord or an injury with potential recovery. To this end it is ideal to have complete and extensive information about the injury and this information must reveal the treatment required to ensure a favorable outcome.

In SCI, the neurological examination brings the first very important information about the lesion and this directs imaging procedures to confirm the lesion. But because of the spinal shock, unstable condition of the patient, attendant injuries, alcohol or drugs etc., the clinical examination immediately following injury, even using the American Spinal Injury Association (ASIA) motor scores or other scales, cannot be considered reliable. These clinical examinations must be repeated, but they offer only static clinical states and no data about possible future development.

The noninvasive imaging techniques used in SCI are the radiographies of the spine, spinal computed tomography (CT) or/and spinal magnetic resonance imaging (MRI), even functional MRI, tractography, or the recent structural volumetric and microstructural MRI protocols of the site of SCI.

All these offer only static images of the stage of the lesion and not an accurate prediction of the severity of SCI and about the development of the secondary spinal cord lesions.

We need a dynamic approach for the lesions; hence, biomarkers were evaluated for their capacity to be sensitive and accurate tools to measure the neuronal injuries and to predict the evolution of these injuries. Biomarkers are measurable features that can be used to confirm the presence or to predict the severity of the disorders. Biomarkers as biochemical indicators in SCI can allow detection of the secondary lesion, can monitor its progress and predict the severity of SCI, and can also indicate the specific treatments required. In SCI, biomarkers detect the severity of injury within the first few hours and can direct the best patient care in a timely manner.

In acute traumatic SCI, the mechanical injuries directly cause axonal destruction in fiber tracts, destruction of the neurons in gray matter, and of the glial cells. Their destruction releases substances—cellular constituents, whose presence, quantity, and dynamics can be lesional biomarkers.

The reactions of partially injured cells and of uninjured cells around the site of injury simultaneously start as response to the biochemical substances released by the destruction. The responses of these cells, that is, the synthesis of new proteins, are secondary to changes in mRNA. Detecting these changes allows us to determine their role at the site of SCI, to stabilize the damaged cells, to stop the spinal cord scar formation, and so on. The correlation of these changes with copied, or transcribed mRNA, from DNA, will establish the responsible genes intervening in the response to the SCI [3].

The assessment of these changes in the damaged spinal cord will allow therapeutic responses, for example:

- to stop the mechanisms by which secondary spinal cord lesion occurs and its progression,

- to understand the mechanisms of formation of a spinal cord scar as mechanical barrier that obstructs the axonal regeneration processes,

- even genetically targeted therapy to stimulate the genes in DNA responsible for neuronal regeneration, stimulating mRNA or to use the necessary proteins for SCI healing, and so on.

Detecting these protein changes, their quantity and dynamics may be biomarkers of response, or reaction biomarkers.

Correlating the lesional biomarkers and the reaction biomarkers with the clinical outcome and with the imaging techniques will enable understanding the complexity of the biological response to SCI and the establishment of appropriate therapies. Obtaining cells from the site of SCI is problematic in patients, therefore most research evaluated the lesional biomarkers in human spinal cord injuries. There are new approaches in the management of acute traumatic SCI that could enable obtaining cells from the site of SCI without adverse consequences for the patient.

The lesional biomarkers appear immediately post injury and their dynamics show the extension of the SCI and after several hours there are both lesional biomarkers and reaction biomarkers, involving the secondary cellular response to injury.

## 2. Current status of biomarkers and the diagnostic value in SCI

In recent years, a number of protein biomarkers have been evaluated to detect neuronal injury and recently there have been studies about their potential diagnostic and predictive value for spinal cord injuries. The concentration of specific proteins in blood or in the cerebrospinal fluid

(CSF) must be compared with the nervous tissue injury and these can be biomarkers for the pathologic processes in SCI.

There are numerous experimental studies and a smaller number of clinical studies for determining and validating biomarkers in SCI: c-Tau, myelin basic protein (MBP), neuron-specific enolase (NSE), glial fibrillar acidic protein (GFAP), and so on [4].

The researches have not been systematized and because the studies have been done at different time interval from the moment of the trauma, they did not differentiate between lesional biomarkers and reaction biomarkers and many of them were not followed to verify the clinical usefulness.

A brief overview of the evolution of these researches is shown below.

van Dongen et al. [5, 6] correlated the concentration of S-100 protein in the CSF with the results of somatosensory and motor-evoked potential monitoring indicating spinal cord ischemia during and after thoracoabdominal aortic aneurysm (TAAA) surgery and concluded that the S-100 protein in CSF seems to be a marker to detect spinal cord ischemia [5, 6], and in 2001 Kunihara et al. [7] found increased levels of S-100β in patients with post-operative SCI caused by spinal cord ischemia too. Basu et al. [8] presented free radicals as an inflammatory response indicator with the role of biomarker during spinal cord ischemia.

In 2003, Guéz et al. evaluated the CSF concentration of light subunits of neurofilaments (NF-L, 68 kDa) and of glial fibrillary acid protein (GFAP) in after trauma to the cervical spine: patients with acute traumatic cervical SCI and whiplash cases, compared to a control group of normal cases. The CSF concentrations of both light subunits of neurofilaments and GFAPs were significantly higher in all the cases with cervical SCI and pronounced neurological deficits [9].

In 2005, Loy et al. [10] reported that serum levels of NSE and S-100β protein are biomarkers in an animal model of traumatic SCI.

Kwon et al. [11] studied as possible biomarkers other inflammatory cytokines and structural proteins: S-100β (a glial-specific calcium-binding β protein), glial fibrillary acidic protein (GFAP), and interleukin 8 (IL-8, also known as neutrophil chemotactic factor), in patients within 24 hours post-SCI. Their concentration in the CSF and blood samples in patients with complete and incomplete SCI showed they could be potential biomarkers to diagnose the severity of SCI [11, 12].

In a literature review from 1966 to 2008, Pouw et al. [13] identified the biomarkers S-100β, NSE, neurofilament light chain, and glial fibrillary acidic protein as significantly higher in cases of experimental SCI in animal models.

New potential biomarkers were reported: the neurofilaments, the major cytoskeletal components in axon fibers. The most important are neurofilament subunit proteins (NF) that coassemble forming the cytoskeletal of axon fibers and they consist of five subunits of neurofilaments, named on the basis of molecular weight: heavy or highest (NF-H, 200–220 kDa), medium or middle (NF-M, 145–160 kDa), and light or lowest (NF-L, 68–70 kDa) subunits,

http://dx.doi.org/10.5772/63035

also alpha-internexin subunit (NF66) discovered later than NF and the intermediate filament protein subunit peripherin [4].

Ueno et al. [14] presented a rat model of acute SCI and they showed that the high molecular weight neurofilament subunit levels in plasma could be a biomarker for evaluating the efficacy of therapies for SCI.

Hayakawa et al. [15] studied the concentration of the phosphorylated neurofilament subunit NF-H (pNF-H) in plasma in patients with acute cervical SCI and concluded pNF-H may be a prognostic biomarker for SCI.

Iencean et al. [16] measured pNF-H concentration by enzyme-linked immunosorbent assay (ELISA) test in CSF in acute SCI patients and correlated the values of pNF-H with the clinical evolution, also they measured the normal values in samples obtained by lumbar puncture from individuals without neurologic disorders. They showed the phosphorylated form of the neurofilament subunit NF-H (pNF-H) is a biomarker in SCI in humans and its increased values are consistent with an unfavorable outcome. The neurofilament subunit NF-H (pNF-H) is a lesional biomarker, it appears after the mechanical injury by axonal destruction in the fibers tracts [16].

By now these studies have identified some potential biomarkers, but these biomarkers have not been validated and they still cannot be used in the clinical setting, for diagnosis, prognosis, and evaluating therapeutic interventions.

## 3. New research on biomarkers in traumatic SCI

The research in traumatic SCI has been focused on the discovery of lesional biomarkers and lesser for reaction biomarkers. Lesional biomarkers can be studied in patients with acute traumatic SCI immediately after injury; reaction biomarkers occur after a short period post injury and after several hours post injury these two types of biomarkers coexist, and it is difficult to differentiate them. The study of reaction biomarkers involves cells around the lesion, which is not possible in patients with SCI. Therefore research is conducted on nerve cell cultures and there are experimental animal models, but the translation into human medicine is difficult because there are important differences. The most important studies on lesional biomarkers concern the neurofilament subunit proteins (NF).

Pouw et al. [17] in a prospective cohort study obtained CSF from sixteen acute traumatic SCI patients within 24 hours post injury and found that the concentrations of glial fibrillary acidic protein, NSE, S-100β, tau and neurofilament heavy chain (NFH) in motor complete patients was significantly higher compared with motor incomplete patients.

Takahashi et al. [18] conducted a study to evaluate pNF-H levels in the CSF of patients with worsening symptoms of cervical compression myelopathy and their results suggest that pNF-H in CSF can act as a biomarker that reflects the severity of acutely worsening compression myelopathy.

Iencean et al. measured the phosphorylated neurofilament subunit NF-H (pNF-H) in the CSF of patients with SCI and demonstrated the correlation between the pNF-H levels and the severity of the injury. They studied 15 subjects with acute traumatic SCI who underwent surgery during the first 24 hours post injury (decompression, stabilization): eight patients with complete SCI and seven patients with incomplete SCI. They measured daily the heavy phosphorylated neurofilament subunit (pNF-H) concentration by sandwich ELISA test in CSF in all patients. The level of CSF pNF-H was ten to a hundred times higher in complete SCI than the level of CSF pNF-H in cases with incomplete SCI, where the level of this biomarker was close to normal [19, 20].

The patients with early surgery in complete SCI and with a favorable outcome had a specific pattern of daily values of pNF-H: a sudden increase up to a maximum value then a gradual decrease to normal; the peak was different in each case, from 10 times up to 170 times higher than normal (**Figure 1**).

The same type of the pattern for the values of pNF-H appears in the incomplete SCI with favorable outcome, but with smaller values of pNF-H.

There are two patterns in cases with unfavorable outcome or neurological stationary after the same early surgery and treatment:

- the second unfavorable pattern had a progressive increase up to a peak and then was followed by a progressive decrease to normal values, the peak was a hundred times higher than normal values (**Figure 2**),

- an increase to a plateau of pNF-H values, with increased values five or ten times higher than normal (**Figure 3**).

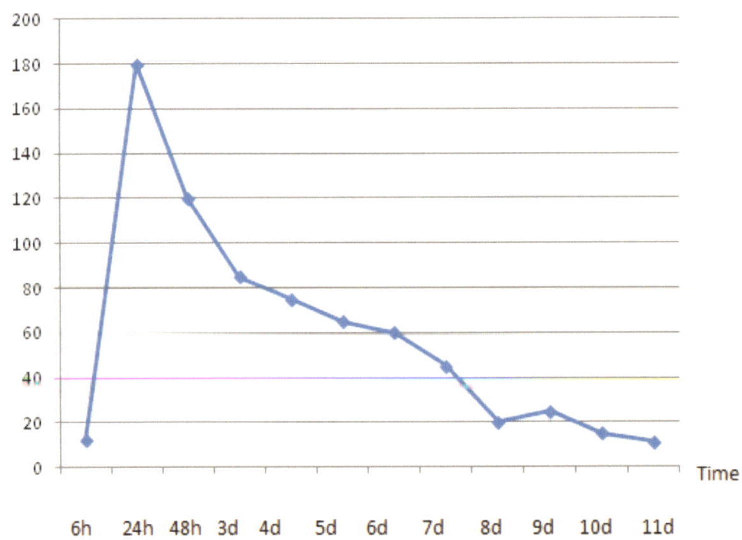


**Figure 1.** Pattern of daily value of pNF-H in patients with favorable outcome.

http://dx.doi.org/10.5772/63035

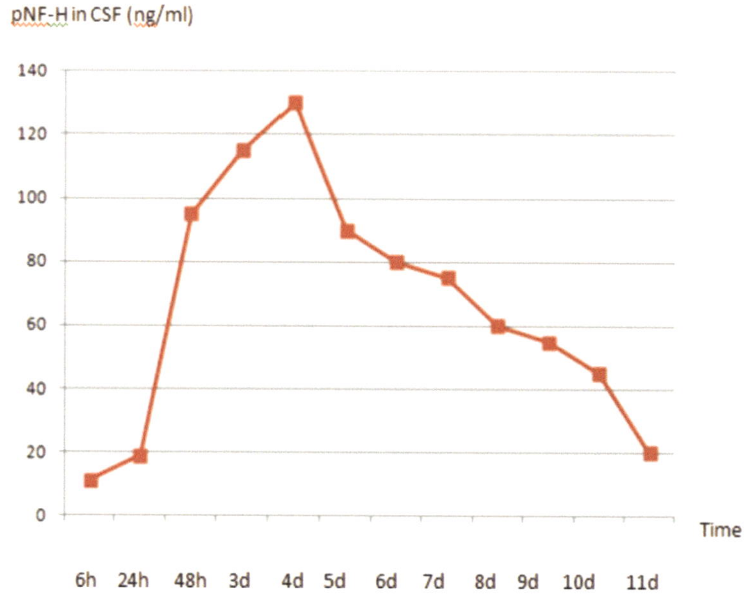


**Figure 2.** Pattern with progressive increase of pNF-H.

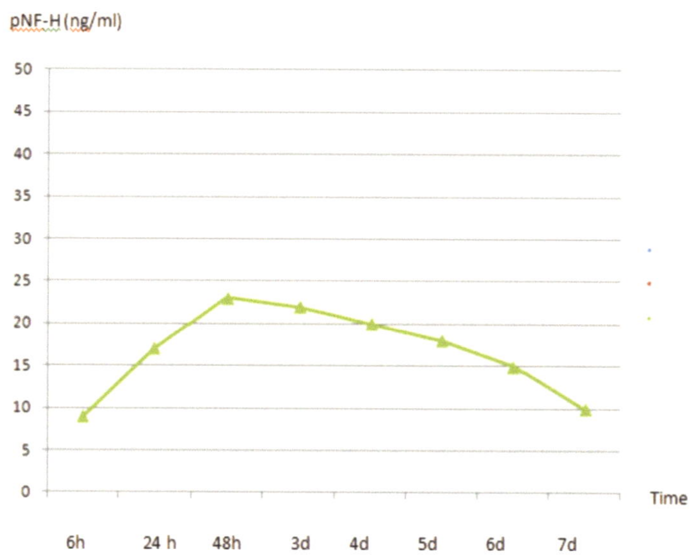


**Figure 3.** Pattern with increase up to a plateau of pNF-H.

The authors found that in patients with favorable development the progressive decrease of pNF-H values after the initial sudden increase, without extension of increased values in plateau or without a second peak, signifies a reduction or even a stop of the secondary lesion with evident effect on the favorable outcome in the SCI (**Figure 4**).

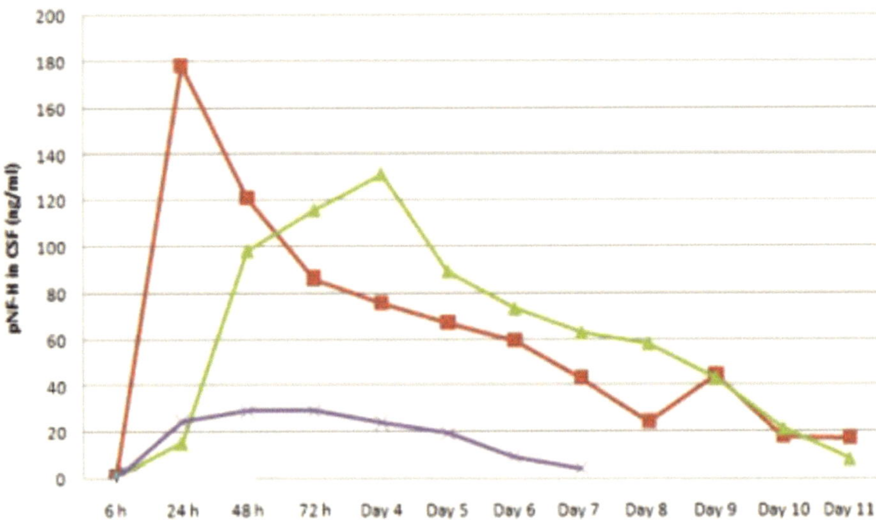


**Figure 4.** The three specific and predictive patterns of daily values of pNF-H in traumatic SCI.

Kato et al. [21] investigated the phosphorylated form of the high molecular weight neurofilament subunit (pNF-H) levels in the serum in patients with cervical compressive myelopathy and they found an elevated serum level of pNF-H only in acute worsening of myelopathy and this study confirms that pNF-H is a lesional biomarker.

Kuhle et al. [22] presented their results on a study of serum neurofilament light chain (pNF-L) in human SCI. They concluded that serum neurofilament light subunit (pNF-L) concentration in SCI patients has a close correlation with acute severity and neurological outcome and it is of predictive value in SCI patients.

The presentation of these studies on biomarkers in SCI highlights that the most important ones and those with significant results relate to lesional biomarkers, and first are the phosphorylated neurofilament subunits, light or heavy (pNF-L or pNF-H), resulting from the axonal neurofilament destruction. The research showed that the phosphorylated neurofilament subunit, light or heavy (pNF-L or pNF-H) in SCI is a specific lesional biomarker for SCI and it can distinguish the severity of SCI (Hayakawa, Iencean, and Kuhle).

The heavy phosphorylated neurofilament subunit (pNF-H) is a predictive lesional biomarker because its values pattern can show the reducing or stopping of the secondary lesions and the favorable outcome. The complete SCI patients with a favorable development had a specific pattern of daily values of pNF-H: a sudden increase up to a maximum value then a progressive decrease to normal. The patients with unfavorable outcome or neurological stabilization had two patterns: an increase to a plateau of pNF-H values or a progressive increase up to a peak followed by a progressive decrease to quasi-normal values.

http://dx.doi.org/10.5772/63035

## 4. Conclusion and future perspectives. Ethics

These studies on biomarkers in spinal cord injuries highlight that the most important lesional biomarkers are the phosphorylated neurofilament subunits, light or heavy (pNF-L or pNF-H). The phosphorylated neurofilament subunits (pNF-L or pNF-H) are specific lesional biomarkers for SCI and they can distinguish the severity of SCI.

The heavy phosphorylated neurofilament subunit (pNF-H) is a predictive lesional biomarker; its values pattern shows the reducing or stopping of the secondary lesions and the favorable outcome.

There is a specific pattern of daily values of pNF-H in complete SCI patients with a favorable outcome: a sudden increase up to a maximum value then a progressive decrease to normal. Also there are two patterns in the patients with unfavorable outcome: an increase to a plateau of pNF-H values or a progressive increase up to a peak followed by a progressive decrease to quasi-normal values.

These specific patterns could be used to aid clinicians with making a diagnosis and establishing a prognosis, and evaluating therapeutic interventions. These studies should continue on larger groups of patients to prove the clinical usefulness.

Also the studies on reaction biomarkers are very important, but obtaining cells from the site of SCI is problematic in humans. A new approach in the management of acute traumatic SCI has been proposed that could enable obtaining cells from the site of SCI without adverse consequences for the patient. In the cases with a predictive pattern of unfavorable outcome or neurological stationary after decompression and stabilization during the first 24 hours, a new approach was proposed based on the predictive pattern of daily values of pNF-H. If the clinical neurologic evolution is unfavorable and imaging techniques (MRI) show a complete SCI and the daily values of NFP-H as lesional biomarker form predictive unfavorable pattern, a second microneurosurgery in the SCI site can create favorable conditions for functional recovery of the remaining spinal cord: opening the spinal cord in the midline and microsurgical debridement of the necrotic tissue. At the same time this second microneurosurgical approach in the SCI site could enable obtaining cells from the site of SCI without adverse consequences for the patient. The use of these cells (neurons and glial cells around the lesion) for cell culture techniques will allow the study of the changes in the spinal cord at the molecular and structural levels in humans.

Diagnosis, prognosis, and treatment guidance based on biomarker used as a predictive indicator can determine ethical difficulties by differentiated therapies in patients with SCI.

It is difficult to stop or to limit the treatment of neurological recovery in patients with complete SCI, with paraplegia or tetraplegia, with complete spinal cord lesions on imaging techniques and unfavorable patterns of predictive lesional biomarkers. We do not currently know the value of the lesional predictive biomarkers for the neurological outcome several years after the injury. At the moment, we cannot take a decision limiting the treatment of neurological recovery in patients with complete SCI because we do not know the complexity of the biological response to SCI.

This requires extensive and profound research both on lesional biomarkers and on reaction biomarkers correlated with genetic and molecular response in SCI and we hope further research will deliver effective treatments.

## Acknowledgements

This work was funded by the CNCS– UEFISCDI Romania, grant: "Immediate neuroprotective therapy in acute traumatic spinal cord injury", grant number: PN-II-IDPCE-2011-3-0569.

## Author details

Stefan Mircea Iencean[1] and Andrei Stefan Iencean[2*]

*Address all correspondence to: mirceasteffan@yahoo.com

1 Neurosurgery, "GrT Popa" University of Medicine and Pharmacy, Iasi, Romania

2 Neurosurgery, Emergency "Prof N Oblu" Hospital, Iasi, Romania

## References

[1] Burns AS, Marino RJ, Flanders AE, Flett H. Clinical diagnosis and prognosis following spinal cord injury. In: Verhaagen J, McDonald JW, editors. Spinal Cord Injury. Handbook of Clinical Neurology. Volume 109, Elsevier B.V. Philadelphia 2012. p. 47–62. ISBN: 978-0-444-52137-8.

[2] Tator CH, Fehlings MG. Review of the secondary injury theory of acute spinal cord trauma with emphasis on vascular mechanisms. J Neurosurg. Sp. Suppl. 2010; 112(2): 15–26.

[3] Liverman CT, Altevogt BM, Joy JE, Johnson RT, editors. Spinal Cord Injury. Progress, Promise, and Priorities. The National Academic Press, Washington DC,USA; 2005. 344 p. ISBN: 0-309-09585-9.

[4] Yokobori S, Zhang Z, Moghieb A, Mondello S, Gajavelli S, Dietrich WD, Bramlett H, Hayes RL, Wang M, Wang KK, Bullock MR. Acute diagnostic biomarkers for spinal cord injury: review of the literature and preliminary research report. World Neurosurg. 2015; 83(5):867–78. doi: 10.1016/j.wneu.2013.03.012.

[5] van Dongen EP1, Ter Beek HT, Boezeman EH, Schepens MA, Langemeijer HJ, Aarts LP. Normal serum concentrations of S-100 protein and changes in cerebrospinal fluid concentrations of S-100 protein during and after thoracoabdominal aortic aneurysm

surgery: Is S-100 protein a biochemical marker of clinical value in detecting spinal cord ischemia? J Vasc Surg. 1998; 27(2):344–6.

[6] van Dongen EP, ter Beek HT, Schepens MA, Morshuis WJ, Haas FJ, de Boer A, Boezeman EH, Aarts LP. The relationship between evoked potentials and measurements of S-100 protein in cerebrospinal fluid during and after thoracoabdominal aortic aneurysm surgery. J Vasc Surg. 1999; 30(2):293–300.

[7] Kunihara T, Shiiya N, Yasuda K.Changes in S100beta protein levels in cerebrospinal fluid after thoracoabdominal aortic operations. J Thorac Cardiovasc Surg. 2001; 122(5): 1019–20.

[8] Basu S, Hellberg A, Ulus AT, Westman J, Karacagil S. Biomarkers of free radical injury during spinal cord ischemia. FEBS Lett. 2001; 508(1):36–8.

[9] Guéz M, Hildingsson C, Rosengren L, Karlsson K, Toolanen G. Nervous tissue damage markers in cerebrospinal fluid after cervical spine injuries and whiplash trauma. J Neurotrauma. 2003; 20(9):853–8.

[10] Loy DN1, Sroufe AE, Pelt JL, Burke DA, Cao QL, Talbott JF, Whittemore SR. Serum biomarkers for experimental acute spinal cord injury: rapid elevation of neuron-specific enolase and S-100beta. Neurosurgery. 2005; 56(2):391–7.

[11] Kwon BK, Casha S, Hurlbert RJ, Yong VW. Inflammatory and structural biomarkers in acute traumatic spinal cord injury. Clin Chem Lab Med. 2011; 49(3):425–33. doi: 10.1515/CCLM.2011.068.

[12] Kwon BK, Stammers AM, Belanger LM, Bernardo A, Chan D, Bishop CM, Slobogean GP, Zhang H, Umedaly H, Giffin M, Street J, Boyd MC, Paquette SJ, Fisher CG, Dvorak MF. Cerebrospinal fluid inflammatory cytokines and biomarkers of injury severity in acute human spinal cord injury. J Neurotrauma. 2010; 27(4):669–82. doi: 10.1089/neu.2009.1080.

[13] Pouw MH, Hosman AJ, van Middendorp JJ, Verbeek MM, Vos PE, van de Meent H. Biomarkers in spinal cord injury. Spinal Cord. 2009; 47(7):519–25. doi: 10.1038/sc.2008.176.

[14] Ueno T, Ohori Y, Ito J, Hoshikawa S, Yamamoto S, Nakamura K, Tanaka S, Akai M, Tobimatsu Y, Ogata T. Hyperphosphorylated neurofilament NF-H as a biomarker of the efficacy of minocycline therapy for spinal cord injury. Spinal Cord. 2011; 49(3):333–6. doi: 10.1038/sc.2010.116.

[15] Hayakawa K, Okazaki R, Ishii K, Ueno T, Izawa N, Tanaka Y et al. Phosphorylated neurofilament subunit NF-H as a biomarker for evaluating the severity of spinal cord injury patients, a pilot study. Spinal Cord. 2012; 50:493–496. doi: 10.1038/sc.2011.184.

[16] Iencean StM, Adam D, Ungureanu D, Tascu Al, Cuciureanu D, Costachescu B, Iencean ASt, Poeata I. Preliminary results of CSF phosphorylated neurofilament subunit NF-H as biomarkers of acute spinal cord injury. Romanian Neurosurg. 2013; XX(4):351–6.

[17] Pouw MH, Kwon BK, Verbeek MM, Vos PE, van Kampen A, Fisher CG, Street J, Paquette SJ, Dvorak MF, Boyd MC, Hosman AJ, van de Meent H. Structural biomarkers in the cerebrospinal fluid within 24 h after a traumatic spinal cord injury: a descriptive analysis of 16 subjects. Spinal Cord. 2014; 52(6):428–33. doi: 10.1038/sc.2014.26.

[18] Takahashi H, Aoki Y, Nakajima A, Sonobe M, Terajima F, Saito M, Taniguchi S, Yamada M, Watanabe F, Furuya T, Koda M, Yamazaki M, Takahashi K, Nakagawa K. Phosphorylated neurofilament subunit NF-H becomes elevated in the cerebrospinal fluid of patients with acutely worsening symptoms of compression myelopathy. J Clin Neurosci. 2014; 21(12):2175–8.

[19] Ungureanu D, Iencean StM, Dimitriu C, Iencean ASt, TascuAl. Determination of the phosphorylated neurofilament subunit NF-H (pNF-H) in cerebro-spinal fluid as biomarker in acute traumatic spinal cord injuries. Rom Rev Lab Med. 2014; 22(3):377–86.

[20] Iencean StM, Iencean ASt. Cerebrospinal Fluid Phosphorylated Neurofilament Subunit NF-H (pNF-H) is a specific biomarker and its pattern is predictive for spinal cord injury. Glob Spine J. 2015; 5(S 01): A217. doi: 10.1055/s-0035-1554321.

[21] Kato S, Chikuda H, Ohya J, Hayakawa K, Takeshita K, Tanaka S, Ogata T. Phosphorylated neurofilament subunit levels in the serum of cervical compressive myelopathy patients. J Clin Neurosci. 2015; 22(10):1638–42.

[22] Kuhle J, Gaiottino J, Leppert D, Petzold A, Bestwick JP, Malaspina A, Lu CH, Dobson R, Disanto G, Norgren N, Nissim A, Kappos L, Hurlbert J, Yong VW, Giovannoni G, Casha S. Serum neurofilament light chain is a biomarker of human spinal cord injury severity and outcome. J Neurol Neurosurg Psychiatry. 2015; 86(3):273–9.

Chapter 10

# Biomarkers-Directed Strategies to Treat Autism

Afaf El-Ansary and Hussain Al Dera

Additional information is available at the end of the chapter

http://dx.doi.org/10.5772/62566

**Abstract**

Autism is a neurodevelopmental disorder characterized by social, communication, and behavioral symptoms. Recent research has attempted to identify the potential mechanisms that may contribute to the pathogenesis of autism. Biomarkers as noninvasive quantitative biological measures with accurate indication of a specific mechanism can lead to a better understanding of the pathogenesis required to design the most effective treatments of autism. There is also great hope that the discovery of valid and predictive biomarkers for this disorder will help earlier and more targeted methods for diagnosis and intervention. In this chapter, we discuss some of the current theorized mechanisms contributing to autism, including inflammation, oxidative stress, impaired detoxification, glutamate excitotoxicity, gut-microbiota-brain axis, impaired fatty acid profiling, and serotonin (5-HT)/oxytocin (OT) abnormalities as target to treat autism. Moreover, based on our understanding of the role of these mechanisms, selected treatment strategies are suggested. These strategies include nutraceuticals, probiotics/prebiotics and ω-3 supplementation, targeting glutamate transporters or selective 5-HT reuptake inhibitors, and intranasal OT treatment. Of course, the joint efforts of scientists, caregivers, and other stakeholders must combine to identify valid, clinically useful autism biomarkers that may lead to efficient treatment strategy and/or combined strategies.

**Keywords:** autism, biomarkers, excitotoxicity, neuroinflammation, nutraceuticals, ω-3, oxidative stress, probiotic

## 1. Introduction

Autism is a neurodevelopmental disorder characterized by deficits in cognition and learning, behavior, social interaction, and communication. Among the challenging behaviors that negatively affect the child with autism is the social interaction impairment. Social interaction is defined as how an individual uses verbal and nonverbal communication during interpersonal exchanges. Children with autism usually present difficulty in recognizing the thoughts and feelings of others, and this is described as "mind blindness," which can lead to ineffective communication [1]. Cognitive differences are also prevalent in children with autism. As a result, academic differences often exist due in part to weaknesses with executive functioning. The current management strategies, practice, and methods are put into place by professionals, researchers, and parents to compensate for the deficits in these areas. They are designed and selected in hopes of producing the maximum improvement in autistic behavior. Genetic heterogeneity was recorded earlier in twin, family, and linkage studies. The autism-related genes seem to be contributed on few etiological pathways related to detoxification, synaptic function, and neurogenesis [2–5]. As genes and environment rarely act independently to induce autism, the interaction between both at various developmental times usually plays an important role in the pathology of this disorder. Because development is a dynamic process, a constant interplay between genes and environment usually occurs [6]. Although the progressive increase in the prevalence of autism can be attributed to the increase in public awareness and the broadening of diagnostic construct, of course, it can be also related to the incidence of environmental factors [7, 8] and their interactions with yet unknown genetic vulnerability. Nutrients, heavy metal pollution, medications, and pesticides as the most commonly examined exposures during pregnancy are among the environmental neurotoxic insult on developing brains. Understanding how low-level chemical exposures influence the molecular, cellular, and behavioral outcomes relevant to autism will provide insight regarding gene-environment interactions and possibly yield novel intervention strategies. There is no metabolic biomarker or panel of markers that can precisely define autism, but examining different signaling pathways to identify any abnormalities in autistic patients compared to their normal peers can be enhanced to treat autism through the amelioration of these defected pathways.

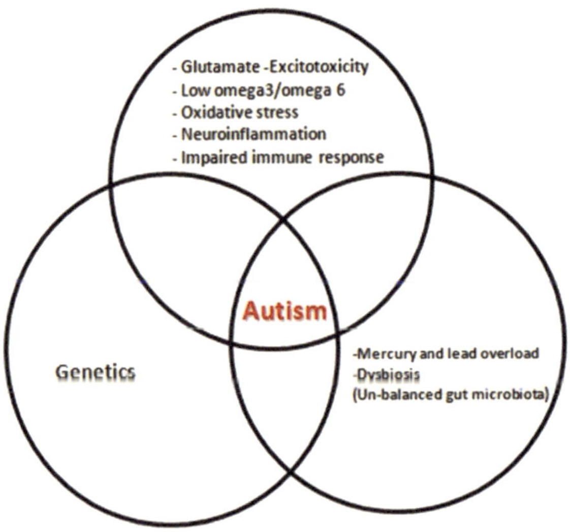


**Figure 1.** Role of genetic, environmental, and biological mechanisms in the etiology of autism.

http://dx.doi.org/10.5772/62566

Many studies related to the screening of biomarkers of autism were successful enough and reproducible to ascertain the role of oxidative stress, environmental toxicants, mitochondrial dysfunction, and immunology/inflammation as four main etiopathological mechanisms of autism. In addition, there is accumulating evidence pointing to the contribution of lipid abnormalities, gut microbiota, and glutamate excitotoxicity in generating biomarkers related to autism. **Figure 1** demonstrates the relationship between genetic, environmental, and biological mechanisms in the etiology of autism.

## 2. Biomarkers related to autism

Screening for antioxidants includes the measurement of glutathione (GSH) as the primary antioxidant entrusted with the protection against oxidative stress, neuroinflammation, and mitochondrial damage. GSH is critically important in regulating the detoxification mechanism and modulating the production of oxidative stress-related parameters. Measuring reduced GSH, oxidized GSH (GSSG), or GSH status (GSH/GSSG) proves to be of great use in the determination of the patient's oxidation status. In a trial that evaluated the detoxification mechanism in autism, a systematic review of 39 studies was conducted. It proved that many patients with autism have lower GSH/GSSG, indicating poor antioxidant and detoxification mechanisms [9]. Among the recorded detoxification markers that are studied in autism are *p*-hydroxyphenyllactate, pyroglutamate, benzoate, and hippurate. Elevated levels of hippurate and benzoate are related to impaired phase II detoxification via glycine conjugation [10]. Abnormal levels of pyroglutamate can indicate an impairment of GSH metabolism and a depleted GSH status.

In more recent studies, serum thioredoxin levels and $F_2$-isoprostane are related to cognitive and social impairment severity in autistic patients [measured by Childhood Autism Rating Scales (CARS) or Social Responsiveness Scale (SRS), respectively] [11–13]. A negative correlation between GSH peroxidase and CARS has also been reported [11]. Many studies prove that oxidative stress can easily be related to chronic inflammation, glutamate excitotoxicity, and increased mitochondrial dysfunction as etiological mechanisms in autism [14]. Additionally, the observed cellular damage in these patients may range from structural damage and mitotic arrest to apoptosis and cell necrosis depending on the severity of oxidative stress.

**Figure 2** demonstrates the suggested relationship between these etiological mechanisms and apoptosis of neurons that might lead to abnormal brain maturation that presents as autistic features and behavioral deficits. Glutamate excitotoxicity, oxidative stress, and neuroinflammation are signaling pathways that might cause an increase and/or decrease of proapoptotic and antiapoptotic proteins, respectively. Under the effect of genetic change or the environment (e.g., heavy metal toxicity and altered gut microbiota), the activation of pathological apoptosis (elevation of caspases) impairs normal brain maturation and induces autistic phenotype.

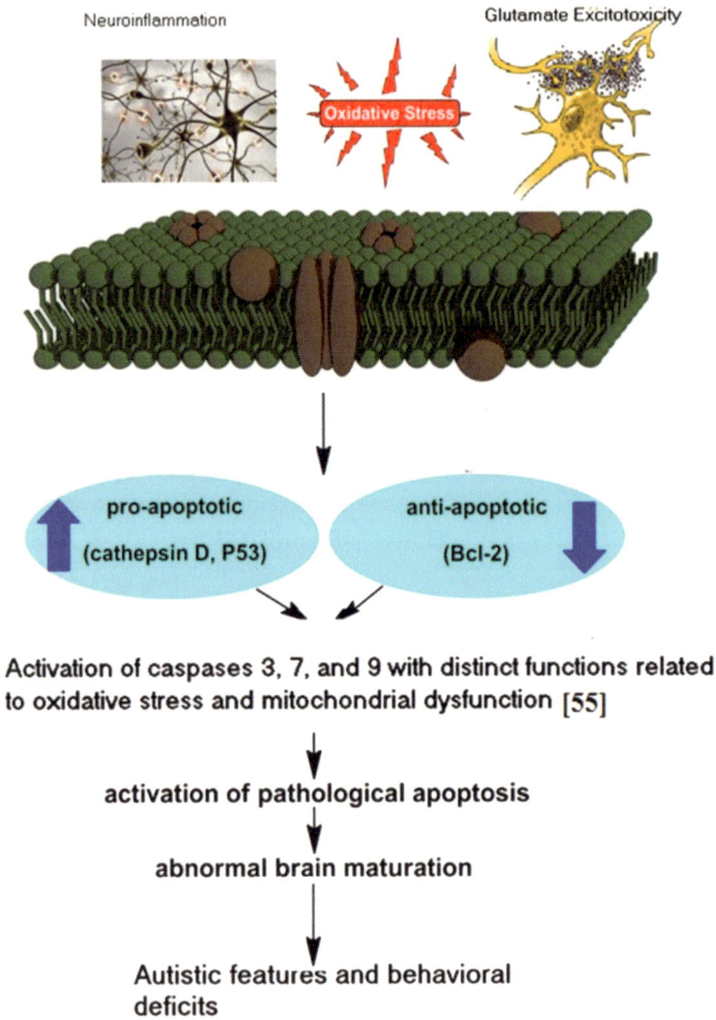


**Figure 2.** Suggested relationship between oxidative stress, glutamate excitotoxicity, neuroinflammation, and pathological apoptosis leading to autistic phenotype.

The realization that the microbiota-gut-brain axis plays a critical role in the etiology of autism has recently emerged. The regulation of this axis is essential for maintaining homeostasis, including that of the central nervous system (CNS). Nowadays, understanding microbiota-brain interactions has become exciting area of research, which may contribute new insights into individual variations in cognition, social interaction, mood, and sleep disorders as characteristic features of patients with autism [15, 16]. The ability of gut microbiota to communicate with the brain and in turn induce behavioral changes is emerging as an interesting concept in autism. The brain-gut axis is a bidirectional communication system composed of neural pathways, such as the enteric nervous system (ENS), vagus, sympathetic, and spinal nerves, as well as humoral pathways, which include cytokines, hormones, and neuropeptides

http://dx.doi.org/10.5772/62566

as signaling molecules [16]. Brain excitotoxicity, oxidative stress, and neuroinflammation can directly or indirectly affect the composition of the gut microbiota. On the contrary, microbial overgrowth and their metabolites can modulate the brain normal function. **Figure 3** demonstrates the suggested bidirectional interaction between the gut-microbiota and the brain as an etiological mechanism in autism.

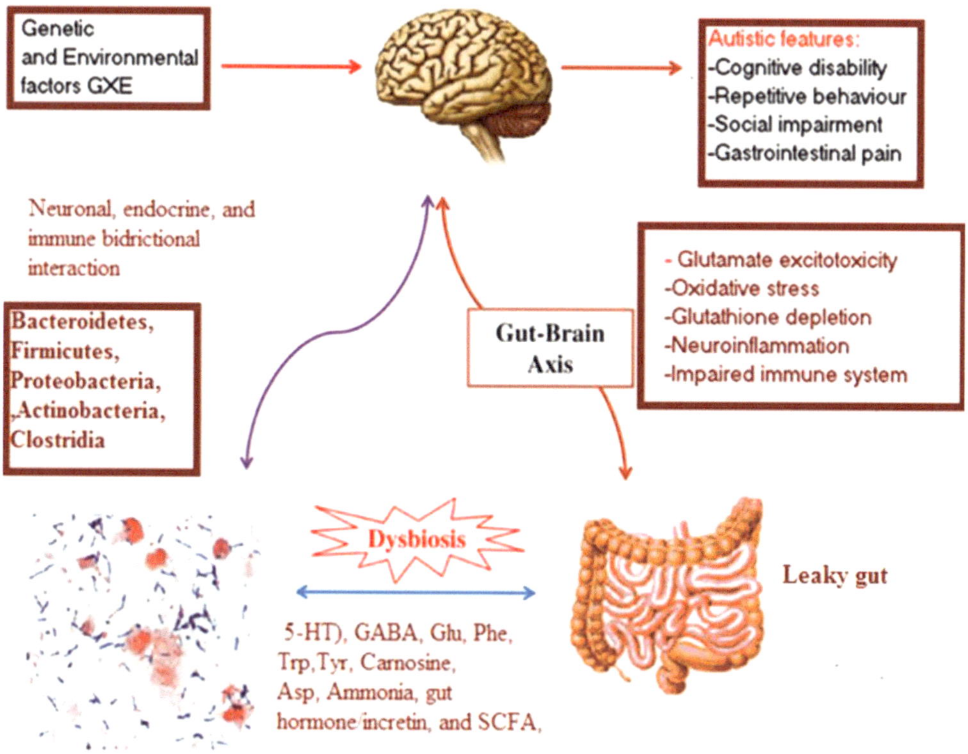


**Figure 3.** Gut-brain axis: pathways of communication between brain and gut microbiota.

This fact was confirmed by a study that has suggested a significant risk of autism in children born to mothers with severe infections during pregnancy [17]. Additionally, offspring of pregnant female monkeys exposed to antibodies produced postinfection usually develop pathologies of the CNS and exhibited behavioral changes similar to those seen in autistic children [18]. Autoantibodies triggered by systemic inflammation are generated during pregnancy and are now accepted to play a role in abnormal neurological and impaired blood-brain barrier (BBB) development in the fetus with a concomitant increased risk of autism [19]. The molecular trigger for autoantibody generation is poorly understood, but there is a possibility that autoantibodies against receptors for key microbiota metabolites, such as serotonin (5-HT), γ-aminobutyric acid (GABA), glutamate, tryptophan, and short-chain fatty acids (SCFA), may be directed by the immune system under conditions of aberrant metabolite accumulation in the blood as well as inappropriate immune system in early life or mimicry by gut bacteria [20].

These early observations provide a potential explanation for the gastrointestinal problems suffered by patients with autism. In support of this line of thinking, children with autism are shown to have increased permeability of the gastrointestinal tract, called "leaky gut," causing microbial products to escape into the bloodstream and possibly reach the brain [21]. These products alter the immune system, resulting in a progression of the disease [22]. Differences in the gut microbiota between maternal infection activated (MIA) offspring and controls are observed due primarily to changes in the diversity of Clostridia and Bacteroidia [23]. The intestines of some autistic patients with intestinal abnormalities are known to bear *Sutterella* and *Clostridium bolteae* [24], organisms lacking in control populations with similar gastrointestinal problems, together with lower *Bifidobacterium* and *Lactobacillus* species. **Table 1** demonstrates altered gut microbiota in individuals with autism in relation to social impairment.

| **Autism** |
|---|
| Significantly ↑ in *Clostridium histolyticum* [24] |
| Significantly ↑ in Bacteroidetes [25] |
| Significantly ↓ in species of *Bifidobacterium* and ↑ in *Lactobacillus* [26] |
| Significantly ↓ in species of *Bifidobacterium* spp. [27] |
| Significantly ↓ in Bacteroidetes, ↑ in Firmicutes: Bacteroidetes, ↑ in Betaproteobacteria [28] |
| Significant ↑ in *Sutterella* spp. [29] |
| Significant ↑ in *Clostridium* [30] |
| ↑ in *Clostridium*, Bacteroidetes, *Prophyromonas, Prevotella, Pseudomonas, Aeromonas,* and Enterobacteriaceae; ↓ in *Enterococcus, Lactobacillus, Streptococcus,* and *Staphylococcus* [31] |

**Table 1.** Association between gut microbiota altered composition and social impairment as core symptom in autistic patients.

The metabolomic studies of urine from patients with autism have identified molecules associated with the microbiome, such as dimethylamine, hippuric acid, and phenylacetylglutamine [24, 32]. Decreased plasma levels of *p*-hydroxyphenyllactate, the metabolite of *Bifidobacterium* and *Lactobacillus,* which is known to serve as an antioxidant both in the circulation and tissues, were also detected in urine of patients with autism [33].

SCFA, such as acetate, propionate, and butyrate, are neuroactive microbial metabolites that can cross the BBB and induce remarkable changes in brain function during development and thus lead to behavior abnormalities [34–36]. Increased levels of total as well as individual SCFA levels have been associated with autism [37]. Propionate has also been shown to induce behavioral changes similar to autism when infused interventricularly to the brain [35]. It was also reported that increased butyrate levels in valproic acid (VPA) *in utero*-exposed male offspring could contribute to deficits in social behavior. Both butyrate and VPA neurotoxicity are associated with the impairment of fatty acids transport by the carnithine pathway. This

http://dx.doi.org/10.5772/62566

can easily be related to mitochondrial dysfunction as an etiological mechanism in autism [34]. Both acids can also relate to intestinal inflammatory phenotype common in autistic patients through their inhibitory effects on histone deacetylase in the gut of exposed animals [38]. Modulating intestinal mucus composition through MUC-2 gene expression can affect epithelial protection, gut morphology, and gut microbiota composition [39]. Moreover, if blood butyrate levels are increased, it can affect various neuronal cells directly and thereby affect the maturation of oligodendrocytes and hippocampal neuronal cells in the brain during postnatal development and induce autistic features in treated animals [40, 41].

In the case of neurodevelopmental disorders, such as autism, the neuroimmune system could affect not only function but also brain development [42]. The inflammatory response elicited during pregnancy in the mother can induce inflammation in the fetus through the placenta [43].

Clinical and postmortem studies have shown that neuroinflammatory processes induced during the prenatal period usually remain altered throughout autism pathology. Abnormal inflammatory response to infection of different blood cell populations has been described in autistic children, and such patients usually suffer from chronic gastrointestinal disturbances [24, 37, 44]. It is well known that their mononuclear cells and lymphoblasts produce excessive proinflammatory cytokines, such as tumor necrosis factor-$\alpha$ (TNF-$\alpha$), interleukin (IL)-6, and IL-1$\beta$, both basally [45] and after being stimulated with lipopolysaccharides (LPS) [46],

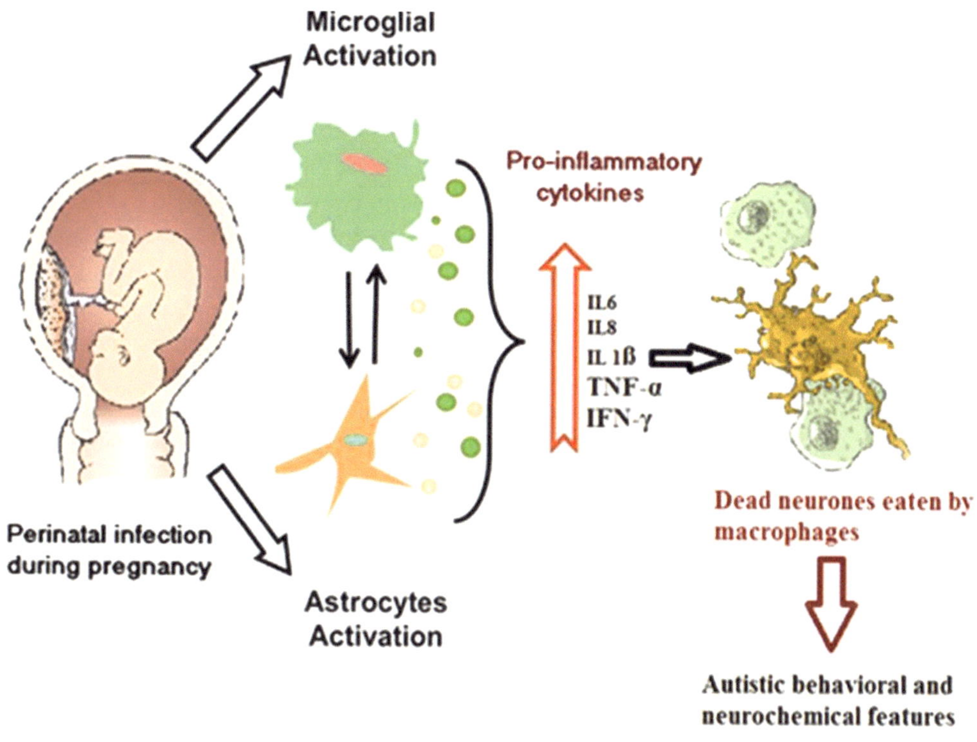


**Figure 4.** Early inflammation as an etiological mechanism in autism.

compared to healthy controls. Astrogliosis and microglial activation, together with the overexpression of cytokines in different regions of the autistic brain, show that autistic patients demonstrate an altered neuroinflammatory response throughout their lives; they also show increased astrocyte and microglia inflammatory response in the cortex and the cerebellum [47, 48]. Moreover, increased expression of interferon-$\gamma$ (IFN-$\gamma$), monocyte chemoattractant protein-1 (MCP-1), transforming growth factor-$\beta$1 (TGF-$\beta$1), IL-8, IL-6, and TNF-$\alpha$ and other genes associated with the immune response have been reported in those brain regions and in the cerebrospinal fluid [48–50] (**Figure 4**).

In a 2D gel-based proteomic analysis of urine, a total of 250 protein spots were detected in autistic samples compared to 195 in normal control subjects. Whereas 10 proteins were overexpressed, others were found to be underexpressed. Out of the significantly different urine analysis, three overexpressed peptides were identified as kininogen-1 (KNG-1)-50, IgG1 heavy chain variable region, and mannan-binding lectin serine protease-2 isoform-2 precursor-45. The abnormal formation of KNG-1 as an important regulator of urokinase plasminogen activator receptor is involved in cell migration and proliferation [51]. The increase of urinary KNG-1 levels in all the tested autistic children highlights the possibility of using this protein as a diagnostic marker.

Significant changes in the levels of aspartate, citrate, creatinine, hydroxyphenyllactate, indoleacetate, isoleucine, glutamate, and glutarate between autistic and control individuals were identified by West et al. [52]. They identified a decreased level of blood homocitrulline as a new biomarker in autism. Homocitrulline is a poorly understood molecule that is known to be formed inside the mitochondria from lysine and carbamoyl phosphate. The decreased blood level of this marker also suggests that its metabolism in the brain may also be disrupted. Homocitrulline levels are increased in urine and blood in patients with ornithine translocase deficiency, which diverts the reaction between carbamyl phosphate and lysine. Patients with ornithine translocase deficiency exhibit behavioral abnormalities similar to autism, such as developmental delay, spasticity, learning, and cognitive abnormalities, together with frequent seizures [53]. In addition, disrupted brain redox status and energy metabolism were reported in rats that received homocitrulline intraventricularly [54, 55]. These observations suggest that elevated brain levels of homocitrulline are deleterious; however, additional studies are needed to define the brain levels of homocitrulline and its potential role in the development of autism.

The role of polyunsaturated fatty acids (PUFA) in neurodevelopment is becoming clear. The brain and nervous tissue usually depend on $\omega$-3 fatty acids, specifically docosahexaenoic acid (DHA) and eicosapentaenoic acid (EPA), for structural cell signaling purposes [56]. Among the ascertained and reproducible markers in autism are the elevated $\omega$-6 PUFA, LA ($n$-6) together with $\omega$-6:$\omega$-3 ratio ($n$-6:$n$-3). Elevated $n$-6:$n$-3 ratios above 4–6:1 have been associated with neuroinflammation as an etiopathogenesis mechanism in autism [57]. In several studies, patients with autism exhibited elevated $n$-6:$n$-3 ratio and decreased $n$-3 fatty acid compared to intellectually impaired control [58, 59]. Fombonne et al. [60] reported that the absence of incidence of autism from 1991 to 2006 among an Inuit population was attributed to the consumption of large amount of fish.

http://dx.doi.org/10.5772/62566

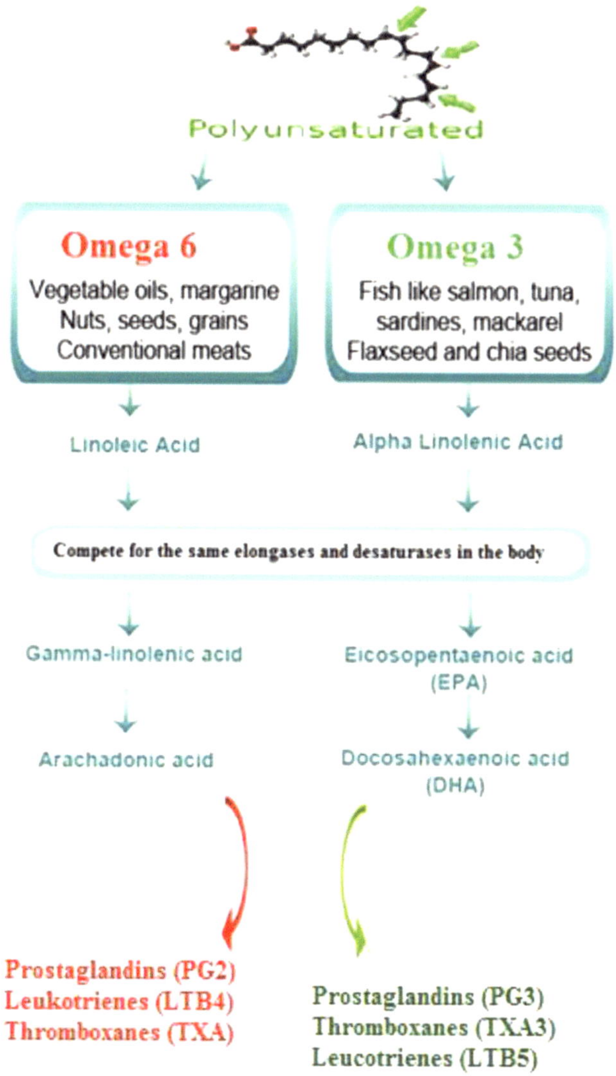


**Figure 5.** Unbalance between ω-6/ω-3 fatty acids as etiological mechanism in autism.

Glutamate and GABA as the main excitatory and inhibitory neurotransmitters in the human brain, respectively, have important roles during prenatal or postnatal brain development. Upon excitation of the presynaptic neuron, glutamate is released from the synaptic vesicles into the synaptic cleft. This is followed by the binding of the released glutamate to ionotropic (NMDAR and AMPAR) or metabotropic receptors (mGluR) on the postsynaptic neurons. The binding of glutamate to mGluRs triggers the activation of G-protein-dependent intracellular signaling cascade. The activation of ionotropic glutamate receptors AMPA, kainate, and NMDA by glutamate induces the opening of $Na^+$ and $Ca^{2+}$ ion channels. The overactivation of glutamate receptors by excessive glutamate results in the influx of high levels of calcium ions

($Ca^{2+}$) into the postsynaptic cells, which in turn activate a cascade of proteases, lipases, nitric oxide synthase, and a number of enzymes that damage cell structures leading to cell death.

Early studies described the neurotoxic effect of the excitatory neurotransmitter glutamate [61]. In 1969, Olney [62] found that the subcutaneous injection of monosodium glutamate resulted in necrotic brain lesions in the hypothalamus of newborn mice, leading to a number of developmental abnormalities. These reports led to the introduction of the term "excitotoxicity," describing cell damage induced by an excess of glutamate as the most important excitatory amino acids. The control of extracellular glutamate level at the synapse relatively depends on $Na^+$-dependent glutamate transporters located perisynaptically on astrocytes or neurons. Dysfunction of these transporters usually contributed to severe excitotoxicity [63]. It is also true that the activity of glutamate transporters is regulated by the extracellular concentration of glutamate.

Glutamic acid decarboxylase (GAD) as a rate-limiting enzyme in glutamate/GABA cycle catalyzes the conversion of glutamate to GABA. GAD65 and GAD67 are two isoforms of GAD, expressed from two unlinked genes in the adult brain [64]. GAD67 is localized in chromosome 2q31.1, which is related to susceptibility for autism, so it might be a potential biomarker for GABAergic abnormalities demonstrated in autistic patients [65]. The reduction in the number of cerebellar Purkinje cells that express GAD67 abundantly has also been widely reported in autism [66]. A high percentage decrease of mRNA expression for GAD67 was observed in Purkinje cells of autistic individuals compared to control brains [67]. These findings suggest that the reduction in the GABA input to cerebellar nuclei disrupts the output to cerebral cortex and can be related to the motor and cognitive abnormalities seen in autistic patients. An early study has also reported the reduction of GAD65 and GAD67 protein in the parietal cortex and in the cerebellum of autistic brains [68]. There are also reports of increased glutamate levels in the blood and platelets of autistic patients [69, 70]. In addition, a significantly lower glutamate/glutamine ratio was reported by Abu-Shmais et al. [71]. Other studies have also shown that an increased release from presynaptic neurons can also contribute to excitotoxicity. Moreover, increased frequencies and amplitudes of action potential-evoked excitatory synaptic potentials have been observed in mouse models of autism. Therefore, many studies were conducted to clarify and analyze the functional status of glutamatergic and GABAergic neurotransmission in the autistic brain [72, 73]. Based on these studies, strong evidence indicates that dysfunctional excitatory and inhibitory synaptic activities underlie several of the characteristics of autism and support a hyperglutamatergic hypothesis of autism. This was attributed in some studies highlighting an imbalance between GABAergic and glutamatergic as inhibitory and excitatory neurotransmitters, respectively [73]. Another potential source of glutamate excitotoxicity is either the abnormal high release of glutamate or the decrease of glutamate transporters as proteins on the presynaptic neurons and astrocytes playing an important role in the reuptake and removal of glutamate from the synaptic cleft. Raghavendra Rao et al. [74] showed that glutamate transporter-1 (GLT-1) expression was significantly reduced (38–47%) in the rat brain 24 h after fluid percussion injury. The resulting decrease in transport leads to an excess of glutamate in the synaptic cleft. Either increased glutamate release from the presynaptic neuron or removal by glutamate transporters, as two mechanisms that might be related to glutamate excitotoxicity, has been proven in rodent models of autism [75, 76]. Purcell et al. [77] used 10 brain postmortem samples from individuals with autism to identify genes that were significantly up-regulated or down-regulated. These researchers found abnormalities in the AMPA-type glutamate receptors and glutamate transporters in the cerebellum of autistics compared to control involving these transporters directly in the pathogenesis of this disorder. This was ascertained when the down-regulation of glial glutamate transporters, GLT-1 and GLAST, was found effective in the generation of animal models of autism in which glutamate receptors are overstimulated [76].

Glutamate excitotoxicity can easily be related to low GSH level and this has been repeatedly reported in autistic patients. It is well known that more than 80% of extracellular glutamate is transported into astrocytes [78]. This in turn stimulates both GSH synthesis and cysteine inward flow as a prerequisite for the maintenance of high GSH level in astrocytes [79]. On the contrary, neurons import cysteine through EAAT2 and EAAT3 and this process is competitively inhibited by glutamate. Based on this, glutamate excitotoxicity will starve neurons of cysteine in favor of ensuring high GSH level in astrocytes.

Several reproducible studies have ascertained that individuals with autism demonstrate an abnormal brain 5-HT system [80, 81]. This was clinically presented as hyperserotonemia [80], altered 5-HT synthesis or 5-HT receptor affinity, and dystrophic serotonergic [82–84]. In a recent study on postmortem brains, a significant decrease in both 5-$HT_{2A}$ and 5-$HT_{1A}$ binding was reported in autism [85]. Some researchers suggested an association of 5-HT dysfunction with repetitive and self-injurious behaviors [86–88]. This gives support to the idea that peripheral alterations in the 5-HT system may be an important marker of central abnormalities in autism.

Oxytocin (OT) as a neuropeptide of great interest has been known to play important roles in social behavior in both animals and humans [89, 90]. OT-related studies in autism have repeatedly reported lower blood OT level in autistic patients compared to age- and gender-matched control subjects [12, 81, 91, 92]. The faulty processing of the OT prohormone to the active OT neuropeptide was also found [93] together with abnormalities and polymorphism in the OT receptor (OTR) gene, raising the possibility of OT resistance in autism [94–98]. Multiple intersections of the 5-HT and OT systems have been ascertained and were found to influence behaviors such as sociability, aggression, and anxiety that are relevant to autism [99, 100].

With the move toward the development of disease treatment strategy, there is a great need for more specific diagnostic criteria of autism as a heterogeneous disorder. The diagnostic accuracy of biomarkers is most commonly measured by calculating its sensitivity and specificity. Receiver operating characteristic (ROC) curve analysis is a useful tool in the assessment of biomarker accuracy. The accuracy of a biomarker depends on how well it separates the groups being tested into those with and without the disease in question. In ROC analysis, the ratio of the abnormals found by the marker to the total number of abnormals known to have the disease is the true positive rate (or sensitivity), whereas the ratio of the normals found by the test to the total number of normals is the true negative rate (or specificity). The ROC curve is a graph of sensitivity ($y$-axis) versus 1-specificity ($x$-axis). Accuracy is measured by the area under the ROC curve. An area of 0.9 to 1 represents a perfect marker, an area of 0.8 to 0.6 represents good-fair marker, and an area of 0.5 represents a worthless marker [101]. More recently, combined ROC was introduced as a simple clinical method with great potential for assisting the diagnosis of autism through the increase of the AUC, specificity, and sensitivity and the diagnostic value of combined markers [102].

## 3. Biomarkers-directed treatment strategies

Positive roles between selected nutraceuticals or vitamins/minerals-based treatment strategies and the improvement of autistic features have been reported. In a comparative case-control treatment strategies, two groups each of 44 autistic patients, with an age range of 2 to 28 years, were given either micronutrient supplement containing (14 vitamins, 16 dietary minerals, 3 amino acids, and 3 antioxidants) without any autism medication or conventional medication without supplementation. Patients in both groups improved, but the level of improvement was remarkably higher in micronutrient recommended group than in the conventional medication group [103].

Similarly, in an observatory study, the administration of vitamin B12 and GSH along with low fructose and food additive/color organic diet of 10 children (4–10 years of age) for 3 to 6 months resulted in a significant improvement in the social interaction, concentration, writing, language, and behavior [104]. A meta-analysis of 18 studies revealed that the supplementation of vitamin B6, especially in combination with magnesium, improved the health of autistic patients [105, 106].

Complementary alternative medicine (CAM) treatments are usually recommended to promote health, to avoid side the effects of conventional drugs, or to ameliorate the core symptoms of autism. Prenatal exposure to VPA induces a rearrangement of early microbial colonization, leading to an increase of butyrate levels in the gastrointestinal tract of male offspring. Consequently, increased levels of butyrate in the gut may interfere directly with gene expression in intestinal cells or indirectly with gene expression of neuronal cells after crossing the BBB. This is usually accompanied with induced deleterious changes in the intestinal and brain functions that might explain certain autistic features. These results open the road to a novel strategy to treat autism through gut microbiome manipulation. The administration of probiotic or prebiotic may provide an excellent tool to treat autism based on our understanding of the role of gut-brain axis and microbial metabolites in the pathology of this disorder.

Clinical studies have shown that prenatal supplementation with *n*-3 PUFA may be beneficial for healthy neural development in both preterm and full term infants [107–109]. Regarding preterm infants, the timing of supplementation is of critical importance because these infants cannot fully use accumulated long-chain PUFA that usually start in the last trimester of gestation. Studies in full-term infants show that both prenatal and postnatal supplementations cause an improvement in cognition [110, 111]. Moreover, in humans, the outcome of infant *n*-3 PUFA supplementation on long-term brain development appears to be subtle [112–114] compared to the rodent model studies [115], which demonstrate more pronounced beneficial effects of $n$-3 PUFA supplementation [115–117]. Overall, our adequate dietary $n$-3 PUFA levels starting early in life may support optimal neural development in healthy full-term infants.

In a randomized, double-blind, placebo-controlled 6-week pilot study, Amminger et al. [118] investigated the effects of 1.5 g/d ω-3 fatty acids (0.84 g/d EPA and 0.7 g/d DHA) supplementation given in the form of seven pale-yellow, 1 g gelatin capsules of fish oil, each containing 120 mg EPA and 100 mg DHA plus 1 mg vitamin E to 13 autistic children (aged 5–17 years). The placebo was seven gelatin capsules of coconut oil that were of similar shape and size and also contained 1 mg vitamin E as well as 1 mg fish oil to mimic fish taste. The experimental daily dose of 1.5 g ω-3 fatty acids is based on a study in children with developmental coordination disorder by Richardson and Montgomery [119]. The findings of their trial suggested that ω-3 fatty acids may be effective in treating the aggression and impulsivity in autistic patients. The underlying mechanism of action is not fully understood but may be related to the modulation of serotonergic and dopaminergic neurotransmission [120]. This can be ascertained by considering the phenomenon that DHA or the EPA/ARA ratio might control aggression by depressing the noradrenergic system [112]. The more recent work of El-Ansary et al. [116] supports that the essential fatty acids/long-chain PUFA and ω-3/ω-6 ratios, phosphatidylethanolamine, phosphatidylserine, and phosphatidylcholine could be used as potential biomarkers that point to specific mechanisms in the development of autism and may help tailor treatment or prevention strategies (**Figure 5**). In the recent study of Weiser et al. [121], DHA supplementation greatly reduced the level of IL-6 as an acute inflammatory marker induced in the rodent model of autism exposed to the viral mimetic polyriboinosinic-polyribocytidylic acid during gestation. This gives preliminary evidence that ω-3 fatty acids may be an effective treatment strategy for children with autism.

A recent report by the Autism Genome Project Consortium identified a new linkage peak for autism in the region of chromosome 11 where the gene for EAAT2 is located [122]. Signs of astroglial, oligodendroglial, and microglial dysfunction were reported in the autistic brain, suggesting that all these cellular processes may represent presumptive targets for novel therapeutic strategies [123]. Additionally, a study investigating the effects of ceftriaxone and cefixime, activators of GLT-1, demonstrated that these drugs improved some symptoms of autism and decreased epilepsy seizures by increasing the expression of the GLT-1, which reduces extracellular glutamate levels [124].

Elevated levels of glutamate are present in high proteins, including wheat gluten and milk casein. This can explain the sensitivity of autistic children to both proteins as a rich source of glutamate. Some parents of autistic children try gluten/casein-restricted diet in an attempt to improve their child's behavior, but evidence is lacking that following such diet improves the child's challenging behaviors, cognitive and social functioning as core symptoms of autism [125]. Furthermore, following a gluten casein-free diet may place children at risk for suboptimal bone development [126].

Several animal models and research in typically developing volunteers suggest that the manipulation of the OT system may have a potential therapeutic effect in treating social deficits in autistic patients. Twelve weeks of intranasal treatment with OT (0.4 IU/kg/dose) was found effective in improving social impairment, repetitive behavior, and anxiety in children and adolescents with autism. Some measures suggest the safety and maintenance of the effect for 3 months after the discontinuation of intranasal OT treatment [127]. Meziane et al. [128] reported that an early OT treatment just after birth could be a novel therapeutic approach for the treatment of autism.

In a recent study, Carminati et al. [129] tested the therapeutic efficacy of venlafaxine, an antidepressant drug that inhibits the reuptake of 5-HT, and proved that venlafaxine at a low dose represents a substantial improvement in repetitive behaviors, restricted interests, social impairment, communication, and language. Venlafaxine probably acts via serotonergic mechanisms by affecting the selective 5-HT reuptake inhibitors. **Figure 6** summarizes the biomarkers directed to treat autism.

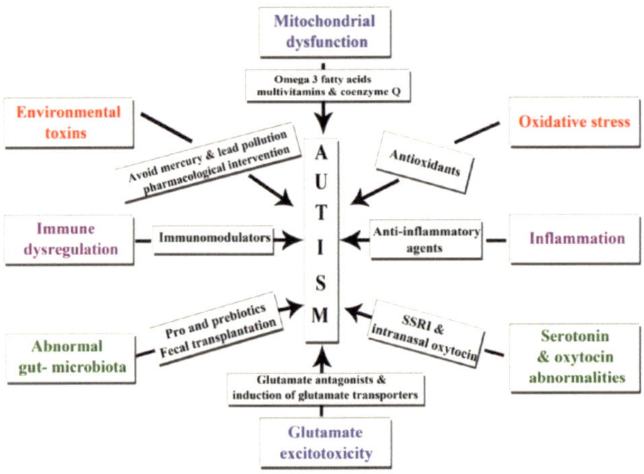


**Figure 6.** Biomarkers-directed strategies to treat autism.

## Author details

Afaf El-Ansary[1,2*] and Hussain Al Dera[3,4]

*Address all correspondence to: afafkelansary@gmail.com

1 Therapuetic Chemistry Department, National Research Centre, Dokki, Cairo, Egypt

2 Biochemistry Department, Science College, King Saud University, Riyadh, Saudi Arabia

3 Basic Medical Department, College of Medicine, King Saud bin Abdul Aziz University for Health Sciences, Riyadh, Saudi Arabia

4 King Abdullah International Medical Research Center (Kaimrc), Ministry of National Guard, Riyadh, Saudi Arabia

## References

[1] Aspy R, Grossman BG. *Designing Comprehensive Interventions for High-Functioning Individuals with Autism Spectrum Disorders: The Ziggurat Model*. USA, AAPC Publishing; 2011.

[2] Berkel S, Marshall CR, Weiss B, Howe J, Roeth R, Moog U, Endris V, Roberts W, Szatmari P, Pinto D. Mutations in the SHANK2 synaptic scaffolding gene in autism spectrum disorder and mental retardation. *Nat Genet* 2010;42:489–491.

[3] Pinto D, Pagnamenta AT, Klei L, Anney R, Merico D, Regan R, Conroy J, Magalhaes TR, Correia C, Abrahams BS. Functional impact of global rare copy number variation in autism spectrum disorders. *Nature* 2010;466:368–372.

[4] Gilman SR, Iossifov I, Levy D, Ronemus M, Wigler M, Vitkup D. Rare *de novo* variants associated with autism implicate a large functional network of genes involved in formation and function of synapses. *Neuron* 2011;70:898–907.

[5] State MW, Šestan N. The emerging biology of autism spectrum disorders. *Science* 2012;337:1301.

[6] Sanders SJ, Ercan-Sencicek AG, Hus V, Luo R, Murtha MT, Moreno-De-Luca D, Chu SH, Moreau MP, Gupta AR, Thomson SA. Multiple recurrent *de novo* CNVs, including duplications of the 7q11. 23 Williams syndrome region, are strongly associated with autism. *Neuron* 2011;70:863–885.

[7] Fombonne E. Epidemiology of pervasive developmental disorders. *Pediatr Res* 2009;65:591–598.

[8] Kim YS, Leventhal BL, Koh Y-J, Fombonne E, Laska E, Lim E-C, Cheon K-A, Kim S-J, Kim Y-K, Lee H. Prevalence of autism spectrum disorders in a total population sample. *Am J Psychiatry* 2011;168:904–912.

[9] Main P, Angley MT, O'Doherty CE, Thomas P, Fenech M. The potential role of the antioxidant and detoxification properties of glutathione in autism spectrum disorders: a systematic review and meta-analysis. *Nutr Metab (Lond)* 2012;9:35.

[10] Lord RS, Bralley JA. Clinical applications of urinary organic acids. Part I: detoxification markers. *Altern Med Rev* 2008;13:205–215.

[11] Mostafa GA, El-Hadidi ES, Hewedi DH, Abdou MM. Oxidative stress in Egyptian children with autism: relation to autoimmunity. *J Neuroimmunol* 2010;219:114–118.

[12] Alabdali A, Al-Ayadhi L, El-Ansary A. Association of social and cognitive impairment and biomarkers in autism spectrum disorders. *J Neuroinflamm* 2014;11.

[13] Q-b Zhang, Gao S-j, H-x Zhao. Thioredoxin: a novel, independent diagnosis marker in children with autism. *Int J Dev Neurosci* 2015;40:92–96.

[14] Rossignol D, Frye R. Mitochondrial dysfunction in autism spectrum disorders: a systematic review and meta-analysis. *Mol Psychiatry* 2012;17:290–314.

[15] Mulle JG, Sharp WG, Cubells JF. The gut microbiome: a new frontier in autism research. *Curr Psychiatry Rep* 2013;15:1–9.

[16] Burokas A, Moloney RD, Dinan TG, Cryan JF. Chapter one—microbiota regulation of the mammalian gut-brain axis. *Adv Appl Microbiol* 2015;91:1–62.

[17] Smith SE, Li J, Garbett K, Mirnics K, Patterson PH. Maternal immune activation alters fetal brain development through interleukin-6. *J Neurosci* 2007;27:10695–10702.

[18] Libbey JE, Fujinami RS. Role for antibodies in altering behavior and movement. *Autism Res* 2010;3:147–152.

[19] Angelidou A, Asadi S, Alysandratos K-D, Karagkouni A, Kourembanas S, Theoharides TC. Perinatal stress, brain inflammation and risk of autism-Review and proposal. *BMC Pediatr* 2012;12:89.

[20] Fetissov SO, Sinno MH, Coëffier M, Bole-Feysot C, DucrottéP, Hökfelt T, Déchelotte P. Autoantibodies against appetite-regulating peptide hormones and neuropeptides: putative modulation by gut microflora. *Nutrition* 2008;24:348–359.

[21] de Magistris L, Familiari V, Pascotto A, Sapone A, Frolli A, Iardino P, Carteni M, De Rosa M, Francavilla R, Riegler G. Alterations of the intestinal barrier in patients with autism spectrum disorders and in their first-degree relatives. *J Pediatr Gastroenterol Nutr* 2010;51:418–424.

[22] Turner JR. Intestinal mucosal barrier function in health and disease. *Nat Rev Immunol* 2009;9:799–809.

[23] Hsiao EY, Mc Bride SW, Hsien S, Sharon G, Hyde ER, McCue T, Codelli JA, Chow J, Reisman SE, Petrosino JF. Microbiota modulate behavioral and physiological abnormalities associated with neurodevelopmental disorders. *Cell* 2013;155:1451–1463.

[24] Parracho HM, Bingham MO, Gibson GR, McCartney AL. Differences between the gut microflora of children with autistic spectrum disorders and that of healthy children. *J Med Microbiol* 2005;54:987–991.

[25] Finegold SM, Dowd SE, Gontcharova V, Liu C, Henley KE, Wolcott RD, Youn E, Summanen PH, Granpeesheh D, Dixon D. Pyrosequencing study of fecal microflora of autistic and control children. *Anaerobe* 2010;16:444–453.

[26] Adams JB, Johansen LJ, Powell LD, Quig D, Rubin RA. Gastrointestinal flora and gastrointestinal status in children with autism—comparisons to typical children and correlation with autism severity. *BMC Gastroenterol* 2011;11:22.

[27] Wang L, Christophersen CT, Sorich MJ, Gerber JP, Angley MT, Conlon MA. Low relative abundances of the mucolytic bacterium *Akkermansia muciniphila* and *Bifidobacterium* spp. in feces of children with autism. *Appl Environ Microbiol* 2011;77:6718–6721.

[28] Williams BL, Hornig M, Buie T, Bauman ML, Cho Paik M, Wick I, Bennett A, Jabado O, Hirschberg DL, Lipkin WI. Impaired carbohydrate digestion and transport and mucosal dysbiosis in the intestines of children with autism and gastrointestinal disturbances. *PLoS One* 2011;6:e24585.

[29] Williams BL, Hornig M, Parekh T, Lipkin WI. Application of novel PCR-based methods for detection, quantitation, and phylogenetic characterization of *Sutterella* species in intestinal biopsy samples from children with autism and gastrointestinal disturbances. *MBio* 2012;3:e00261–00211.

[30] Finegold SM, Molitoris D, Song Y, Liu C, Vaisanen M-L, Bolte E, McTeague M, Sandler R, Wexler H, Marlowe EM. Gastrointestinal microflora studies in late-onset autism. *Clin Infect Dis* 2002;35:S6–S16.

[31] De Angelis M, Piccolo M, Vannini L, Siragusa S, De Giacomo A, Serrazzanetti DI, Cristofori F, Guerzoni ME, Gobbetti M, Francavilla R. Fecal microbiota and metabolome of children with autism and pervasive developmental disorder not otherwise specified. *PLoS One* 2013;8:e76993.

[32] Yap IK, Angley M, Veselkov KA, Holmes E, Lindon JC, Nicholson JK. Urinary metabolic phenotyping differentiates children with autism from their unaffected siblings and age-matched controls. *J Proteome Res* 2010;9:2996–3004.

[33] Beloborodova N, Bairamov I, Olenin A, Shubina V, Teplova V, Fedotcheva N. Effect of phenolic acids of microbial origin on production of reactive oxygen species in mitochondria and neutrophils. *J Biomed Sci* 2012;19:89.

[34] MacFabe DF. Short-chain fatty acid fermentation products of the gut microbiome: implications in autism spectrum disorders. *Microb Ecol Health Dis* 2012;23. doi: 10.3402/mehd.v23i0.19260.

[35] MacFabe DF, Cain DP, Rodriguez-Capote K, Franklin AE, Hoffman JE, Boon F, Taylor AR, Kavaliers M, Ossenkopp K-P. Neurobiological effects of intraventricular propionic acid in rats: possible role of short chain fatty acids on the pathogenesis and characteristics of autism spectrum disorders. *Behav Brain Res* 2007;176:149–169.

[36] MacFabe DF, Cain NE, Boon F, Ossenkopp K-P, Cain DP. Effects of the enteric bacterial metabolic product propionic acid on object-directed behavior, social behavior, cognition, and neuroinflammation in adolescent rats: relevance to autism spectrum disorder. *Behav Brain Res* 2011;217:47–54.

[37] Wang LW, Tancredi DJ, Thomas DW. The prevalence of gastrointestinal problems in children across the United States with autism spectrum disorders from families with multiple affected members. *J Dev Behav Pediatr* 2011;32:351–360.

[38] Kataoka S, Takuma K, Hara Y, Maeda Y, Ago Y, Matsuda T. Autism-like behaviours with transient histone hyperacetylation in mice treated prenatally with valproic acid. *J Neuropsychopharmacol* 2013;16:91–103.

[39] Burger-van Paassen N, Vincent A, Puiman P, Van Der Sluis M, Bouma J, Boehm G, van Goudoever J, Van Seuningen I, Renes I. The regulation of intestinal mucin MUC2 expression by short-chain fatty acids: implications for epithelial protection. *Biochem J* 2009;420:211–219.

[40] D'Souza A, Onem E, Patel P, La Gamma EF, Nankova BB. Valproic acid regulates catecholaminergic pathways by concentration-dependent threshold effects on TH mRNA synthesis and degradation. *Brain Res* 2009;1247:1–10.

[41] Liu H, Hu Q, Kaufman A, D'Ercole AJ, Ye P. Developmental expression of histone deacetylase 11 in the murine brain. *J Neurosci Res* 2008;86:537–543.

[42] Patterson PH. Maternal infection: window on neuroimmune interactions in fetal brain development and mental illness. *Curr Opin Neurobiol* 2002;12:115–118.

[43] Stolp H, Dziegielewska K. Review: role of developmental inflammation and blood-brain barrier dysfunction in neurodevelopmental and neurodegenerative diseases. *Neuropathol Appl Neurobiol* 2009;35:132–146.

[44] Hornig M, Briese T, Buie T, Bauman ML, Lauwers G, Siemetzki U, Hummel K, Rota PA, Bellini WJ, O'Leary JJ. Lack of association between measles virus vaccine and autism with enteropathy: a case-control study. *PLoS One* 2008;3:e3140.

[45] Malik M, Sheikh AM, Wen G, Spivack W, Brown WT, Li X. Expression of inflammatory cytokines, Bcl2 and cathepsin D are altered in lymphoblasts of autistic subjects. *Immunobiology* 2011;216:80–85.

[46] Jyonouchi H, Sun S, Le H. Proinflammatory and regulatory cytokine production associated with innate and adaptive immune responses in children with autism spectrum disorders and developmental regression. *J Neuroimmunol* 2001;120:170–179.

[47] Morgan JT, Chana G, Pardo CA, Achim C, Semendeferi K, Buckwalter J, Courchesne E, Everall IP. Microglial activation and increased microglial density observed in the dorsolateral prefrontal cortex in autism. *Biol Psychiatry* 2010;68:368–376.

[48] Vargas DL, Nascimbene C, Krishnan C, Zimmerman AW, Pardo CA. Neuroglial activation and neuroinflammation in the brain of patients with autism. *Ann Neurol* 2005;57:67–81.

[49] Chez MG, Guido-Estrada N. Immune therapy in autism: historical experience and future directions with immunomodulatory therapy. *Neurotherapeutics* 2010;7:293–301.

[50] Garbett K, Ebert PJ, Mitchell A, Lintas C, Manzi B, Mirnics K, Persico AM. Immune transcriptome alterations in the temporal cortex of subjects with autism. *Neurobiol Dis* 2008;30:303–311.

[51] Suganya V, Geetha A, Sujatha S. Urine proteome analysis to evaluate protein biomarkers in children with autism. *Clin Chim Acta* 2015;450:210–219.

[52] West PR, Amaral DG, Bais P, Smith AM, Egnash LA, Ross ME, Palmer JA, Fontaine BR, Conard KR, Corbett BA. Metabolomics as a tool for discovery of biomarkers of autism spectrum disorder in the blood plasma of children. *PLoS One* 2014;9:e112445.

[53] Palmieri F. The mitochondrial transporter family (SLC25): physiological and pathological implications. *Pflügers Arch* 2004;447:689–709.

[54] Viegas CM, Busanello ENB, Tonin AM, de Moura AP, Grings M, Ritter L, Schuck PF, da CostaFerreira G, Sitta A, Vargas CR. Dual mechanism of brain damage induced in vivo by the major metabolites accumulating in hyperornithinemia-hyperammonemia-homocitrullinuria syndrome. *Brain Res* 2011;1369:235–244.

[55] Sokoro AA, Lepage J, Antonishyn N, McDonald R, Rockman-Greenberg C, Irvine J, Lehotay DC. Diagnosis and high incidence of hyperornithinemia-hyperammonemia-homocitrullinemia (HHH) syndrome in northern Saskatchewan. *J Inherit Metab Dis* 2010;33:275–281.

[56] Brenna JT, Carlson SE. Docosahexaenoic acid and human brain development: evidence that a dietary supply is needed for optimal development. *J Hum Evol* 2014;77:99–106.

[57] Simopoulos AP. Evolutionary aspects of diet: the ω-6/ω-3 ratio and the brain. *Mol Neurobiol* 2011;44:203–215.

[58] Vancassel S, Durand G, Barthelemy C, Lejeune B, Martineau J, Guilloteau D, Andres C, Chalon S. Plasma fatty acid levels in autistic children. *Prostaglandins Leukot Essent Fatty Acids* 2001;65:1–7.

[59] Ghezzo A, Visconti P, Abruzzo PM, Bolotta A, Ferreri C, Gobbi G, Malisardi G, Manfredini S, Marini M, Nanetti L. Oxidative stress and erythrocyte membrane alterations in children with autism: correlation with clinical features. *PLoS One* 2013;8:e66418.

[60] Fombonne E, Morel J, Macarthur J. No autism amongst Inuits from northern Quebec. In *Fifth International Meeting for Autism Research*, Montreal, Quebec; 2006.

[61] Lucas D, Newhouse J. The toxic effect of sodium L-glutamate on the inner layers of the retina. *AMA Arch Ophthalmol* 1957;58:193–201.

[62] Olney JW. Brain lesions, obesity, and other disturbances in mice treated with monosodium glutamate. *Science* 1969;164:719–721.

[63] Blaylock R, Strunecka A. Immune-glutamatergic dysfunction as a central mechanism of the autism spectrum disorders. *Curr Med Chem* 2009;16:157–170.

[64] Bu D-F, Erlander MG, Hitz BC, Tillakaratne N, Kaufman DL, Wagner-McPherson CB, Evans GA, Tobin AJ. Two human glutamate decarboxylases, 65-kDa GAD and 67-kDa GAD, are each encoded by a single gene. *Proc Natl Acad Sci U S A* 1992;89:2115–2119.

[65] Rabionet R, Jaworski JM, Ashley-Koch AE, Martin ER, Sutcliffe JS, Haines JL, DeLong GR, Abramson RK, Wright HH, Cuccaro ML. Analysis of the autism chromosome 2 linkage region: GAD1 and other candidate genes. *Neurosci Lett* 2004;372:209–214.

[66] Kern JK. Purkinje cell vulnerability and autism: a possible etiological connection. *Brain Dev* 2003;25:377–382.

[67] Yip J, Soghomonian J-J, Blatt GJ. Decreased GAD67 mRNA levels in cerebellar Purkinje cells in autism: pathophysiological implications. *Acta Neuropathol* 2007;113:559–568.

[68] Fatemi SH, Halt AR, Stary JM, Kanodia R, Schulz SC, Realmuto GR. Glutamic acid decarboxylase 65 and 67 kDa proteins are reduced in autistic parietal and cerebellar cortices. *Biol Psychiatry* 2002;52:805–810.

[69] Aldred S, Moore KM, Fitzgerald M, Waring RH. Plasma amino acid levels in children with autism and their families. *J Autism Dev Disord* 2003;33:93–97.

[70] Shinohe A, Hashimoto K, Nakamura K, Tsujii M, Iwata Y, Tsuchiya KJ, Sekine Y, Suda S, Suzuki K, Sugihara G-I. Increased serum levels of glutamate in adult patients with autism. *Prog Neuro-psychopharmacol Biol Psychiatry* 2006;30:1472–1477.

[71] Abu-Shmais GA, Al-Ayadhi LY, Al-Dbass AM, El-Ansary AK. Mechanism of nitrogen metabolism-related parameters and enzyme activities in the pathophysiology of autism. *J Neurodev Disord* 2012;4:4.

[72] Uzunova G, Pallanti S, Hollander E. Excitatory/inhibitory imbalance in autism spectrum disorders: implications for interventions and therapeutics. *World J Biol Psychiatry* 2015:1–13.

[73] El-Ansary A, Al-Ayadhi L. Neuroinflammation in autism spectrum disorders. *Neuroinflammation* 2012;9:265.

[74] Raghavendra Rao VL, Başkaya MK, Doğan A, Rothstein JD, Dempsey RJ. Traumatic brain injury down-regulates glial glutamate transporter (GLT-1 and GLAST) proteins in rat brain. *J Neurochem* 1998;70:2020–2027.

[75] Wei H, Ding C, Jin G, Yin H, Liu J, Hu F. Abnormal glutamate release in aged BTBR mouse model of autism. *Int J Clin Exp Pathol* 2015;8:10689.

[76] Tanaka K. Role of glutamate transporters in the pathophysiology of major mental illnesses. *Nihon Shinkei Seishin Yakurigaku Zasshi* 2009;29:161–164.

[77] Purcell A, Jeon O, Zimmerman A, Blue M, Pevsner J. Postmortem brain abnormalities of the glutamate neurotransmitter system in autism. *Neurology* 2001;57:1618–1628.

[78] Hertz L, Peng L. Energy metabolism at the cellular level of the CNS. *Can J Physiol Pharmacol* 1992;70:S145–S157.

[79] Bannai S, Tateishi N. Role of membrane transport in metabolism and function of glutathione in mammals. *J Membr Biol* 1986;89:1–8.

[80] Gabriele S, Sacco R, Persico AM. Blood serotonin levels in autism spectrum disorder: a systematic review and meta-analysis. *Eur Neuropsychopharmacol* 2014;24:919–929.

[81] Yang C-J, Tan H-P, Yang F-Y, Wang H-P, Liu C-L, He H-Z, Sang B, Zhu X-M, Du Y-J. The cortisol, serotonin and oxytocin are associated with repetitive behavior in autism spectrum disorder. *Res Autism Spectr Disord* 2015;18:12–20.

[82] Chugani DC, Muzik O, Rothermel R, Behen M, Chakraborty P, Mangner T, Da Silva EA, Chugani HT. Altered serotonin synthesis in the dentatothalamocortical pathway in autistic boys. *Ann Neurol* 1997;42:666–669.

[83] Makkonen I, Riikonen R, Kokki H, Airaksinen MM, Kuikka JT. Serotonin and dopamine transporter binding in children with autism determined by SPECT. *Dev Med Child Neurol* 2008;50:593–597.

[84] Nakamura K, Sekine Y, Ouchi Y, Tsujii M, Yoshikawa E, Futatsubashi M, Tsuchiya KJ, Sugihara G, Iwata Y, Suzuki K. Brain serotonin and dopamine transporter bindings in adults with high-functioning autism. *Arch Gen Psychiatry* 2010;67:59–68.

[85] Oblak A, Gibbs TT, Blatt GJ. Reduced serotonin receptor subtypes in a limbic and a neocortical region in autism. *Autism Res* 2013;6:571–583.

[86] Kolevzon A, Newcorn JH, Kryzak L, Chaplin W, Watner D, Hollander E, Smith CJ, Cook EH, Silverman JM. Relationship between whole blood serotonin and repetitive behaviors in autism. *Psychiatry Res* 2010;175:274–276.

[87] Sacco R, Curatolo P, Manzi B, Militerni R, Bravaccio C, Frolli A, Lenti C, Saccani M, Elia M, Reichelt KL. Principal pathogenetic components and biological endophenotypes in autism spectrum disorders. *Autism Res* 2010;3:237–252.

[88] Veenstra-VanderWeele J, Muller CL, Iwamoto H, Sauer JE, Owens WA, Shah CR, Cohen J, Mannangatti P, Jessen T, Thompson BJ. Autism gene variant causes hyperserotonemia, serotonin receptor hypersensitivity, social impairment and repetitive behavior. *Proc Natl Acad Sci U S A* 2012;109:5469–5474.

[89] Insel TR. The challenge of translation in social neuroscience: a review of oxytocin, vasopressin, and affiliative behavior. *Neuron* 2010;65:768–779.

[90] Meyer-Lindenberg A, Domes G, Kirsch P, Heinrichs M. Oxytocin and vasopressin in the human brain: social neuropeptides for translational medicine. *Nat Rev Neurosci* 2011;12:524–538.

[91] Modahl C, Green LA, Fein D, Morris M, Waterhouse L, Feinstein C, Levin H. Plasma oxytocin levels in autistic children. *Biol Psychiatry* 1998;43:270–277.

[92] Andari E, Duhamel J-R, Zalla T, Herbrecht E, Leboyer M, Sirigu A. Promoting social behavior with oxytocin in high-functioning autism spectrum disorders. *Proc Natl Acad Sci U S A* 2010;107:4389–4394.

[93] Green L, Fein D, Modahl C, Feinstein C, Waterhouse L, Morris M. Oxytocin and autistic disorder: alterations in peptide forms. *Biol Psychiatry* 2001;50:609–613.

[94] Wu S, Jia M, Ruan Y, Liu J, Guo Y, Shuang M, Gong X, Zhang Y, Yang X, Zhang D. Positive association of the oxytocin receptor gene (OXTR) with autism in the Chinese Han population. *Biol Psychiatry* 2005;58:74–77.

[95] Jacob S, Brune CW, Carter C, Leventhal BL, Lord C, Cook EH. Association of the oxytocin receptor gene (OXTR) in Caucasian children and adolescents with autism. *Neurosci Lett* 2007;417:6–9.

[96] Lerer E, Levi S, Salomon S, Darvasi A, Yirmiya N, Ebstein R. Association between the oxytocin receptor (OXTR) gene and autism: relationship to Vineland Adaptive Behavior Scales and cognition. *Mol Psychiatry* 2008;13:980–988.

[97] Yrigollen CM, Han SS, Kochetkova A, Babitz T, Chang JT, Volkmar FR, Leckman JF, Grigorenko EL. Genes controlling affiliative behavior as candidate genes for autism. *Biol Psychiatry* 2008;63:911–916.

[98] Ebstein RP, Knafo A, Mankuta D, ChewSH, SanLai P. The contributions of oxytocin and vasopressin pathway genes to human behavior. *Horm Behav* 2012;61:359–379.

[99] Dölen G, Darvishzadeh A, Huang KW, Malenka RC. Social reward requires coordinated activity of nucleus accumbens oxytocin and serotonin. *Nature* 2013;501:179–184.

[100] Dölen G. Autism: oxytocin, serotonin, and social reward. *Soc Neurosci* 2015;10:450–465.

[101] Pepe M, Longton G, Janes H. Estimation and comparison of receiver operating characteristic curves. *Stata J* 2009;9:1.

[102] Yang CJ, Liu CL, Sang B, Zhu XM, Du YJ. The combined role of serotonin and interleukin-6 as biomarker for autism. *Neuroscience* 2015;284:290–296.

[103] Mehl-Madrona L, Leung B, Kennedy C, Paul S, Kaplan BJ. Micronutrients versus standard medication management in autism: a naturalistic case-control study. *J Child Adolesc Psychopharmacol* 2010;20:95–103.

[104] Patel K, Curtis LT. A comprehensive approach to treating autism and attention-deficit hyperactivity disorder: a prepilot study. *J Altern Complement Med* 2007;13:1091–1098.

[105] Kidd PM. Autism, an extreme challenge to integrative medicine. Part II: medical management. *Altern Med Rev* 2002;7:472–499.

[106] Cornish S, Mehl-Madrona L. The role of vitamins and minerals in psychiatry. *Integr Med Insights* 2008;3:33.

[107] Henriksen C, Haugholt K, Lindgren M, Aurvåg AK, Rønnestad A, Grønn M, Solberg R, Moen A, Nakstad B, Berge RK. Improved cognitive development among preterm infants attributable to early supplementation of human milk with docosahexaenoic acid and arachidonic acid. *Pediatrics* 2008;121:1137–1145.

[108] Isaacs EB, Ross S, Kennedy K, Weaver LT, Lucas A, Fewtrell MS. 10-year cognition in preterms after random assignment to fatty acid supplementation in infancy. *Pediatrics* 2011;128:e890–e898.

[109] Makrides M, Gibson RA, McPhee AJ, Yelland L, Quinlivan J, Ryan P. Effect of DHA supplementation during pregnancy on maternal depression and neurodevelopment of young children: a randomized controlled trial. *JAMA* 2010;304:1675–1683.

[110] Dunstan J, Simmer K, Dixon G, Prescott S. Cognitive assessment of children at age 2½ years after maternal fish oil supplementation in pregnancy: a randomised controlled trial. *Arch Dis Child* 2008;93:F45–F50.

[111] Smithers LG, Gibson RA, Makrides M. Maternal supplementation with docosahexaenoic acid during pregnancy does not affect early visual development in the infant: a randomized controlled trial. *Am J Clin Nutr* 2011;93:1293–1299.

[112] Wurtman RJ. Synapse formation and cognitive brain development: effect of docosahexaenoic acid and other dietary constituents. *Metabolism* 2008;57:S6–S10.

[113] Bouwstra H, Dijck-Brouwer DJ, Decsi T, Boehm G, Boersma ER, Muskiet FA, Hadders-Algra M. Relationship between umbilical cord essential fatty acid content and the quality of general movements of healthy term infants at 3 months. *Pediatr Res* 2006;59:717–722.

[114] Fewtrell MS, Morley R, Abbott RA, Singhal A, Isaacs EB, Stephenson T, MacFadyen U, Lucas A. Double-blind, randomized trial of long-chain polyunsaturated fatty acid supplementation in formula fed to preterm infants. *Pediatrics* 2002;110:73–82.

[115] Carrié I, Guesnet P, Bourre J-M, Francès H. Diets containing long-chain *n*-3 polyunsaturated fatty acids affect behaviour differently during development than ageing in mice. *Br J Nutr* 2000;83:439–447.

[116] El-Ansary AK, Al-Daihan SK, El-Gezeery AR. On the protective effect of ω-3 against propionic acid-induced neurotoxicity in rat pups. *Lipids Health Dis* 2011;10:19.

[117] Coluccia A, Borracci P, Renna G, Giustino A, Latronico T, Riccio P, Carratù MR. Developmental ω-3 supplementation improves motor skills in juvenile-adult rats. *Int J Dev Neurosci* 2009;27:599–605.

[118] Amminger GP, Berger GE, Schäfer MR, Klier C, Friedrich MH, Feucht M. ω-3 fatty acids supplementation in children with autism: a double-blind randomized, placebo-controlled pilot study. *Biol Psychiatry* 2007;61:551–553.

[119] Richardson AJ, Montgomery P. The Oxford-Durham study: a randomized, controlled trial of dietary supplementation with fatty acids in children with developmental coordination disorder. *Pediatrics* 2005;115:1360–1366.

[120] Hibbeln JR, Linnoila M, Umhau JC, Rawlings R, George DT, Salem N. Essential fatty acids predict metabolites of serotonin and dopamine in cerebrospinal fluid among

healthy control subjects, and early-and late-onset alcoholics. *Biol Psychiatry* 1998;44:235–242.

[121] Weiser MJ, Wynalda K, Salem N, Butt CM. Dietary DHA during development affects depression-like behaviors and biomarkers that emerge after puberty in adolescent rats. *J Lipid Res* 2015;56:151–166.

[122] Szatmari P, Paterson AD, Zwaigenbaum L, Roberts W, Brian J, Liu X-Q, Vincent JB, Skaug JL, Thompson AP, Senman L. Mapping autism risk loci using genetic linkage and chromosomal rearrangements. *Nat Genet* 2007;39:319–328.

[123] Zeidán-Chuliá F, Salmina AB, Malinovskaya NA, Noda M, Verkhratsky A, Moreira JCF. The glial perspective of autism spectrum disorders. *Neurosci Biobehav Rev* 2014;38:160–172.

[124] Ghanizadeh A, Michael B. β-Lactam antibiotics as a possible novel therapy for managing epilepsy and autism: a case report and review of literature. *Iran J Child Neurol* 2015;9:99.

[125] Millward C, Ferriter M, Calver S, Connell-Jones G. Gluten-and casein-free diets for autistic spectrum disorder. *Cochrane Database Syst Rev* 2008;2.

[126] Geraghty ME, Depasquale GM, Lane AE. Nutritional intake and therapies in autism a spectrum of what we know: part 1. *Infant Child Adolesc Nutr* 2010;2:62–69.

[127] Anagnostou E, Soorya L, Brian J, Dupuis A, Mankad D, Smile S, Jacob S. Intranasal oxytocin in the treatment of autism spectrum disorders: a review of literature and early safety and efficacy data in youth. *Brain Res* 2014;1580:188–198.

[128] Meziane H, Schaller F, Bauer S, Villard C, Matarazzo V, Riet F, Guillon G, Lafitte D, Desarmenien MG, Tauber M. An early postnatal oxytocin treatment prevents social and learning deficits in adult mice deficient for Magel2, a gene involved in Prader-Willi syndrome and autism. *Biol Psychiatry* 2014.

[129] Carminati GG, Gerber F, Darbellay B, Kosel MM, Deriaz N, Chabert J, Fathi M, Bertschy G, Ferrero F, Carminati F. Using venlafaxine to treat behavioral disorders in patients with autism spectrum disorder. *Prog Neuro-psychopharmacol Biol Psychiatry* 2016;65:85–95.

Chapter 11

# Biomarkers in Rare Genetic Diseases

Chiara Scotton and Alessandra Ferlini

Additional information is available at the end of the chapter

http://dx.doi.org/10.5772/63354

**Abstract**

Biomarkers offer a way to speed up medical research by shedding light on the physiopathological mechanisms of disease. Furthermore, biomarkers are considered invaluable tools for monitoring disease progression, prognosis, and response to drugs, especially in clinical trials, where they can be used to assess the efficacy, efficiency, and side effects of novel drugs.

Biomarkers also pave the way to personalised medicine, a rapidly developing field that is of particular interest in rare diseases (RDs), i.e. those with a prevalence of less than 5/10,000, which are often genetic in origin. Although rare genetic diseases may be less appealing targets for pharmaceutical companies, they are nevertheless in urgent need of research into their diagnosis, prevention, treatment, and standards of care.

Here we summarise the state of the art in RDs, genetic diagnosis, and novel strategies aimed at accurately identifying and defining gene mutations, and review the evidence emerging from the latest research and clinical trials. We focus in particular on novel biomarkers, describing the different types discovered so far, highlighting their importance and indicating how they may be translated into research, diagnostics, treatment, and preventative applications in personalised strategies for RDs.

**Keywords:** biomarker, rare disease, genetic disease, genomics, transcriptomics, proteomics

## 1. Introduction

As each rare disease (RD) only affects a relatively small number of individuals across the globe, there are often great obstacles to their research, diagnosis, treatment, and prevention. In Europe, a disease is considered to be rare, or orphan, when it affects fewer than 5 people in 10,000, in line with the definitions adopted by the European Committee (EC) in their Orphan

Drugs Regulation N° 141/2000 and Commission Communication COM (2008) 679/2 on RDs: Europe's challenges [1]. However, RDs are often chronic, progressive, degenerative, life-threatening and/or severely disabling in terms of a patient's quality of life, frequently leading to a lack or loss of autonomy.

Although infections, allergies, and environmental factors, linked in particular to degenerative and proliferative processes (i.e. auto-immunity or cancer), may be implicated in the onset of RDs, the vast majority, approximately 80%, is caused by genetic defects (though not all RDs are genetic diseases). The signs and symptoms of many RDs may therefore be observed at birth or during childhood, and, indeed, roughly 75% of RDs affect children, including chondrodysplasia, neurofibromatosis, osteogenesis imperfecta, proximal spinal muscular atrophy and Rett syndrome. The RDs that manifest in adulthood, on the contrary, include amyotrophic lateral sclerosis (ALS), and Charcot-Marie-Tooth, Crohn, and Huntington diseases.

Although each individual condition may fit the definition of rare, about 7000 distinct RDs have been identified so far, affecting 6–8% of the global population. In fact, it is estimated that 350 million people worldwide suffer from even rarer conditions, suggesting that one in 20 patients will be affected by an orphan disease [2]. Therefore, collectively, RDs are not at all rare, and as a whole, they generate a considerable socioeconomic burden.

In addition to there being a wide spectrum of RDs, they are also characterised by great variability in the age of onset, signs and symptoms, and patterns of tissue/organ involvement. To further complicate the issue, molecular testing and phenotype analysis reveal that mutations occurring in the same gene can be associated with different clinical diagnoses, and marked intra- and interfamilial phenotype variability has been documented. RDs are therefore often extremely difficult to diagnose, and only about 4000 genes have been identified for the 7000 RDs described in the OMIM database [3]. Understandably, therefore, the IRDiRC [4] has set its members the challenge of diagnosing most, if not all, RDs by 2020, and discovering at least 200 new therapeutic options for their patients.

Nevertheless, without early diagnosis and effective treatment strategies, it is impossible to guarantee any improvement in the quality of life and/or life expectancy of such patients. Furthermore, our lack of knowledge regarding the causes, physiopathological mechanisms, and clinical progression of RDs makes it difficult to apply available treatments and to develop novel therapeutic strategies. In addition, the small number of patients complicates the recruitment of an adequate sample for clinical trials, especially in children, which make up an even smaller percentage of the overall RD population. This is an obvious deterrent to the pharmaceutical industry, which has only limited interest in developing and marketing products for this small consumer base. In order to counter some of these problems, both national and the EU governments have made orphan drug laws and funding a priority, but, despite this recent interest, treatment options are currently only available for 5% of RDs [2].

It is not only RDs that could benefit from more activity in this area, as RD research is also considered pivotal for many common diseases, and has in some cases revealed mechanisms and pathways that have been subsequently associated with other rare or common diseases [5]. Indeed, several RDs have been linked to a high degree of genetic and phenotypic heterogeneity;

for example, mutations occurring in the LMNA gene can cause different disease types by affecting different tissues, such as (i) striated muscle (muscular dystrophy such as Emery-Dreifuss muscular dystrophy and limb-girdle muscular dystrophy or dilated cardiomyopathy), (ii) adipose tissue (lipodystrophy syndromes), (iii) peripheral nerve (peripheral neuropathy such as Charcot-Marie-Tooth disorder) or (iv) accelerated ageing (progeria diseases). There are also clinical signs that can be associated with both genetic and acquired disease. For instance, renal cell carcinoma is characterised by the dysregulation of metabolic pathways (oxygen, iron, and nutrient sensing) which are also manifestations of rare hereditary syndromes such as Von Hippel-Lindau (VHL, OMIM 193300) and Birt-Hogg-Dubé (BHD, OMIM 135150) syndromes, as well as hereditary leiomyomatosis and renal cell carcinoma (HLRCC, OMIM 150800) [5]. It is therefore essential for the research being carried out worldwide to focus on identifying characteristic determinants able to discriminate between specific disease states, stages, and probabilities of responding to particular treatments—put simply, biomarkers.

## 2. Biomarker: definition and utility

Biomarkers were first described and defined in 2001 by two different review papers [6, 7], both of which suggested that they would be the key to understanding the physiopathology of disease and discovering novel treatment strategies. The classic definition of a biomarker is 'a characteristic that is objectively measured and evaluated as an indicator of normal biological processes, pathogenic processes, or pharmacological responses to a therapeutic intervention'. In other words, biomarkers are 'measurables' that rely on tools and technologies for assessing body fluids or tissue (blood, urine, cell, skin, etc.), such as DNA analysis [point variants, copy number variation (CNV), translocations, methylation analysis], RNA analysis [expression profile and microRNA (miRNA) characterisation], protein analysis (quantification of circulating proteins), and imaging technologies, or other means of physiological measurement [8].

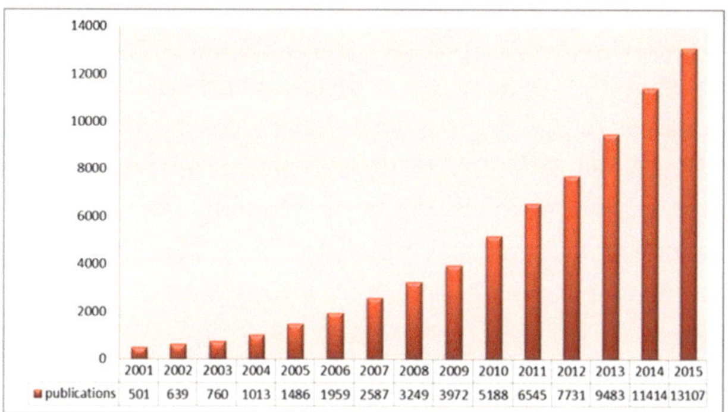


**Figure 1.** Literature survey. Number of citations in PubMed in which the keyword 'biomarker' is present in 'title' and/or 'abstract' from 2001 to 2015.

From their definition, the number of published papers related to biomarker discovery has increased more than 20-fold (**Figure 1**), and the discovery and development of novel biomarkers have kept pace with technical advances, in particular the advent of high-throughput analysis technologies. Moreover, the large number of grant projects set up over the last 5 years to fund biomarker research, including BIO-NMD [9] and NeurOmics [10], has begun to yield considerable fruits in this field.

The BIO-NMD project is a Europe-wide research network whose aim is to identify and validate biomarkers for rare neuromuscular diseases, such as dystrophinopathies (Becker muscular dystrophy, OMIM 300376; Duchenne muscular dystrophy OMIM 310200; dilated cardiomyopathy, OMIM 302045) and COL6-related myopathies (Bethlem myopathy, OMIM 158810; Ullrich congenital muscular dystrophy, OMIM 254090). Funded by the EU (2009–2012), BIO-NMD set out to investigate different human tissues/cells/fluids using multiple -omic strategies (genomics, transcriptomics, and proteomics), an approach that led to the identification of several biomarkers. Thanks to this project, both plasma and tissue biomarkers that will be useful for monitoring disease progression, prognosis, and treatment response have been described and will ultimately help to pinpoint appropriate options for personalised treatment [11, 12].

In a similar vein, the EU's NeurOmics project is still ongoing and aims to revolutionise diagnostics and develop new treatments for 10 major neuromuscular and neurodegenerative diseases by using sophisticated -omics technologies. To do this, it has brought together leading European research groups, five highly innovative SMEs, and experts from outside the EU, who are all working to identify genes and develop biomarkers for clinical application, as well as to identify drug targets and improve understanding of the physiopathology of the diseases in question.

This research activity has been largely prompted by the versatility of biomarkers. Indeed, the classical view of biomarkers as a clinical end-point, an objective snapshot that reflects how a patient feels, functions or survives, is extremely reductive. In addition to numerous applications in clinical settings, biomarkers may also serve as a surrogate end-point, a predictor of clinical benefit (or lack thereof) based on epidemiological, therapeutic, physiopathological, or other scientific evidence [13]. In other words, a biomarker may act as a clinically meaningful end-point in clinical trials. Such surrogate end-point biomarkers are foreseeably of particular benefit in RDs, in which a high percentage of diseases without a genetic cause, slow disease progression, chronic nature of the diseases, high heterogeneity of signs and symptoms within the same phenotype, and the difficulty in objectively measuring any change in symptoms dramatically increase the expense of clinical trials. Not only the cost but also the difficulty in undertaking trials based on conventional end-points severely curtails their number, and the lack of sensitive, specific, and timely outcome measures hinders the discovery and development of novel treatments.

However, a biomarker can lessen the burden of the clinical trial process by providing information about the safety and efficacy of treatments before the collection of definitive clinical data, which provides the opportunity for mid-course re-appraisal, and even interruption if the intervention being investigated is revealed as potentially harmful to participants [14]. Indeed,

http://dx.doi.org/10.5772/63354

biomarkers are far superior to subjective measurements, which may not be directly associated to a disease characteristic, or able to detect small changes, especially in the short term. Biomarkers, on the other hand, can provide an objective measurement of aspects precisely correlated to a specific disease condition, potentially enabling small changes in status to be identified, the disease progression to be assessed, and the likely effects of the therapeutic intervention to be predicted [1] while the trial is ongoing, as well as in real-world settings.

Considering the versatility of biomarkers, the European Medicines Agency (EMA) has attempted to standardise them by drawing up a list of the features of an 'ideal' biomarker, namely [15]:

- Analytical validity. Like a fingerprint, a biomarker should enable measurement, within a specific range, of a parameter able to accurately and clearly distinguish between altered/normal status or treatment response/non-response. The test(s) used to detect a biomarker should be accurate, reliable, and reproducible, and their technological limits clearly defined. As the analytical accuracy depends on laboratory procedures, such as sample preparation and technology application, these should be reported in order to ensure reproducibility of biomarker discovery and validation.

- Clinical validity. Like a mirror, a biomarker should accurately reflect the features of a disease (or treatment), detecting even small changes, and not be influenced by circumstantial factors such as diet, exercise, stress, age, sex, or the environment, i.e. an alteration in the disease features should always be reflected by the biomarker, and a difference in the biomarker should always reflect a change in the disease. In other words, an ideal biomarker will identify *specific* disease parameters and be *sensitive* to any change in them. Likewise, to be clinically valid, a biomarker must display a high degree of *accuracy* (indicating correctly whether a patient has or does not have the disease or treatment effects in the vast majority of cases).

- Clinical utility. Like a prophet, a biomarker should herald the outcome of a given situation/intervention. In other words, biomarkers should predict the members of a population who will develop a disease, manifest a disease progression, or respond to a specific treatment. The clinical utility of a biomarker in an appropriate population can be measured by two predictive values, the PPV and NPV, which are respectively used to quantify the probability that a person with a positive test for that biomarker will manifest the outcome predicted by the test, and the probability that a person with negative test will not respond to the intervention/treatment.

- Non-invasiveness. Like an open door, a biomarker should grant *accessibility*, i.e. enable an early, sensitive measurement, of disease severity etc., via the simple collection of body fluids (urine/blood) or scanned images (e.g. MRI or PET, etc.). This will allow a disorder to be monitored at different time points, without recourse to invasive procedures such as biopsies or tissue analysis.

- Feasibility. Like the passage of time, a biomarker should be practical to identify and measure, as well as invariable, irrespective of the type of sample collection, processing procedures, or methods used in its detection.

- Time and cost-effectiveness. Like a moneybox, a biomarker should be quick and easy to use and not be so expensive and time-consuming to measure that it cannot be used as a surrogate endpoint in clinical trials or to aid diagnostics and disease monitoring.

Biomarkers that possess all these features will inevitably lead to improvements in clinical trials, especially in the field of personalised medicine. Personalised medicine shifts the current 'one-size-fits-all' approach to a more individual line of attack or defence, centred on giving 'the right drug to the right patients at the right time' [16]. This is particularly crucial in RDs, in which successful treatment development is generally hindered by the small number of patients and short runs that characterise trials for novel interventions.

## 3. Strategies for biomarker discovery

In recent years, novel techniques and strategies have emerged for biomarker discovery, and there are currently two major approaches being applied:

- **Candidate approach**. This is a hypothesis-driven method based on knowledge of the relevant physiopathological processes, disease pathway(s), or key molecule(s). It analyses the known gene/protein and their linking products in order to discover a qualitative or quantitative variation in diseased samples (fluids, cells, tissues) with respect to normal ones.

- **High-throughput approach**. This is a hypothesis-free strategy that takes advantage of the development of novel techniques for generating very large amounts of data to compare pathological and normal status. This 'big-data' approach is extremely powerful, although it is cost-intensive and requires significant time for validation and clinical definition of the biomarkers identified.

### 3.1. Discovery of genetic variations

Next-generation sequencing (NGS) techniques are based on high-throughput genomic and transcriptomic sequencing. In brief, target regions can be isolated from the entire genome by hybridisation to complementary sequences. This 'capturing' is performed on demand, to isolate sequences that may consist of protein-coding regions only (whole exome sequencing), a specifically targeted gene region (focusing on a limited number of known genes), or the entire genome (whole-genome sequencing). The captured region can then be sequenced by one of several methods (pyrosequencing, 454 Roche; sequencing by reversible termination, Illumina; sequencing by ligation, Solid; semiconductor sequencing, Ion Torrent), and the resulting output is composed of several sequence reads, which are then computationally aligned to the known genome in order to unravel any variations, such as small insertions or deletions [17]. Unlike traditional Sanger sequencing, which reads a sequence base by base, NGS is very time-efficient, enabling the simultaneous analysis of millions of base pairs organised in multiple aligned reads. Despite its efficiency, however, NGS is unable to detect dynamic mutations (e.g. triplet expansions) and still has limited capability to identify CNVs. Nevertheless, while we await the development of specific algorithms to overcome these limitations, NGS can be integrated with DNA profiling tools, such as array-CGH, for the detection of CNVs and other genetic imbalances.

The methylation profile of genes can also be explored via epigenomics. In fact, the recent advent of methylomic profiling now allows us to determine the DNA methylation status of the entire genome, and thereby to identify an increasing number of genes that are methylated in disease states, particularly cancer [18].

### 3.2. Discovery of RNA variations

Complementary genome-wide information technologies can be used to identify qualitative and quantitative variations at the RNA level. For example, a gene expression microarray or high-throughput technology such as RNA sequencing (RNAseq) can be used to perform transcriptome analysis. Transcriptome profiling can be performed on samples from biopsy or cell cultures from specific affected tissues, or, less invasively, from different body fluids such as urine, blood, or saliva [1]. The technique enables the generation of enriched RNA/cDNA libraries that cover the entire transcribed region, or, alternatively, a catalogue of genes of interest that can be used to evaluate gene expression or identify novel transcripts, alternative splicing, and/or gene fusion products.

Although transcript sequencing is heavily influenced by the tissue/cell type analysed, transcription and RNA editing being profoundly tissue specific, it is highly versatile. Indeed, in addition to mRNAs, transcriptomics can be extended to non-coding RNAs such as miRNA—single-strand sequences of 18–25 nucleotides regulating the expression of target genes already known for their role as biomarkers.

Gene expression profiling is also considered a very powerful method of identifying biomarkers of pathological status, disease progression, and/or drug response, with the advantage of exploring specific tissue behaviour [19]. Microarray technologies may be used to quantify and compare the DNA levels/configurations of many transcripts in diseased and healthy samples, or at different time points (e.g. pre- and post-treatment).

### 3.3. Discovery of protein biomarkers

The evolution of mass spectrometry (MS)-based technologies and the development of other proteomic strategies such as two-dimensional gel electrophoresis (2D-DIGE) have considerably advanced our understanding of the nature of the proteome. This can be analysed to explore specific cellular functions and the control of specific biological processes, although the complexity and size of the human proteome pose larger challenges than those encountered in genomic and transcriptomic research [20]. Indeed, the individual proteome can change markedly over the course of a lifetime, and a single gene often produces very different isoforms, by alternative splicing or post-translational modifications such as phosphorylation, glycosylation, acetylation, and ubiquitination. However, proteins are often a target for pharmacological intervention, and proteomic technologies able to evaluate the expression level of soluble proteins are emerging, thereby paving the way to the discovery and validation of protein biomarkers.

The most common novel high-throughput approaches currently being used in discovery proteomics are those based on MS. These technologies enable the analysis of complex mixtures of proteins, measuring the mass-to-charge ratio of charged particles in order to determine their mass, quantity, and elemental composition. There are essentially two different types of MS approaches, namely top-down experiments, which analyse the whole protein, and bottom-up, which analyse proteins previously digested by proteases. For characterisation purposes, the resulting peptide mixtures may then be separated using different strategies, such as liquid chromatography (LC), gas chromatography, or ion mobility spectrometry, and then the identified proteins can be quantified. To achieve this, samples can be isotopically labelled by different methods, such as stable isotope labelling by amino acids (SILAC), isotype-coded affinity tagging (ICAT), isobaric tags for relative and absolute quantification (iTRAQ), and mass tags for relative and absolute quantification (mTRAQ) [21]. A typical MS protocol would therefore consist of sample loading (of intact or digested protein), vaporisation, ionisation, and separation of the ionised sample by mass-to-charge ratio, detection in an MS instrument, and generation of a detailed profile of the exact chemical composition of a sample.

By these means, it is possible to differentially analyse proteins from different biological processes or disease states in order to discover candidate biomarkers. Many biomarkers used in existing clinical practice are assays to quantify proteins, and proteomics techniques such as 2D-DIGE can be used to separate non-digested proteins within a biological sample based upon either apparent molecular mass (by gel electrophoresis) or charge (via isoelectric focusing). Such strategies thereby provide a measure of protein abundance and enable the identification of isoforms and post-translational modifications [21]. Validation of such potential biomarkers can be performed using a common protein expression method such as Western blotting and/or antibody-based assays.

As shown in the workflow illustrated in **Figure 2**, biomarker discovery can be facilitated by using a strategy combining two or more of the above approaches, for example

- **High-throughput/candidate approach**. This strategy exploits the benefits of both the techniques by filtering the high-throughput data beforehand using a candidate list or a functional interactome map. This provides better applicability to the disease/treatment response but, considering the large amount of data generated by the high-throughput method, is very labour-intensive.

- **Multiple -omics approach**. This is a highly demanding method based on the simultaneous use of genomics, transcriptomics, proteomics, etc., to analyse the interactome and define interactome and functional pathways. If performed on the same individual at different times, or disease or treatment stage, such analyses are able to monitor changes in an individual's -omic profile, thereby lending themselves to the development of personalised medicine strategies.

The benefit of multiple -omics approaches has been clearly demonstrated by Finkel et al., in their recent 'BforSMA' cross-sectional study aimed at identifying novel biomarkers in spinal muscular atrophy (SMA, OMIM: 253300). SMA is a neuro-degenerative motor neuron disorder caused by homozygous/compound heterozygous mutations in the motor neuron 1 (SMN1) gene [22]. It is characterised by the degeneration of the anterior horn cells of the spinal cord and leads to symmetrical muscle weakness and atrophy. The SMN protein plays a crucial role in RNA biosynthesis in all tissues, forming a large, multiprotein complex that drives the assembly of small nuclear ribonucleoproteins (snRNPs) of the spliceosomes. Through functions in RNP assembly, the SMN complex is required for the expression of essentially all protein-coding genes [23]. Preliminary results from the 'BforSMA' project—based on proteomics, metabolomics, and transcriptomics discovery platforms—indicate the discovery of a total of 200 candidate biomarkers, including 97 plasma proteins, 59 plasma metabolites, and 44 urine metabolites that could potentially be used to address clinical trial design and identify novel therapeutic targets in SMA [22].

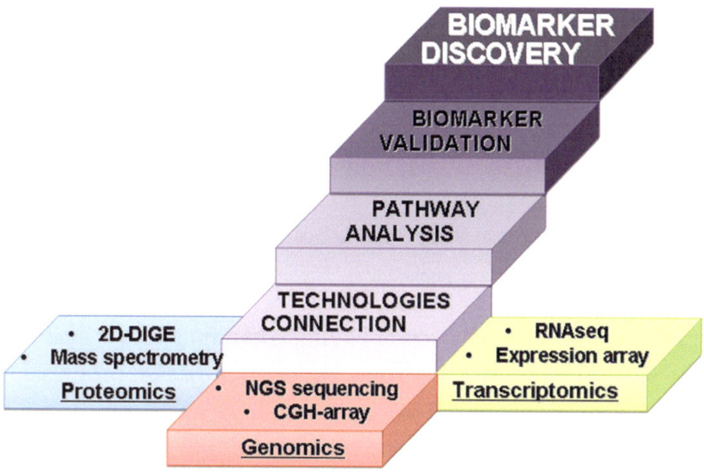


**Figure 2.** Flowchart of biomarker discovery. Different technologies from genomic, transcriptomic, and proteomic levels are able to detect potential biomarkers; subsequently the connection between the three approaches and validation may confirm the biomarker identification.

## 4. Molecular biomarkers

### 4.1. Genomic biomarkers

New molecular biomarkers could be detected at different levels. According to the Food and Drug Administration/EMA definition, genomic biomarkers include both DNA and RNA determinants, and genomic biomarkers therefore include DNA methylation status and sequence variations, such as single-nucleotide polymorphisms (SNPs), insertions, deletions, translocations, CNV, as well as RNA alterations such as differential gene expression and miRNAs (**Figure 3**). The current research focus has shifted somewhat, from SNP to haplotype analysis, which it is hoped will furnish useful disease, prognostic, or predictive biomarkers.

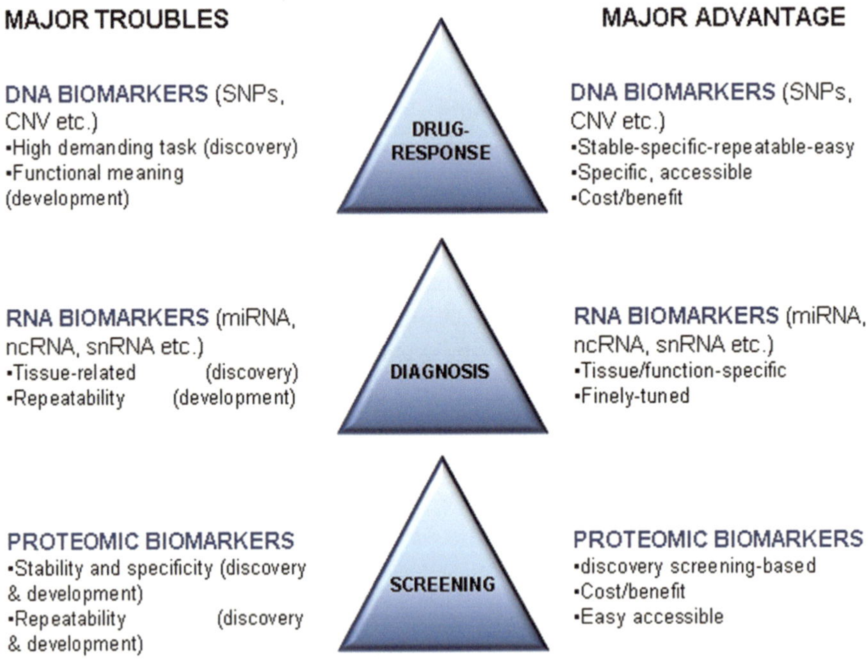


**Figure 3.** Schematic representation of the main features (applications, troubles, and advantages) of biomarker types, in terms of stability, specificity, repeatability, and accessibility.

Indeed, DMD patients, for example, despite having common features such as the absence of dystrophin in the striated muscles, show different rates of disease progression, especially in terms of the age of loss of ambulation. This supports the idea that genetic modifiers exist and can influence both the phenotype and the clinical severity of the disease. To this end, Flanigan et al. identified SNPs located within the LTBP4 gene, which encodes for the latent transforming growth factor (TGF) b binding protein (LTBP), in more than 200 patients, showing that individuals homozygous for the IAAM LTBP4 haplotype remained ambulatory significantly longer than those heterozygous or homozygous for the VTTT haplotype [24]. Furthermore, in long QT syndrome (LQTS)—a rare hereditary cardiac disorder characterised by a prolongation of the QT interval due to mutations in genes encoding ion channels responsible for the generation of electrical impulses—it appears that the haplotype group C-G-T of the heat shock protein HSP-70 gene is strongly related to the disease condition and may therefore represent a diagnostic biomarker [25].

An example of potential RNA biomarkers has been provided in a study by Harten et al. into Hutchinson-Gilford progeria syndrome (HGPS, OMIM: 176670). This is a rare, fatal, autosomal dominant premature-aging disease (prevalence: <1/1,000,000) caused by splicing mutations in the LMNA gene that creates cryptic splice sites and leads to the production of progerin, a toxic, permanently farnesylated splicing variant [26]. In their study, the authors analysed the expression profile of several matrix metalloproteinases, identifying a donor-age-dependent reduction in the expression of MMP-3 mRNA in HGPS primary dermal fibroblast cultures, suggesting that a fall in MMP-3 correlates with disease severity in vivo [26].

RNAseq can be used in conjunction with new technologies such as NGS to analyse the whole transcriptome both quantitatively and qualitatively and thereby provide information about alterations in gene expression. This approach can potentially speed up the process of genomic biomarker discovery and was used to good effect in a recent study aimed at tracing a detailed RNA profile in both collagen VI myopathy (ColVI) patients and an animal model of the same. Collagen VI myopathies are genetic disorders arising from mutations in the collagen VI genes; they range from the severe Ullrich congenital muscular dystrophy (UCMD, OMIM: 254090, prevalence: 1–9/1,000,000) to the milder Bethlem myopathy (BTHLM1, OMIM: 158810, prevalence: <1/1,000,000), which can both be inherited via both dominant and recessive models. Generally speaking, neither the type of mutation nor the effect of the mutation on the protein structure/function allows precise discrimination between two phenotypes. However, by a combined RNAseq approach, the authors identified the potential involvement of circadian genes, reporting a marked deregulation of the CLOCK gene in UCMD patients alone, suggesting it as a candidate biomarker of disease severity in ColVI [27].

miRNAs also make quite appealing biomarkers, and a recent study by Eisenberg et al. found that the levels of muscle-specific miRNAs (myomirs) are correlated with disease severity in several muscular dystrophies, including limb girdle and Duchenne/Becker muscular dystrophies [28]. miRNA studies have also been extended to other RDs, such as cystic fibrosis (CF, OMIM: 219700). This is a recessive genetic disorder (prevalence: 1–9/100,000) characterised by eccrine gland dysfunction, chronic obstructive lung disease, and exocrine pancreatic dysfunction. It is caused by mutations in the cystic fibrosis conductance regulator gene (CFTR), and it appears that miR-494 and miR-145 are significantly over-expressed in CF tissues with respect to those of healthy individuals, suggesting their role as disease biomarkers [29].

As mentioned above, genomic biomarkers also include epigenomics modifications such as DNA methylation. Recent studies on Friedreich ataxia (FRDA, OMIM 229300), the most common ataxia, which is caused by an expanded GAA repeat in the first intron of FXN, have demonstrated that hypermethylation of the gene region upstream of the expanded GAA repeat correlates with clinical severity, while hypomethylation of the downstream region correlates with the age at onset [30]. It is evident, therefore, that genomic biomarkers may have a wide spectrum of functions as clinical and research outcome measures.

### 4.2. Proteomic biomarkers

Proteomic studies have several advantages over genomic analysis, not least the potential identification of biomarkers more closely related to biological function/dysfunction. Furthermore, proteomic biomarkers are more readily accessible than genomic biomarkers, being detectable in body fluids such as blood and urine (**Figure 3**). This makes them potentially useful in clinical trials as early indicators of the disease condition, disease progression, or treatment effects (drug response or adverse effects).

As an example, Martell et al. have provided a clear indication of biomarker accessibility and utility in Morquio A syndrome, also named mucopolysaccharidosis IVA (MPS, OMIM: 253000, prevalence: 1–9/1,000,000). This recessive lysosomal storage disorder is caused by a mutation in N-acetylgalactosamine-6-sulfatase gene (GALNS), which codes for keratan sulphate and chondroitin-6-sulphate. The mutation results in a wide spectrum of clinical features involving skeletal, cardiac, pulmonary, corneal, and hearing impairment, and the identification of biomarkers able to monitor the response to enzyme replacement therapy during clinical trials is long past due. To this end, the authors measured the plasma levels of 88 candidate proteins, finding that three of them (alpha-1-antitrypsin, lipoprotein a, and serum amyloid P) may be suitable surrogate end-points for clinical trials [31].

The main advantage of techniques that can assess biomarkers in body fluids is, of course, their lack of invasiveness. In this regard, a new protein technology, the SOMA scan assay—an aptamer-based method able to recognise specific protein epitopes—has been used to evaluate protein levels in the sera of DMD patients. By using this technology to compare serum samples from two independent DMD cohorts with healthy individuals, 44 serum biomarkers were identified [32]. Similarly, Auray-Blais et al. have recently applied novel MS-based high-throughput technologies to protein biomarker discovery in the urine samples of patients affected by Fabry disease, succeeding in identifying the lyso-Gb3/related analogue profile as a diagnostic biomarker [33].

Low invasiveness is also a feature of the most commonly used method of measuring and validating protein biomarkers, the immunoassay. Immunoassays are based on the ability of monoclonal antibodies to capture and detect specific protein domains and enable the simultaneous investigation of several proteins using very low amounts of samples. For example, in idiopathic pulmonary fibrosis (IPF, OMIM 178500), a rare lethal lung disease (prevalence: 1–5/10,000) of unknown aetiology and variable and unpredictable course, a multiplexed assay has been used to simultaneously evaluate 92 proteins in plasma samples from more than 200 patients. By these means, three biomarkers predictive of IPF outcome were identified [34]. Other studies have used the ELISA immunoassay to evaluate serum levels of an extracellular matrix glycoprotein, tenascin-C (TN-C), in Emery-Dreifuss muscular dystrophy (EMD, OMIM 310300), a rare neuromuscular disorder (1–9/1,000,000) characterised by muscular weakness and atrophy, with early joint contractures and cardiomyopathy, finding an association between elevated circulating TN-C levels and an increased risk of developing dilated cardiomyopathy [35].

Due to the low invasiveness of the methods involved, proteomic biomarkers are also very appealing as surrogate end-points in clinical trials and/or screening (e.g. neonatal testing).

### 4.3. Other biomarkers

As mentioned earlier, imaging technologies, and indeed any diagnostic test that is able to measure the disease status in patients, are useful for measuring, and therefore for investigating certain biomarkers. Magnetic resonance imaging (MRI), for example, is a safe and non-invasive method of analysing muscle, connective tissue, fat, and bone. Indeed, Kinali and co-workers have demonstrated that the MRI scan, focused on particular muscles, can serve as a biomarker

http://dx.doi.org/10.5772/63354

for disease progression in Duchenne muscular dystrophy (DMD, OMIM: 310200), a rare neuromuscular disease (affecting 1/3300 male births) characterised by rapidly progressive muscle weakness and wasting due to degeneration of skeletal, smooth, and cardiac muscles. MRI can be used to accurately identify which type of muscles is sufficiently preserved in DMD, making it a reliable tool for use in clinical trials. Similarly, MRI scans of muscle biopsies are currently being used to correlate the clinical features of muscle diseases with the structure and morphology of muscle fibres [36].

Neurophysiological measurements can also be exploited as imaging biomarkers. For instance, Vucic and colleagues have reported that transcranial magnetic stimulation (TMS) is a useful and non-invasive method of assessing the functional integrity of the motor cortex and its corticomotoneuronal projections in ALS. Despite their similarities, TMS was able to reliably distinguish between ALS and similar peripheral disorders, thereby demonstrating its potential diagnostic utility [37].

In fact, imaging biomarkers are generally considered very appealing, generating a large amount of intensive research in recent years. The ultimate aim of such research is the development of innovative methods of using imaging tools for the detection and monitoring of the signs and symptoms of RDs.

## 5. Applications and clinical translation of biomarkers

### 5.1. Diagnostic/prognostic biomarkers

A diagnostic, or prognostic, biomarker is one that identifies a disease or quantifies its pathogenic factors (**Figure 4**). Essentially, they are signatures that divide the population into healthy and diseased individuals, but in some cases they can finely stratify the disease phenotype into different degrees of severity or sub-phenotypes. The routine diagnostic markers classically used in clinical practice are temperature, blood pressure, and cholesterol levels, among others, whereas in genetic diseases, according to the IRDiRC statement [4], all gene mutations known to cause a Mendelian disease have to be considered their primary genetic biomarkers. For example, DMD, the most common fatal genetic disorder diagnosed during early childhood, arises through mutations in the causative dystrophin (*DMD*) gene, which are therefore considered disease biomarkers, and can accordingly be used to select patients for enrolment in clinical trials [38].

In some cases, mutations in causative genes can be considered biomarkers of disease severity. This is the case in fragile X syndrome (FXS, OMIM: 300624), a rare intellectual disability disorder with an estimated prevalence about 1 in 2500 to 5000 men and 1 in 4000 to 6000 women. FXS is caused by an expanded CGG triple-repeat located within the 5' UTR of the FMR1 gene. The triplet expansion variability defines four different phenotypes, ranging from healthy to a severe phenotype, and can therefore be used to distinguish between them [39].

In ALS (OMIM 105400), the situation is less clear cut. ALS is a devastating neurodegenerative disease with an incidence of 1/50,000 per year. Although several mutated genes have been identified in ALS (DCTN1, OMIM 601143; PRPH, OMIM 170710; SOD1 OMIM 147450; NEFH OMIM 162230), the vast majority of patients do not show a defined genetic defect. This would seem to indicate that the causative gene is still missing [40], and research in this area has therefore focused on the discovery of specific biomarkers able to assist clinical diagnosis and monitor the disease progression. In this regard, Hwang et al. have correlated an increased level of HMGB1, non-histone architectural protein, in serum samples with the onset of ALS, even in early stages of the disease. This increased level of HMGB1 could also be useful as a severity biomarker, since they also found higher HMGB1 levels in patients with a severe disease status [41]. Moreover, the same group has recently correlated a reduction in the protein level of LG72 gene, activator of D-amino acid oxidase, to the pathogenesis of ALS [42].

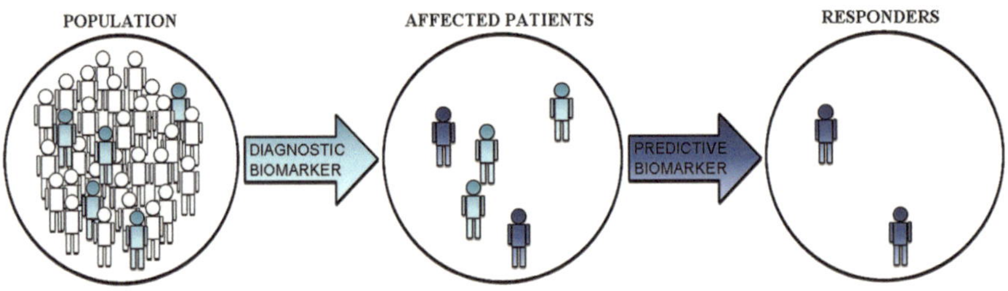


**Figure 4.** Schematic representation of biomarker application. Biomarker may identify, within a population, the individuals affected by a specific disease and then select patients able to respond to treatment/intervention.

Another example of a diagnostic biomarker has been found in Alexander disease (ALXDRD, OMIM: 203450), a very rare neurodegenerative disorder (incidence of 1/2.7 million per year) characterised by varying degrees of macrocephaly, spasticity, ataxia, and seizures. It ultimately leads to psychomotor regression and death, and causative mutations have been identified in Glial Fibrillary Acidic Protein (GFAP), the major intermediate filament protein of astrocytes, which result in toxic accumulation of the protein. Animal model studies have demonstrated that transactivation of the GFAP promoter is an early indicator of the disease process, and that GFAP level in the CSF could be a potential biomarker in human patients [43].

Biomarkers used in clinical practice to improve disease progression monitoring or disease-risk prediction are defined as prognostic. Simply put, a prognostic biomarker provides information on the course of a disease in an untreated individual, and an example has been identified for Marfan syndrome (MFS, OMIM: 154700), a systemic disease of the connective tissue characterised by a wide spectrum of cardiovascular, skeletal muscular, ophthalmic, and pulmonary manifestations. With an estimated prevalence of around 1/5000, patients affected by MFS suffer from an increased risk of cardiovascular complications that lead to premature death, and a correlation has been demonstrated between the larger aortic root diameters, coupled to a faster aortic root growth, and high serum levels of transforming growth factor-β (TGF-β). Increasing levels of TGF-β predict cardiovascular events and thereby possesses significant prognostic value [44].

Another biomarker for cardiac muscular involvement has been found in Fabry disease (FD, OMIM: 301500), a rare systematic disease (prevalence 1–5/10 000) characterised by the

http://dx.doi.org/10.5772/63354

accumulation of globotriaosylceramide in the plasma and cellular lysosomes of vessels, nerves, tissues, and organs throughout the body. This accumulation leads to progressive skin lesions, renal failure, cardiac and cerebrovascular involvement, and peripheral neuropathy. Continuously elevated cardiac troponin I (cTNI), a laboratory parameter well known to reflect acute and chronic cardiac muscle damage, has been demonstrated in a substantial proportion of patients with FD, suggesting that raised cTNI levels could be a useful laboratory marker for assessing myocardial damage in FD [45].

Finally, a recent study on DMD has indicated the matrix metalloproteinase-9 (MMP-9) as both a diagnostic and prognostic biomarker. Indeed, DMD patients showed a higher serum level of MMP-9 protein and tissue inhibitors of metalloproteinase-1 (TIMP-1) proteins with respect to controls, with MMP-9 levels being even higher in older, non-ambulant patients than in ambulant patients [46].

### 5.2. Predictive/therapeutic biomarker

Considering the heterogeneous nature of RDs, not all patients are expected to benefit from a newly available treatment. Hence the identification of a sub-group of patients likely to respond to a novel treatment is important both in terms of health, and in terms of cost-effectiveness [12]. To this end, a predictive, or therapeutic, marker must be able to discriminate between drug responders (patients gaining benefit from the therapy) and poor/low responders (**Figure 4**). Predictive biomarkers will therefore enable the most appropriate and efficacious treatments or interventions to be selected for each patient, thereby underpinning a personalised approach to treatment.

There are a few examples of therapeutic biomarkers useful in RDs, generally SNPs, as in typical pharmacogenetics, although some protein studies have also been reported. For instance, a pharmacological predictive biomarker has been reported in idiopathic nephrotic syndrome, a RD affecting the kidneys. Specifically, Wen et al. [47] found a significant difference in the serum proteome of steroid-sensitive nephrotic syndrome (SSNS) and steroid-resistant nephrotic syndrome (SRNS, OMIM 256370) patients, predictive of their respective responses to treatment.

Another example of a predictive biomarker has been found for Gaucher disease (GD, OMIM: 230800), a rare recessive genetic disorder (approximate prevalence 1/100,000) caused by mutations in the GBA gene, which codes for a lysosomal enzyme, glucocerebrosidase. Although the clinical manifestations of this disease are extremely variable, ranging from non-neurological manifestations such as organomegaly, bone anomalies, and cytopenia to acute neurological forms, a recent time-course analysis of ferritin, chitotriosidase, haemoglobin, and platelets showed that the levels of these biomarkers undergo variation during the course of enzyme replacement therapy [48].

Sometimes the same biomarker can be useful in multiple scenarios and, for example TGF-c, in addition to serving a prognostic function in Marfan syndrome, could feasibly be used as a therapeutic biomarker in the same condition. Indeed, in a recent study, patients who responded to losartan used to reduce the aortic root dilatation rate, had higher baseline TGF-β levels but exhibited lower plasma TGF-β concentrations during losartan therapy [49].

Predictive biomarkers such as these are likely to play an increasingly important role in clinical practice, since evaluating the efficacy of a treatment/intervention is fundamental to making decisions about treatment choices, and therefore determining therapy outcomes.

## 6. Conclusions

Since the definition of biomarkers in 2001, their importance in clinical and research settings has increased dramatically due to their diagnostic/prognostic functions and their ability to monitor/predict disease stage, treatment response, and/or adverse effects. Indeed, the creation of an exhaustive catalogue of approved biomarkers may be the single most important innovation in healthcare, bringing considerable clinical and economic benefits. Although current research, both academic and corporate, is heavily focused on the development of drugs and companion diagnostic tests, in the future, biomarker discovery and development will be vital for tailoring medical care to individual patients. This will be especially important in the field of RDs, in which the discovery of efficacious biomarkers is likely to greatly facilitate the process of EMA approval and development of novel orphan drugs. In addition to being both and time and cost-effective, biomarker research also provides exciting opportunities to expand our knowledge of the physiopathological mechanisms behind rare and other diseases, helping to discriminate between distinct disease presentations and comorbidities, as well as predict the different impacts of concomitant medication, and various important demographic parameters such as gender, age, and ethnicity. In short, biomarker discovery represents a giant leap towards the ultimate goal of truly personalised medicine.

## Acknowledgements

The BIO-NMD (http://www.bio-nmd.eu/) (European Union FP7 #241665) and Neuromics (European Union FP7 #305121) projects are acknowledged.

## Author details

Chiara Scotton and Alessandra Ferlini*

*Address all correspondence to: fla@unife.it

Medical Genetics Unit, Department of Medical Sciences, University of Ferrara, Ferrara, Italy

## References

[1] Ferlini A, Scotton C, Novelli G. Biomarkers in rare diseases. Public Health Genomics. 2013;16:313–321. DOI: 10.1159/000355938

[2] 2005–2015: a decade of innovation in rare diseases. Available from: http://www.phrma.org/reportscharts/2005-2015-Decade-of-Innovation-In-Rare-Diseases [Accessed: 2016-02-28].

[3] OMIM database. Available from: http://www.ncbi.nlm.nih.gov/omim [Accessed: 2016-02-28].

[4] International Rare Diseases Research Consortium. Available from: http://www.irdirc.org/ [Accessed: 2016-28].

[5] Roubertoux PL, de Vries PJ. From molecules to behavior: lessons from the study of rare genetic disorders. Behav Genet. 2011;41:341–348. DOI: 10.1007/s10519-011-9469-y

[6] Lesko LJ, Atkinson AJ Jr. Use of biomarkers and surrogate endpoints in drug development and regulatory decision making: criteria, validation, strategies. Annu Rev Pharmacol Toxicol. 2001;41:347–366.

[7] Biomarkers Definitions Working Group. Biomarkers and surrogate endpoints: preferred definitions and conceptual framework. Clin Pharmacol Ther. 2001;69:89–95.

[8] Jain K. The handbook of biomarkers. New York: Springer, 2010. ISBN 978-1-60761-684-9.

[9] BIO-NMD European Project. Available from: http://www.bio-nmd.eu [Accessed: 2016-02-28].

[10] NeurOmics European Project. Available from: http://rd-neuromics.eu [Accessed: 2016-02-28].

[11] Kotelnikova E, Shkrob MA, Pyatnitskiy MA, Ferlini A, Daraselia N. Novel approach to meta-analysis of microarray datasets reveals muscle remodeling-related drug targets and biomarkers in Duchenne muscular dystrophy. PLoS Comput Biol. 2012;8:e1002365. DOI: 10.1371/journal.pcbi.1002365

[12] Scotton C, Passarelli C, Neri M, Ferlini A. Biomarkers in rare neuromuscular diseases. Exp Cell Res. 2014;325:44–49. DOI: 10.1016/j.yexcr.2013.12.020

[13] Salter H, Holland R. Biomarkers: refining diagnosis and expediting drug development – reality, aspiration and the role of open innovation. J Intern Med. 2014;276:215–228. DOI: 10.1111/joim.12234

[14] Strimbu K, Tavel JA. What are biomarkers? Curr Opin HIV AIDS. 2010;5:463–466. DOI: 10.1097/COH.0b013e32833ed177

[15] EMA. (2011) Committee for Medicinal Products for Human Use (CHMP): Reflection paper on methodological issues associated with pharmacogenomic biomarkers in

relation to clinical development and patient selection. (Draft) EMA/446337/2011. Available from: http://www.ema.europa.eu/docs/en_GB/document_library/Scientific_guideline/2011/07/WC500108672.pdf [Accessed: 2016-02-28].

[16] Poste G, Compton CC, Barker AD. The national biomarker development alliance: confronting the poor productivity of biomarker research and development. Expert Rev Mol Diagn. 2015;15:211–218. DOI: 10.1586/14737159.2015.974561

[17] Ku CS, Cooper DN, Polychronakos C, Naidoo N, Wu M, Soong R. Exome sequencing: dual role as a discovery and diagnostic tool. Ann Neurol. 2012;71:5–14. DOI: 10.1002/ana.22647

[18] Wang K, Huang C, Nice EC. Proteomics, genomics and transcriptomics: their emerging roles in the discovery and validation of colorectal cancer biomarkers. Expert Rev Proteomics. 2014;11:179–205. DOI: 10.1586/14789450.2014.894466

[19] Caberlotto L, Lauria M. Systems biology meets -omic technologies: novel approaches to biomarker discovery and companion diagnostic development. Expert Rev Mol Diagn. 2015;15:255–265. DOI: 10.1586/14737159.2015.975214

[20] Mallick P, Kuster B. Proteomics: a pragmatic perspective. Nat Biotechnol. 2010;28:695–709. DOI: 10.1038/nbt.1658

[21] Becnel LB, McKenna NJ. Minireview: progress and challenges in proteomics data management, sharing, and integration. Mol Endocrinol. 2012;26:1660–1674

[22] Finkel RS, Crawford TO, Swoboda KJ, Kaufmann P, Juhasz P, Li X, Guo Y, Li RH, Trachtenberg F, Forrest SJ, Kobayashi DT, Chen KS, Joyce CL, Plasterer T, Pilot Study of Biomarkers for Spinal Muscular Atrophy Trial Group. Candidate proteins, metabolites and transcripts in the Biomarkers for Spinal Muscular Atrophy (BforSMA) clinical study. PLoS One. 2012;7:e35462. DOI: 10.1371/journal.pone.0035462

[23] Li DK, Tisdale S, Lotti F, Pellizzoni L. SMN control of RNP assembly: from post-transcriptional gene regulation to motor neuron disease. Semin Cell Dev Biol. 2014;32:22–9. DOI: 10.1016/j.semcdb.2014.04.026

[24] Flanigan KM, Ceco E, Lamar KM, Kaminoh Y, Dunn DM, Mendell JR, King WM, Pestronk A, Florence JM, Mathews KD, Finkel RS, Swoboda KJ, Gappmaier E, Howard MT, Day JW, McDonald C, McNally EM, Weiss RB; United Dystrophinopathy Project. LTBP4 genotype predicts age of ambulatory loss in Duchenne muscular dystrophy. Ann Neurol. 2013;73:481–8. DOI: 10.1002/ana.23819

[25] Ali A, Qureshi SF, Medikare V, Venkateshwari A, Calambur N, Rao H, Jayakrishnan MP, Shenthar J, Thangaraj K, Nallari P. Heat shock protein 70 gene polymorphisms' influence on the electrophysiology of long QT syndrome. J Interv Card Electrophysiol. 2016;45:119–130.

[26] Harten IA, Zahr RS, Lemire JM, Machan JT, Moses MA, Doiron RJ, Curatolo AS, Rothman FG, Wight TN, Toole BP, Gordon LB. Age-dependent loss of MMP-3 in

Hutchinson-Gilford progeria syndrome. J Gerontol A Biol Sci Med Sci. 2011;66:1201–1207. DOI: 10.1093/gerona/glr137

[27] Scotton C, Bovolenta M, Schwartzb E, Martoni E, Falzarano MS, Passarelli C, Armaroli A, Osman H, Rodolico C, Messina S, Pegoraro E, D'Amico A, Bertini E, Gualandi F, Neri M, Selvatici R, Boffi P, Maioli MA, Lochmüller H, Straub V, Bushby K, Castrignanò T, Pesole G, Sabatelli P, Merlini L, Braghetta P, Bonaldo P, Bernardi P, Foley R, Cirak S, Zaharieva I, Muntoni F, Capitanio D, Gelfi C, Kotelnikova E, Yuryev A, Lebowitz M, Zhang X, Hodge B, Esser KA, Ferlini A. Deep RNA profiling identified Clock and molecular clock genes as pathophysiological signatures in collagen VI myopathy. J Cell Sci. 2016;129:1671–1684. DOI: 10.1242/jcs.175927.

[28] Eisenberg I, Alexander MS, Kunkel LM. miRNAs in normal and diseased skeletal muscle. J Cell Mol Med. 2009;13:2–11. DOI: 10.1111/j.1582-4934.2008.00524.x

[29] Megiorni F, Cialfi S, Cimino G, De Biase RV, Dominici C, Quattrucci S, Pizzuti A. Elevated levels of miR-145 correlate with SMAD3 down-regulation in cystic fibrosis patients. J Cyst Fibros. 2013;12:797–802. DOI: 10.1016/j.jcf.2013.03.007

[30] Evans-Galea MV, Carrodus N, Rowley SM, Corben LA, Tai G, Saffery R, Galati JC, Wong NC, Craig JM, Lynch DR, Regner SR, Brocht AF, Perlman SL, Bushara KO, Gomez CM, Wilmot GR, Li L, Varley E, Delatycki MB, Sarsero JP. FXN methylation predicts expression and clinical outcome in Friedreich ataxia. Ann Neurol. 2012;71:487–497. DOI: 10.1002/ana.22671

[31] Martell L, Lau K, Mei M, Burnett V, Decker C, Foehr ED. Biomarker analysis of Morquio syndrome: identification of disease state and drug responsive markers. Orphanet J Rare Dis. 2011;6:84. DOI: 10.1186/1750-1172-6-84

[32] Hathout Y, Brody E, Clemens PR, Cripe L, DeLisle RK, Furlong P, Gordish-Dressman H, Hache L, Henricson E, Hoffman EP, Kobayashi YM, Lorts A, Mah JK, McDonald C, Mehler B, Nelson S, Nikrad M, Singer B, Steele F, Sterling D, Sweeney HL, Williams S, Gold L. Large-scale serum protein biomarker discovery in Duchenne muscular dystrophy. Proc Natl Acad Sci U S A. 2015;112:7153–7158. DOI: 10.1073/pnas.1507719112

[33] Auray-Blais C, Blais CM, Ramaswami U, Boutin M, Germain DP, Dyack S, Bodamer O, Pintos-Morell G, Clarke JT, Bichet DG, Warnock DG, Echevarria L, West ML, Lavoie P. Urinary biomarker investigation in children with Fabry disease using tandem mass spectrometry. Clin Chim Acta. 2015;438:195–204. DOI: 10.1016/j.cca.2014.08.002

[34] Richards TJ, Kaminski N, Baribaud F, Flavin S, Brodmerkel C, Horowitz D, Li K, Choi J, Vuga LJ, Lindell KO, Klesen M, Zhang Y, Gibson KF. Peripheral blood proteins predict mortality in idiopathic pulmonary fibrosis. Am J Respir Crit Care Med. 2012;185:67–76. DOI: 10.1164/rccm.201101-0058OC

[35] Niebroj-Dobosz I, Madej-Pilarczyk A, Marchel M, Sokołowska B, Hausmanowa-Petrusewicz I. Circulating tenascin-C levels in patients with dilated cardiomyopathy

in the course of Emery-Dreifuss muscular dystrophy. Clin Chim Acta. 2011;412:1533–1538. DOI: 10.1016/j.cca.2011.04.033

[36] Kinali M, Arechavala-Gomeza V, Cirak S, Glover A, Guglieri M, Feng L, Hollingsworth KG, Hunt D, Jungbluth H, Roper HP, Quinlivan RM, Gosalakkal JA, Jayawant S, Nadeau A, Hughes-Carre L, Manzur AY, Mercuri E, Morgan JE, Straub V, Bushby K, Sewry C, Rutherford M, Muntoni F. Muscle histology vs MRI in Duchenne muscular dystrophy. Neurology. 2011;76:346–353. DOI: 10.1212/WNL.0b013e318208811f

[37] Vucic S, Ziemann U, Eisen A, Hallett M, Kiernan MC. Transcranial magnetic stimulation and amyotrophic lateral sclerosis: pathophysiological insights. J Neurol Neurosurg Psychiatry. 2013;84:1161–1170. DOI: 10.1136/jnnp-2012-304019

[38] Ferlini A, Neri M, Gualandi F. The medical genetics of dystrophinopathies: molecular genetic diagnosis and its impact on clinical practice. Neuromuscul Disord. 2013;23:4–14. DOI: 10.1016/j.nmd.2012.09.002

[39] Bagni C, Tassone F, Neri G, Hagerman R. Fragile X syndrome: causes, diagnosis, mechanisms, and therapeutics. J Clin Invest. 2012;122:4314–4322. DOI: 10.1172/JCI63141

[40] Agrawal M, Biswas A. Molecular diagnostics of neurodegenerative disorders. Front Mol Biosci. 2015;2:54. DOI: 10.3389/fmolb.2015.00054

[41] Hwang CS, Liu GT, Chang MD, Liao IL, Chang HT. Elevated serum autoantibody against high mobility group box 1 as a potent surrogate biomarker for amyotrophic lateral sclerosis. Neurobiol Dis. 2013;58:13–18. DOI: 10.1016/j.nbd.2013.04.013

[42] Hwang CS, Tsai CH, Liu GT, Li W, Chang HT. Decreased level of serum autoantibody against LG72 is a biosignature of amyotrophic lateral sclerosis. Biomark Med. 2016;10:73–79. DOI: 10.2217/bmm.15.80

[43] Jany PL, Hagemann TL, Messing A. GFAP expression as an indicator of disease severity in mouse models of Alexander disease. ASN Neuro. 2013;5:e00109.

[44] Franken R, den Hartog AW, de Waard V, Engele L, Radonic T, Lutter R, Timmermans J, Scholte AJ, van den Berg MP, Zwinderman AH, Groenink M, Mulder BJ. Circulating transforming growth factor-beta as a prognostic biomarker in Marfan syndrome. Int J Cardiol. 2013;168:2441–2446. DOI: 10.1016/j.ijcard.2013.03.033

[45] Feustel A, Hahn A, Schneider C, Sieweke N, Franzen W, Gündüz D, Rolfs A, Tanislav C. Continuous cardiac troponin I release in Fabry disease. PLoS One. 2014;9:e91757. DOI: 10.1371/journal.pone.0091757

[46] Nadarajah VD, van Putten M, Chaouch A, Garrood P, Straub V, Lochmüller H, Ginjaar HB, Aartsma-Rus AM, van Ommen GJ, den Dunnen JT, 't Hoen PA. Serum matrix metalloproteinase-9 (MMP-9) as a biomarker for monitoring disease progression in Duchenne muscular dystrophy (DMD). Neuromuscul Disord. 2011;21:569–578. DOI: 10.1016/j.nmd.2011.05.011

[47] Wen Q, Huang LT, Luo N, Wang YT, Li XY, Mao HP, Zhang L, Dong XQ, Yu XQ. Proteomic profiling identifies haptoglobin as a potential serum biomarker for steroid-resistant nephrotic syndrome. Am J Nephrol. 2012;36:105–113. DOI: 10.1159/000339755

[48] Vigan M, Stirnemann J, Caillaud C, Froissart R, Boutten A, Fantin B, Belmatoug N, Mentré F. Modeling changes in biomarkers in Gaucher disease patients receiving enzyme replacement therapy using a pathophysiological model. Orphanet J Rare Dis. 2014;30:95. DOI: 10.1186/1750-1172-9-95

[49] Franken R, Radonic T, den Hartog AW, Groenink M, Pals G, van Eijk M, Lutter R, Mulder BJ, Zwinderman AH, de Waard V; COMPARE Study Group. The revised role of TGF-β in aortic aneurysms in Marfan syndrome. Neth Heart J. 2015;23:116–121. DOI: 10.1007/s12471-014-0622-0